Nutrition among
Vulnerable Populations

Nutrition among Vulnerable Populations

Editors

Heather Eicher-Miller
Marie Kainoa Fialkowski Revilla

MDPI • Basel • Beijing • Wuhan • Barcelona • Belgrade • Manchester • Tokyo • Cluj • Tianjin

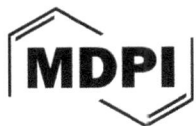

Editors
Heather Eicher-Miller
Purdue University
USA

Marie Kainoa Fialkowski Revilla
University of Hawai'i at Mānoa
USA

Editorial Office
MDPI
St. Alban-Anlage 66
4052 Basel, Switzerland

This is a reprint of articles from the Special Issue published online in the open access journal *Nutrients* (ISSN 2072-6643) (available at: https://www.mdpi.com/journal/nutrients/special_issues/nutrition_vulnerable_population).

For citation purposes, cite each article independently as indicated on the article page online and as indicated below:

LastName, A.A.; LastName, B.B.; LastName, C.C. Article Title. *Journal Name* **Year**, *Article Number*, Page Range.

ISBN 978-3-03943-587-6 (Hbk)
ISBN 978-3-03943-588-3 (PDF)

© 2020 by the authors. Articles in this book are Open Access and distributed under the Creative Commons Attribution (CC BY) license, which allows users to download, copy and build upon published articles, as long as the author and publisher are properly credited, which ensures maximum dissemination and a wider impact of our publications.

The book as a whole is distributed by MDPI under the terms and conditions of the Creative Commons license CC BY-NC-ND.

Contents

About the Editors vii

Heather A. Eicher-Miller and Marie K. Fialkowski
Nutrition among Vulnerable U.S. Populations
Reprinted from: *Nutrients* 2020, 12, 3150, doi:10.3390/nu12103150 1

Heather A. Eicher-Miller, Carol J. Boushey, Regan L. Bailey and Yoon Jung Yang
Frequently Consumed Foods and Energy Contributions among Food Secure and Insecure U.S. Children and Adolescents
Reprinted from: *Nutrients* 2020, 12, 304, doi:10.3390/nu12082304 7

Sally Campbell, John J. Chen, Carol J. Boushey, Heather Eicher-Miller, Fengqing Zhu and Marie K. Fialkowski
Food Security and Diet Quality in Native Hawaiian, Pacific Islander, and Filipino Infants 3 to 12 Months of Age
Reprinted from: *Nutrients* 2020, 12, 2120, doi:10.3390/nu12072120 21

Rachael T. Leon Guerrero, L. Robert Barber, Tanisha F. Aflague, Yvette C. Paulino, Margaret P. Hattori-Uchima, Mark Acosta, Lynne R. Wilkens and Rachel Novotny
Prevalence and Predictors of Overweight and Obesity among Young Children in the Children's Healthy Living Study on Guam
Reprinted from: *Nutrients* 2020, 12, 2527, doi:10.3390/nu12092527 39

Lindsey M. Bryant, Heather A. Eicher-Miller, Irem Korucu and Sara A. Schmitt
Associations between Subjective and Objective Measures of the Community Food Environment and Executive Function in Early Childhood
Reprinted from: *Nutrients* 2020, 12, 1944, doi:10.3390/nu12071944 59

Alexandra E. Cowan, Shinyoung Jun, Janet A. Tooze, Heather A. Eicher-Miller, Kevin W. Dodd, Jaime J. Gahche, Patricia M. Guenther, Johanna T. Dwyer, Nancy Potischman, Anindya Bhadra and Regan L. Bailey
Total Usual Micronutrient Intakes Compared to the Dietary Reference Intakes among U.S. Adults by Food Security Status
Reprinted from: *Nutrients* 2020, 12, 38, doi:10.3390/nu12010038 71

Cindy W. Leung and Megan S. Zhou
Household Food Insecurity and the Association with Cumulative Biological Risk among Lower-Income Adults: Results from the National Health and Nutrition Examination Surveys 2007–2010
Reprinted from: *Nutrients* 2020, 12, 1517, doi:10.3390/nu12051517 83

Julia A. Wolfson and Cindy W. Leung
Food Insecurity and COVID-19: Disparities in Early Effects for US Adults
Reprinted from: *Nutrients* 2020, 12, 1648, doi:10.3390/nu12061648 97

Lamis Jomaa, Muzi Na, Sally G. Eagleton, Marwa Diab-El-Harake and Jennifer S. Savage
Caregiver's Self-Confidence in Food Resource Management Is Associated with Lower Risk of Household Food Insecurity among SNAP-Ed-Eligible Head Start Families
Reprinted from: *Nutrients* 2020, 12, 2304, doi:10.3390/nu12020304 111

Heather A. Eicher-Miller, Rebecca L. Rivera, Hanxi Sun, Yumin Zhang, Melissa K. Maulding and Angela R. Abbott
Supplemental Nutrition Assistance Program-Education Improves Food Security Independent of Food Assistance and Program Characteristics
Reprinted from: *Nutrients* **2020**, *12*, 2636, doi:10.3390/nu12092636 . . . . **127**

Katherine Engel and Elizabeth H. Ruder
Fruit and Vegetable Incentive Programs for Supplemental Nutrition Assistance Program (SNAP) Participants: A Scoping Review of Program Structure
Reprinted from: *Nutrients* **2020**, *12*, 1676, doi:10.3390/nu12061676 . . . . **143**

About the Editors

Heather Eicher-Miller, Associate Professor of Nutrition Science, Purdue University has discovered adverse dietary and health outcomes associated with food insecurity and developed novel interventions to improve food security. She also creates new analytical and methodological techniques to quantify and evaluate the relationship between food insecurity, diet, and health

Marie Kainoa Fialkowski Revilla, Associate Professor of Human Nutrition at the University of Hawai'i at Mānoa, research focuses on gathering more comprehensive diet and health-related information on minority and indigenous populations so that more culturally appropriate health promotion activities may be developed.

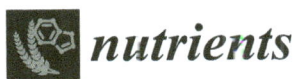 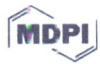

Editorial

Nutrition among Vulnerable U.S. Populations

Heather A. Eicher-Miller [1,*] and Marie K. Fialkowski [2]

[1] Department of Nutrition Science, College of Health and Human Science, Purdue University, West Lafayette, IN 47907, USA
[2] Department of Human Nutrition, Food and Animal Sciences, College of Tropical Agriculture and Human Resources, University of Hawai'i at Mānoa, Honolulu, HI 96822, USA; mariekf@hawaii.edu
* Correspondence: heichnerm@purdue.edu; Tel.: +1-765-494-6815

Received: 2 October 2020; Accepted: 12 October 2020; Published: 15 October 2020

Keywords: food security; food insecurity; low resource; nutrition; diet; health; food access; food environment; interventions; U.S. population

---

Food insecurity and low resources continue to be a burden influencing the health, well-being, growth and development of millions of U.S. children and adults [1–4]. Individuals and families experiencing restrained access to food may be concentrated in certain geographic areas or distributed throughout communities. Sometimes groups managing the situation of little or no food resources are even unknown because of their isolated situations. They include all ages, groups of varying races/ethnicities, diverse household compositions, those living in rural and urban areas and many others [1,2]. Many of these groups, both hidden and visible, have rates of food insecurity well above the national average and are influenced by persistent conditions which are historically resistant to trends of national improvement in food security [1,5,6]. Yet, even national food security estimate trends are currently in flux as environmental influences such as the coronavirus pandemic and economic changes shape the food landscape of the U.S. [7]. Research attention to these subsets of the population and varying environmental influences are imperative to determine U.S. health, well-being and nutritional status associated with food insecurity and to use this information to improve these conditions.

Not enough is known about the nutritional status and dietary intake in the diverse array of low-resource and food insecure groups despite summary information regarding the broad group of U.S. children and adults. Some of these subsets may be missed in national surveillance for reasons such as limited samples to make robust estimates, non-response or attrition [8,9]. Nor are the environments and nutritional barriers of the diversity of vulnerable population groups affected by food insecurity and low resources fully understood [10,11]. Creating interventions that effectively intervene to improve food security and nutritional status, however, are dependent on this knowledge as broad, summary information may not translate to a one-size-fits-all approach to improve food security in such a varied food landscape. Tailored approaches to quantify access to food, the nutrition environment, dietary behaviors and other barriers are necessary to identify the needs in diverse populations and then to build successful interventions that will improve dietary intake, reduce rates of chronic disease and counter negative factors in the environment [12]. In order to begin to fill this gap, this Special Issue on "Nutrition Among Vulnerable Populations" features papers quantifying dietary intake, nutritional status, access to food and food security, barriers to healthful foods and food security and environmental influences experienced by vulnerable groups with a high prevalence of food insecurity. The following sections summarize the findings of the four papers on children [13–16], three papers on adults [17–19] and three papers featuring studies of families or households (Figure 1) [20–22].

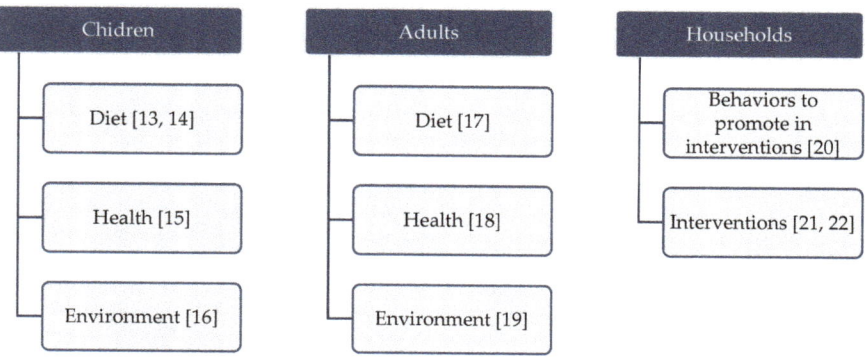

Figure 1. Populations sampled and topical areas of studies included in the Special Issue "Nutrition among Vulnerable Populations".

The diet, health and environmental associations linked with food insecurity or low resources among vulnerable child populations are featured in papers including samples drawn from rarely investigated young children living in Hawai'i, Guam and the Midwestern U.S., while a sample of children and adolescents included in the National Health and Nutrition Examination Survey (NHANES) provided nationally representative contrasts of the diets of food secure and insecure children. Starting with a national scope, the foods and beverages and food groups that were most frequently consumed and contributing most to energy among U.S. children ages 6 to 11 years and 12 to 17 years who were living in situations of food security and food insecurity among household children were determined and compared in a study by Eicher-Miller et al. [14] using NHANES data. Results showed that both the frequency and energy contributions of beverages (including diet, sweetened, juice, coffee and tea) were significantly greater among food insecure compared with food secure children ages 12 to 17 years who had significantly more frequent water intake, while beverage and mixed dish frequency were higher among food insecure children ages 6 to 11 years compared to food secure children who exhibited higher frequency and energy from snacks [14]. Dietary differences by food security status among infants were also investigated by Campbell et al. [13] in a sample from Hawai'i. Surprisingly, findings showed that Native Hawaiian, Pacific Islander and Filipino infants ages 3 to 12 months from food insecure households consumed foods from more food groups and consumed fresh foods on a greater proportion of days compared with infants from food secure households [13]. A community-based sample of children 2 to 8 years old from Guam were the focus of another study evaluating health, lifestyle and dietary intake [15]. Approximately 80% were receiving food assistance, 51% experienced food insecurity and 27.4% were affected by overweight and obesity. Compared with children who had a healthy weight, children who were overweight and obese were more likely to have educated caregivers and to have a higher intake of sugar-sweetened beverages [15]. These dietary and demographic associations with poor health outcomes among young children are important factors to consider in health and food security-promoting interventions. However, broad, environmental-level influences may also be linked with the health and development of young children. The food environment is conceptualized as the availability, affordability and accessibility of grocery stores or other food retail outlets that promote a healthful diet [23]. Parent reports of the community food environment of children ages 3 to 5 years from a Midwestern U.S. state showed that children living in higher quality community food environments had better cognitive ability, specifically executive function, compared with children living in lower quality community food environments [16]. Insights from these child-focused papers contribute new information on the environmental, demographic, lifestyle and behavioral factors of vulnerable groups that influence nutrition, health and development.

Advances in knowledge of the nutrient intake and health risks associated with food security along [17,18] with early effects of the coronavirus pandemic [19] among U.S. adults are featured separately in three articles. Total usual micronutrient intakes from foods, beverages and dietary supplements were compared to the dietary reference intakes among U.S. adults ≥19 years by sex and food security status using nationally representative data from the NHANES [17]. Results showed that both male and female adults living in food insecure households had a higher risk for inadequate intakes of magnesium, potassium and vitamins A, B6, B12, C, D, E and K, while food insecure men also had a higher risk for inadequate phosphorous, selenium and zinc. The risk of inadequacy was not different by food security status for nutrients, calcium, iron (determined in men only), choline or folate. However, the risk for exceeding the tolerable upper intake level was greater among some dietary supplement users [17]. Micronutrient inadequacy may contribute to the risk for chronic disease and poor health, especially when experienced over years into later adulthood [23]. The association of household food insecurity among low-income adults ages 20 to 65 years with cumulative biological risk, a measure of the body's physiological response to chronic stress, was investigated, similarly using NHANES data in a study by Leung et al. [18]. Results showed that women with food insecurity had higher cumulative biological risk scores and higher odds of elevated biological risk, while associations were not observed among men. The authors hypothesized that the chronic stress of food insecurity may facilitate the association with chronic poor health outcomes for women [18]. Another national, although not representative, sample of low-income (<250% of the federal poverty line) U.S. adults ≥18 years old completed a web-based survey to determine the early impact of the COVID-19 pandemic, offering a critical first look at how low-income families are coping with economic and lifestyle changes [19]. Approximately 44% were food insecure, and were significantly more likely to report basic needs challenges compared with food secure adults, with the group experiencing very low food security reporting the most severe difficulties. Food insecure compared with food secure adults were more vulnerable to the economic, dietary and health risks of the pandemic [19]. These current and ongoing effects of the pandemic may compound the micronutrient and cumulative biological risk disparities discovered and documented in these Special Issue articles on U.S. adults.

Clearly, there is a need for interventions that apply knowledge of the barriers, nutrition, health and environmental risks to improve food security and health among low-resource populations. Three studies in this Special Issue focus on interventions or behaviors that may be promoted in future interventions among low-resource families [20–22]. A sample of families with young children in Head Start from a rural area of a northern U.S. state was used to investigate the association of food resource management behaviors, food resource management self-confidence and financial practices with household food insecurity [20]. The participants with high food resource management self-confidence had significantly lower odds of household food insecurity; the inclusion of food resource management self-confidence promotion in nutrition education interventions for the low-resource population may assist management of food dollars to improve household food insecurity [20]. Nutrition education programs like the Supplemental Nutrition Assistance Program Education (SNAP-Ed) have been shown to improve food security and may integrate food resource management self-confidence building to potentially increase the magnitude or sustainability of those changes. Eicher-Miller et al. investigated the characteristics of SNAP-Ed program delivery to determine their role in SNAP-Ed's intervention effect on food insecurity. In addition, the role of participant co-participation in food assistance programs like SNAP was also investigated as a mediator or moderator to food security change due to SNAP-Ed as an intervention [21]. Results of this secondary analysis of data from a longitudinal randomized controlled trial of SNAP-Ed among women ≥18 years from households with children in a Midwestern U.S. state showed that neither variation of program delivery characteristics nor participation or changes in participation in food assistance programs, associated with the impact of SNAP-Ed on change in food security over time, meaning SNAP-Ed directly improved food security among participants [21]. Other interventions among low-income and food insecure participants include incentives to encourage improved fruit and vegetable intake. A scoping review of fruit and vegetable incentive-based interventions was completed to determine structural factors that influenced program effectiveness [22]. Eighteen of the 19 studies reported a positive impact on either participant fruit and vegetable purchases or intake, and most were located at farmers' markets and offered an incentive in the form of a token, coupon or voucher. The summative knowledge may further inform the design, implementation and success of future fruit and vegetable interventions targeted to improve nutrition among low-income populations [22].

In conclusion, the articles in this Special Issue address dietary intake, behaviors and health among low-resource and food insecure groups. Some of the studies feature populations that have not traditionally been included in research and fill gaps, informing knowledge of the characteristics, lifestyles and environments of these groups. Others feature results representative of vulnerable groups in the U.S. population. These contributions may inform future interventions on food security and dietary intake to incorporate confidence-promoting aspects, an evaluation of the program and participation factors of nutrition education interventions, and a summary of the structural factors of successful fruit and vegetable incentive programs. This Special Issue advances knowledge to improve food security and health among vulnerable U.S. populations.

Funding: This work is/was supported by the USDA National Institute of Food and Agriculture, Hatch project 1019736, by the National Institute on Minority Health and Health Disparities of the National Institutes of Health (U54MD00760), and the HMSA Foundation Community Fund grant #CF-021803.

Conflicts of Interest: Unrelated to this submission, HAE-M has served as a consultant to Colletta Consulting, Mead Johnson, the National Dairy Council, the Indiana Dairy Association and the American Egg Board. She has previously received travel support to present research findings from the Institute of Food Technologists and the International Food Information Council. However, the funders listed above (USDA) had no role in this editorial. MKF has no conflicts of interest to report.

References

1. Coleman-Jensen, A.; Rabbitt, M.P.; Gregory, C.A.; Singh, A. *Household Food Security in the United States in 2018*; ERR-237; U.S. Department of Agriculture, Economic Research Service: Washington, DC, USA, 2019.
2. Nord, M. *Food Insecurity in Households with Children: Prevalence, Severity, and Household Characteristics*; EIB-56; U.S. Dept. of Agriculture, Economic Research Service: Washington, DC, USA, 2009.
3. Gundersen, C.; Ziliak, J.P. Food insecurity and health outcomes. *Health Aff.* **2015**, *34*, 1830–1839. [CrossRef] [PubMed]
4. Gregory, C.A.; Coleman-Jensen, A. *Food Insecurity, Chronic Disease, and Health among Working-Age Adults*; ERR-235; U.S. Department of Agriculture, Economic Research Service: Washington, DC, USA, 2017.
5. Kaufman, P.; Dicken, C.; Williams, R. *Measuring Access to Healthful, Affordable Food in American Indian and Alaska Native Tribal Areas*; EIB-131; U.S. Department of Agriculture, Economic Research Service: Washington, DC, USA, 2014.
6. Myers, A.M.; Painter, M.A., II. Food Insecurity in the United States of America: An Examination of Race/Ethnicity and Nativity. *Food Secur.* **2017**, *9*, 1419–1432. [CrossRef]
7. Schanzenbach, D.W.; Pitts, A. How Much Has Food Insecurity Risen? Evidence from the Census Household Pulse Survey. Institute for Policy Research Rapid Research Report. 2020. Available online: https://www.ipr.northwestern.edu/documents/reports/ipr-rapid-researchreports-pulse-hh-data-10-june-2020.pdf (accessed on 30 September 2020).
8. Agency for Healthcare Research and Quality. *Defining Categorization Needs for Race and Ethnicity Data*; Agency for Healthcare Research and Quality: Rockville, MD, USA, 2018. Available online: https://www.ahrq.gov/research/findings/final-reports/iomracereport/reldata3.html (accessed on 30 September 2020).
9. Ver Ploeg, M.; Perrin, E. (Eds.) *Eliminating Health Disparities: Measurement and Data Needs*; U.S. National Research Council; Panel on DHHS Collection of Race and Ethnic Data; National Academies Press: Washington, DC, USA, 2004.
10. Mechanic, D.; Tanner, J. Vulnerable People, Groups, and Populations: Societal View. *Health Aff.* **2007**, *26*, 1220–1230. [CrossRef] [PubMed]

11. Hutch, D.J.; Bouye, K.E.; Skillen, E.; Lee, C.; Whitehead, L.; Rashid, J.R. Potential Strategies to Eliminate Built Environment Disparities for Disadvantaged and Vulnerable Communities. *Am. J. Public Health* **2011**, *101*, 587–595. [CrossRef] [PubMed]
12. U.S. Department of Agriculture. Advisory Report to the Secretary of Health and Human Services and the Secretary of Agriculture. Available online: http://www.health.gov/dietaryguidelines/2015-scientific-report/PDFs/Scientific-Report-of-the-2015-Dietary-Guidelines-Advisory-Committee.pdf (accessed on 10 December 2019).
13. Campbell, S.; Chen, J.; Boushey, C.J.; Eicher-Miller, H.A.; Zhu, F.; Fialkowski, M.K. Food Security and Diet Quality in Native Hawaiian, Pacific Islander, and Filipino Infants 3 to 12 Months of Age. *Nutrients* **2020**, *12*, 2120. [CrossRef] [PubMed]
14. Eicher-Miller, H.A.; Boushey, C.J.; Bailey, R.L.; Yang, Y.J. Frequently Consumed Foods and Energy Contributions among Food Secure and Insecure U.S. Children and Adolescents. *Nutrients* **2020**, *12*, 304. [CrossRef] [PubMed]
15. Leon Guerrero, R.T.; Barber, L.R.; Aflague, T.F.; Paulino, Y.C.; Hattori-Uchima, M.P.; Acosta, M.; Wilkens, L.R.; Novotny, R. Prevalence and Predictors of Overweight and Obesity among Young Children in the Children's Healthy Living Study on Guam. *Nutrients* **2020**, *12*, 2527 [CrossRef] [PubMed]
16. Bryant, L.M.; Eicher-Miller, H.A.; Korucu, I.; Schmitt, S.A. Associations between Subjective and Objective Measures of the Community Food Environment and Executive Function in Early Childhood. *Nutrients* **2020**, *12*, 1944. [CrossRef] [PubMed]
17. Cowan, A.; Jun, S.; Tooze, J.A.; Eicher-Miller, H.A.; Dodd, K.W.; Gahche, J.J.; Guenther, P.M.; Dwyer, J.T.; Potischman, N.; Bhadra, A.; et al. Total Usual Micronutrient Intakes Compared to the Dietary Reference Intakes among U.S. Adults by Food Security Status. *Nutrients* **2020**, *12*, 38. [CrossRef]
18. Leung, C.W.; Zhou, M.S. Household Food Insecurity and the Association with Cumulative Biological Risk among Lower-Income Adults: Results from the National Health and Nutrition Examination Surveys 2007–2010. *Nutrients* **2020**, *12*, 1517. [CrossRef]
19. Wolfson, J.A.; Leung, C.W. Food Insecurity and COVID-19: Disparities in Early Effects for U.S. Adults. *Nutrients* **2020**, *12*, 1648. [CrossRef]
20. Jomaa, L.; Na, M.; Eagleton, S.G.; Diab-El-Harake, M.; Savage, J.S. Caregiver's Self-Confidence in Food Resource Management is Associated with Lower Risk of Household Food Insecurity among SNAP-Ed-Eligible Head Start Families. *Nutrients* **2020**, *12*, 2304. [CrossRef]
21. Eicher-Miller, H.A.; Rivera, R.L.; Sun, H.; Zhang, Y.; Maulding, M.K.; Abbott, A.R. Supplemental Nutrition Assistance Program-Education Improves Food Security Independent of Food Assistance and Program Characteristics. *Nutrients* **2020**, *12*, 2636. [CrossRef] [PubMed]
22. Engel, K.; Ruder, E.H. Fruit and Vegetable Incentive Programs for Supplemental Nutrition Assistance Program (SNAP) Participants: A Scoping Review of Program Structure. *Nutrients* **2020**, *12*, 1676. [CrossRef] [PubMed]
23. U.S. Department of Health and Human Services; U.S. Department of Agriculture. *2015–2020 Dietary Guidelines for Americans*; U.S. Department of Health and Human Services; U.S. Department of Agriculture: Washington, DC, USA, 2015. Available online: http://health.gov/dietaryguidelines/2015/guidelines/ (accessed on 30 September 2020).

Publisher's Note: MDPI stays neutral with regard to jurisdictional claims in published maps and institutional affiliations.

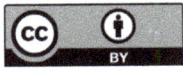

© 2020 by the authors. Licensee MDPI, Basel, Switzerland. This article is an open access article distributed under the terms and conditions of the Creative Commons Attribution (CC BY) license (http://creativecommons.org/licenses/by/4.0/).

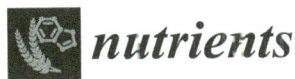

Article

Frequently Consumed Foods and Energy Contributions among Food Secure and Insecure U.S. Children and Adolescents

Heather A. Eicher-Miller [1,*], Carol J. Boushey [1,2], Regan L. Bailey [1] and Yoon Jung Yang [1,3]

1. Department of Nutrition Science, Purdue University, 700 W State St, West Lafayette, IN 47907, USA; cjboushey@cc.hawaii.edu (C.J.B.); reganbailey@purdue.edu (R.L.B.); yang3@purdue.edu (Y.J.Y.)
2. Epidemiology Program, University of Hawaii Cancer Center, 701 Ilalo St, Honolulu, HI 96813, USA
3. Department of Food and Nutrition, Dongduk Women's University, 60 Hwarang-ro 13-gil, Wolgok 2di-dong, Seongbuk-gu, Seoul 136714, Korea
* Correspondence: heicherm@purdue.edu; Tel.: +1-765-494-6815

Received: 24 December 2019; Accepted: 20 January 2020; Published: 23 January 2020

Abstract: Food insecurity is associated with nutritional risk in children. This study identified and compared the most frequently consumed foods, beverages, and food groups and their contributions to energy intake among U.S. children and adolescents (6–11, 12–17 years) by food security status. Dietary intake from the day-1, 24-h dietary recall, and household child food security status were analyzed in the 2007–2014 National Health and Nutrition Examination Survey (n = 8123). Foods and beverages were classified into food categories, ranked, and compared by weighted proportional frequency and energy contribution for food security groups by age. Significant differences between household child food security groups were determined using the Rao-Scott modified chi-square statistic. The weighted proportional frequency of beverages (including diet, sweetened, juice, coffee, and tea) and their energy was significantly higher among food insecure compared with food secure while the reverse was true for water frequency among 12–17 years. Beverage and mixed dish frequency were higher among food insecure compared with food secure 6–11 years while the reverse was true for frequency and energy from snacks. Frequency-differentiated intake patterns for beverages and snacks by food security across age groups may inform dietary recommendations, population-specific dietary assessment tools, interventions, and policy for food insecure children.

Keywords: food group intake; child food security; popularly consumed foods; low-resource children; adolescents; food intake; beverage intake; dietary intake; food insecurity; US children

1. Introduction

The U.S. Dietary Guidelines for Americans Advisory Committee identified many children and adolescents as having low intakes of fruits, vegetables, whole grains, and dairy concomitant with excessive intakes of sodium, saturated fats, added sugars, and refined grains [1]. Such dietary patterns are linked with nutritional risk, or dietary deficiencies that endanger health, as age progresses through childhood. Low micronutrient intakes combined with excessive energy intakes culminate in adolescence, when growth is accelerated and nutrients are at highest demand and yet this age group has the most nutrient shortfalls across the lifespan [2].

Adolescents and children in food insecure households, with "limited or uncertain availability of nutritionally adequate and safe foods or limited or uncertain ability to acquire acceptable foods in socially acceptable ways" [3], may be particularly vulnerable to nutrition risk, increasing the likelihood of suboptimal cognitive and physical health [4–6]. Indeed, iron deficiency anemia and low bone mineral content were associated with food insecurity in childhood as were behavioral and mental health problems, and poorer general health [7–10]. These associations may stem from disparities in dietary intake among food insecure children [11] where the opportunity for divergence from recommended dietary patterns is high considering limited household budget, time, and other resources. For example, a recent systematic review among U.S. children found strong and consistent evidence of higher added sugar intake among food insecure children 6–11 years compared to those who were food secure [11]. Food insecurity is particularly salient in the U.S. as 3.1 million or 8% of households with children in 2016 were food insecure: 7% low food security or "reduced quality and food access problems" and 1% very low food security or "reduced food intake and disrupted eating patterns" because of inadequate food resources [12].

However, little is known about the specific eating patterns and food and beverage exposure patterns among U.S. children and adolescents with regard to food security status. Eating patterns, including frequency and amount of foods and beverages consumed, snacking and meal skipping, time of eating occasions and other eating behaviors, influence energy intake and contribute to dietary quality [13]. Research on these patterns was a data gap in the Scientific Report of the 2015 Dietary Guidelines Advisory Committee along with investigation of foods comprising the U.S. food environments, particularly for food insecure households and low-income individuals [1]. Knowledge of the specific frequently consumed foods is a novel and practical contribution to inform interventions and policies aimed to improve dietary quality and food security among children. For example, results may inform a food package of nutrient-dense foods already known to be familiar and often consumed among food insecure children. Therefore, the purposes of this study were to use the National Health and Nutrition Examination Survey (NHANES) 2007–2014 data to: (1) determine the foods and beverages and categories of foods and beverages most frequently consumed by food security status (food secure, low food secure, and very low food secure) in children (6–11 years) and adolescents (12–17 years), and (2) compare the energy contributions and frequency of reported intake of food and beverage categories by food security status.

2. Materials and Methods

2.1. NHANES Design

NHANES is a nationally representative, cross-sectional survey of the National Center for Health Statistics (NCHS) and Centers for Disease Control and Prevention [14,15]. The non-institutionalized, civilian U.S. population are sampled based on characteristics such as age, sex, race-ethnicity, and income to accommodate the complex, stratified, multistage probability sampling framework [16]. Oversampling of certain sub-groups allows for generation of reliable estimates. NHANES protocol was reviewed and approved by the NCHS Research Ethics Review Board [17].

2.2. Participants

All participants of this secondary analysis completed the dietary component of What We Eat in America (WWEIA)/NHANES 2007–2008, 2009–2010, 2011–2012, and 2013–2014. Children were 6–17 years (n = 8,123, Table 1), having a 24-h dietary recall, dietary weights and scores for the U.S. Household Food Security Survey Module [18]. Socioeconomic characteristics of participants were recorded in participant homes during an in-depth interview for those 16–17 years and a proxy-assisted interview for those 6–15 years. Age (6–11 or 12–17 years), gender (male or female), survey year (2007–2008, 2009–2010, 2011–2012, 2013–2014), poverty-income-ratio (0.00–0.99, 1.00–1.99, 2.00–2.99, 3.00–5.00), race/ethnicity (non-Hispanic white, non-Hispanic black, Hispanic and Mexican American, and "other" race including multi-race), and weight status as indicated by body mass index (underweight, normal weight, overweight), characterized participants. Per NCHS analytic guidelines, "other" race is not representative of race/ethnic population estimates.

Table 1. Characteristics of food secure, low and very low food secure U.S. children and adolescents ages 6–17 years using the National Health and Nutrition Examination Survey 2007–2014 [a].

Characteristic	6–17 Years		6–11 Years (n = 4437)							12–17 Years (n = 3686)						
	n	%	Food Secure		Low Food Secure		Very Low Food Secure		χ² p-value [b]	Food Secure		Low Food Secure		Very Low Food Secure		χ² p-value [b]
			n	%	n	%	n	%		n	%	n	%	n	%	
Total	8123	100	3854	90	510	9	73	1		3178	89	426	10	82	2	
Sex									0.32							0.15
Male	4152	50	1941	51	272	54	40	57		1625	48	233	54	41	39	
Female	3971	50	1913	49	238	46	33	43		1553	52	193	46	41	61	
Survey Year									0.48							0.64
2007–2008	1990	25	939	24	147	25	24	30		738	25	120	31	22	24	
2009–2010	2106	25	1024	26	105	18	15	18		829	25	115	25	18	21	
2011–2012	2011	25	986	25	139	30	19	23		759	25	94	26	14	24	
2013–2014	2016	25	905	25	119	26	15	29		852	25	97	18	28	31	
Poverty-Income-Ratio									<0.0001 *,c							<0.0001 *,c
0.00–0.99	2504	24	1142	23	258	49	48	69		797	18	215	48	44	58	
1.00–1.99	2076	24	948	22	187	40	18	31		766	22	134	37	23	34	
2.00–2.99	1029	16	511	17	41	8	0	0		437	16	36	8	4	8	
3.00–5.00	1977	37	1016	39	12	3	0	0		933	43	16	7	0	0	
Race/Ethnicity									<0.0001 *							0.0004
Mexican American and Other Hispanic	2873	22	1325	21	221	34	41	54		1063	19	180	30	43	44	
Non-Hispanic White	2289	56	1138	57	111	38	9	19		919	60	94	39	18	40	
Non-Hispanic Black	2079	14	983	13	138	21	19	22		805	14	119	21	15	13	
Other-Race including Multi-Racial	882	8	408	8	40	7	4	4		391	7	33	10	6	3	
Body Mass Index Status [d]									0.001 *							0.12
Underweight	280	3	126	4	23	5	1	1		110	3	16	5	4	5	
Normal weight	4819	61	2366	62	264	49	37	52		1877	63	230	54	45	50	
Overweight	1324	16	599	16	99	22	15	18		523	15	69	14	19	26	
Obese	1700	19	763	18	124	24	20	28		668	19	111	27	14	19	

[a] Total numbers do not always add to sample size due to missing values. Percents do not always add to 100 due to rounding. Estimate represents weighted percent. [b] Rao Scott F adjusted χ² p-value is shown, statistical significance for differences among food secure, low food secure, and very low food secure among each respective age groups is indicated when p ≤ 0.02 using a Bonferroni type adjustment for multiple comparisons indicated by "*". Sample weights were appropriately constructed and applied to this analysis as directed by National Center for Health Statistics. Weights were rescaled so that the sum to the weights matched the survey population at the midpoint of the 8 years, 2007–2014. [c] Because of one or more empty cells, food secure and very low food secure were collapsed in order to compute Rao Scott F adjusted χ² p value. [d] Body Mass Index status was classified based on Centers for Disease Control and Prevention values as per: https://www.cdc.gov/nccdphp/dnpao/growthcharts/resources/sas.htm; <5% (underweight), 5 ≥ 85% (normal weight), 85 ≥ 95% (overweight), ≥95% (obese).

2.3. Measures

One adult per household completed the 18-item U.S. Household Food Security Survey Module for households with children <18 years during the household interview. Eight child-focused items determined food security of household children and were used to classify food security, low and very low food security; low and very low categories were also collapsed to classify food insecurity [18]. Food security of household children rather than the entire household was chosen as more directly tied to the child experience and dietary intake of household children. Measures of height and weight were collected during a physical examination at the Mobile Examination Center. Body mass index was calculated as body weight divided by the square of body height and categorized according to age- and sex-specific percentiles of the 2000 Centers for Disease Control and Prevention growth chart such that <5% (underweight), 5 ≥ 85% (normal weight), 85 ≥ 95% (overweight), ≥95% (obese) to indicate weight status [19].

The day-1 dietary recall was completed in person at the Mobile Examination Center using the USDA Automated Multiple Pass Method, designed to enhance food recalls using a 5-step interview process [20,21]. Participants were prompted to recall all types and amounts of foods and beverages (including water) consumed in the 24-h midnight to midnight time frame before the interview. Children 6–11 years reported dietary intake with the assistance of a parent or guardian, those 12–17 years self-reported. Probes queried the time and eating occasion of foods, details about preparation and amounts eaten, and finally, any frequently forgotten foods and foods not mentioned earlier. A USDA food code was assigned to each reported item and linked to a food or beverage in the Food and Nutrient Database for Dietary Studies (version 4.1 released 2010, 5.0 released 2012, 6.0 released 2014, 2013–2014 released 2016) [22], and further sorted and assigned a WWEIA food sub-category/group and broad food category/group [14].

2.4. Statistical Analysis

The data of food secure and food insecure children, including low and very low food secure categories were stratified by ages: 6–11 and 12–17 years because of similar diets within age ranges, food security reporting, known differences in food security by age in the same household and the NHANES methodology of self-reported dietary recall by age groups. Despite small participant n for the very low food secure group, hypothesis testing was included because food category reports were the unit of analysis and $n > 20$ for all food categories except "alcohol" and "other" including infant and baby formula (excluded from Table 2). Food category reports of "water" contributing energy were also <20 but were retained for comparison with frequency. Unadjusted frequencies were assessed for each food code or WWEIA food or beverage category code using: $n\sum i = 1(R_i)$ where n = the sample size, i = each participant, R_i = the number of reports of individual food codes for the ith individual [23]. The weighted sum of each food code was: $n\sum i = 1(R_i w_i)$ where w_i = sample weight for the ith individual was used to determine the weighted proportion of foods to the total foods reported, or the contribution of each food category reported to the total food category reported, given as: $n\sum i = 1(R_i w_i)/n\sum i = 1(T_i w_i)$ (100) where T_i = total number of reports of all food codes for the ith individual. The weighted proportion of reported energy was similarly calculated with substitution of energy for frequency and total energy for total number of reports. Foods were ranked by weighted frequency and contribution to energy individually, by food sub-category and broad category (selected data shown in tables). The Rao-Scott modified chi-square determined significant differences among food secure, low, and very low food secure groups ($p < 0.05/3$ or $p < 0.02$ using a Bonferroni adjustment for multiple comparisons to mitigate the probability of Type 1 error) and among food secure and insecure groups ($p < 0.05$). The results of significant differences among broad food groups were used to focus presentation of the results and discussion. All analyses were completed in SAS version 9.4 using SAS survey procedures with adjustment for survey design elements, non-response, and interview weights to allow inference to U.S. population.

Table 2. What We Eat in America broad food category [a] intake comparisons by frequency and energy among food secure and insecure (low and very low food secure) U.S. children and adolescents 6–11 and 12–17 years using the National Health and Nutrition Examination Survey 2007–2014 [b].

6–11 Years (n = 4437)

WWEIA Broad Food Category [a,c]	Food Secure			Food Insecure			χ^2 p-Value		Low Food Secure			Very Low Food Secure			χ^2 p-Value	
	Wtd % [d] of Reported Foods (SE)		Wtd % [d] of Reported Energy (SE)	Wtd % [d] of Reported Foods (SE)		Wtd % [d] of Reported Energy (SE)	Foods [e]	Energy [e]	Wtd % [d] of Reported Foods (SE)		Wtd % [d] of Reported Energy (SE)	Wtd % [d] of Reported Foods (SE)		Wtd % [d] of Reported Energy (SE)	Foods [f]	Energy [f]
Milk/Dairy [g]	11.6 (0.3)		9.4 (0.3)	12.0 (0.6)		11.0 (0.5)	0.31	0.36	12.0 (0.6)		10.8 (0.6)	11.7 (0.8)		12.7 (1.2)	0.47	0.34
Protein [h]	12.1 (0.3)		12.8 (0.6)	9.6 (0.5)		11.6 (0.7)	0.59	0.57	9.3 (0.5)		11.1 (0.9)	12.0 (0.8)		15.4 (1.0)	0.11	0.14
Mixed Dish [i]	22.1 (0.6)		20.6 (0.7)	9.3 (0.6)		24.8 (1.9)	0.04 *	0.19	9.4 (0.7)		25.3 (2.1)	8.9 (0.9)		20.2 (1.7)	0.05	0.15
Grain [j]	14.3 (0.3)		14.3 (0.5)	11.4 (0.4)		13.7 (0.8)	0.72	0.49	11.4 (0.5)		13.9 (0.8)	10.9 (0.8)		12.8 (1.1)	0.04	0.62
Snack/Sweet [k]	16.1 (0.3)		21.0 (0.5)	14.4 (0.6)		18.3 (0.9)	0.02 *	0.02 *	14.5 (0.6)		18.1 (0.9)	13.9 (1.7)		20.1 (1.8)	0.05	0.02 *
Fruit [l]	5.8 (0.2)		2.8 (0.1)	5.1 (0.4)		2.7 (0.3)	0.17	0.67	4.8 (0.4)		2.5 (0.3)	7.4 (1.1)		4.0 (0.5)	0.07	0.74
Vegetable [m]	6.5 (0.2)		3.6 (0.2)	6.5 (0.7)		4.3 (0.5)	0.98	0.26	6.4 (0.7)		4.4 (0.6)	7.8 (0.9)		3.3 (0.5)	0.72	0.27
Beverage [n]	11.4 (0.2)		8.9 (0.2)	12.7 (0.6)		9.9 (0.6)	0.02 *	0.11	12.8 (0.6)		9.9 (0.7)	12.0 (1.1)		9.8 (1.3)	0.04	0.22
Water [o]	9.0 (0.2)		0.0 (0.0)	8.9 (0.6)		0.0 (0.0)	0.90	0.18	9.0 (0.6)		0.0 (0.0)	8.4 (0.8)		0.0 (0.0)	0.92	0.18
Fat/Oil [p]	3.3 (0.1)		1.5 (0.1)	3.1 (0.3)		1.7 (0.2)	0.56	0.55	3.3 (0.3)		1.8 (0.3)	1.3 (0.2)		0.8 (0.1)	0.03	0.21
Cond'/Sauce [r]	4.2 (0.2)		0.7 (0.0)	4.6 (0.4)		0.8 (0.2)	0.44	0.57	4.7 (0.4)		0.9 (0.2)	3.7 (1.0)		0.5 (0.2)	0.48	0.54
Sugars [s]	2.4 (0.1)		1.1 (0.1)	2.2 (0.2)		1.1 (0.2)	0.46	0.88	2.2 (0.2)		1.2 (0.2)	1.9 (0.6)		0.3 (0.1)	0.70	0.12

12–17 Years (n = 3686)

WWEIA Broad Food Category [a,c]	Food Secure			Food Insecure			χ^2 p-Value		Low Food Secure			Very Low Food Secure			χ^2 p-Value	
	Wtd % [d] of Reported Foods (SE)		Wtd % [d] of Reported Energy (SE)	Wtd % [d] of Reported Foods (SE)		Wtd % [d] of Reported Energy (SE)	Foods [e]	Energy [e]	Wtd % [d] of Reported Foods (SE)		Wtd % [d] of Reported Energy (SE)	Wtd % [d] of Reported Foods (SE)		Wtd % [d] of Reported Energy (SE)	Foods [f]	Energy [f]
Milk/Dairy [g]	10.7 (0.3)		9.8 (0.4)	9.8 (0.4)		8.3 (0.5)	0.06	0.08	9.7 (0.4)		8.1 (0.6)	10.3 (0.5)		9.5 (0.8)	0.17	0.20
Protein [h]	9.6 (0.3)		12.8 (0.5)	9.8 (0.5)		12.7 (0.9)	0.77	0.98	9.7 (0.5)		12.2 (0.9)	10.6 (0.5)		16.2 (0.8)	0.74	0.35
Mixed Dish [i]	8.8 (0.7)		20.6 (0.7)	10.1 (0.7)		23.3 (1.3)	0.09	0.66	10.3 (0.8)		25.8 (1.6)	8.7 (0.3)		21.9 (0.9)	0.08	0.55
Grain [j]	10.6 (0.2)		12.8 (0.3)	10.8 (0.4)		12.7 (0.7)	0.61	0.84	10.9 (0.4)		12.9 (0.7)	10.5 (0.8)		11.3 (1.0)	0.87	0.71
Snack/Sweet [k]	14.3 (0.4)		18.7 (0.6)	13.3 (0.6)		18.6 (1.3)	0.18	0.96	13.5 (0.6)		18.7 (1.3)	12.4 (0.5)		18.5 (0.9)	0.28	0.99
Fruit [l]	4.3 (0.3)		2.0 (0.1)	4.1 (0.4)		2.0 (0.3)	0.66	0.88	4.1 (0.5)		2.0 (0.2)	4.1 (0.5)		2.3 (0.3)	0.92	0.92
Vegetable [m]	7.9 (0.3)		4.2 (0.2)	7.9 (0.6)		3.9 (0.4)	0.96	0.49	7.6 (0.6)		3.8 (0.5)	9.8 (0.7)		4.3 (0.3)	0.63	0.69
Beverage [n]	12.7 (0.2)		11.2 (0.3)	15.4 (0.6)		13.0 (0.7)	<0.0001 *	0.03 *	15.5 (0.5)		13.1 (0.7)	14.4 (0.7)		12.2 (0.7)	0.0001 *	0.05
Water [o]	10.3 (0.3)		0.1 (0.0)	8.7 (0.5)		0.1 (0.0)	0.004 *	0.77	8.6 (0.6)		0.1 (0.1)	8.8 (0.5)		0.1 (0.1)	0.004 *	0.92
Fat/Oil [p]	3.6 (0.2)		1.9 (0.2)	3.5 (0.3)		1.6 (0.2)	0.90	0.18	3.4 (0.3)		1.4 (0.2)	4.0 (0.6)		2.6 (0.2)	0.83	0.10
Cond'/Sauce [r]	5.0 (0.2)		0.9 (0.1)	4.5 (0.5)		0.7 (0.1)	0.32	0.37	4.4 (0.5)		0.8 (0.1)	4.7 (0.4)		0.6 (0.1)	0.60	0.59
Sugars [s]	2.0 (0.1)		1.0 (0.1)	1.8 (0.2)		0.7 (0.1)	0.68	0.08	2.0 (0.3)		0.8 (0.1)	1.4 (0.2)		0.5 (0.1)	0.57	0.06

[a] The What We Eat in America (WWEIA) broad food categories were applied to categorize all foods and beverages reported in a single day to 14 broad food groups. [b] Survey weights and adjustments for the complex survey design were applied to represent the non-institutionalized U.S. population. Total numbers and percentages do not always add up to sample size due to missing values and rounding. [c] "Alcohol" and "Other" WWEIA category removed because of <20 reports. [d] Wtd % stands for the estimated weighted percent of all reports of foods or beverages or energy from reported foods or beverages reported in a single day that are included in a food group; SE = Standard Error. [e] Statistical significance at $p \leq 0.05$ for comparison of food secure vs. food insecure using the Rao–Scott modified chi-square statistic. [f] Statistical significance at $p \leq 0.02$ using a Bonferroni type adjustment for multiple comparisons indicated by "*" for comparison of food secure vs. low food secure and very low food secure using the Rao–Scott modified chi-square statistic. [g] Milk, flavored milk, dairy drinks and substitutes, cheese and yogurt. [h] Meats, poultry, seafood, eggs, cured meats/poultry, and plant-based protein foods. [i] Mixed dishes containing meat, poultry seafood; grain-based; Asian; Mexican; pizza; sandwiches, and soups. [j] Cooked grains, breads, rolls, tortillas, quick breads, and bread products, ready-to-eat cereals, and cooked cereals. [k] Savory snacks, crackers, snack/meal bars, sweet bakery products, candy and other desserts. [l] Fresh fruits, dried fruits, and fruit salads. [m] Vegetables and white potatoes. [n] 100% juice, diet beverages, sweetened beverages, coffee and tea. [o] Plain water and flavored or enhanced water. [p] Butter and animal fats, margarine, cream cheeses, cream, mayonnaise, salad dressings and vegetable oils. [q] Condiment. [r] Tomato based, mustard, olives, pickled vegetables, pasta sauces, dips, gravies, and other sauces. [s] Sugars, honey, jams, syrups, and toppings.

3. Results

Overall, ~90% of U.S. children and adolescents were food secure and 10% food insecure, with the smallest proportion being very low food secure (1–2%). Household poverty-income-ratio and race/ethnicity differed among 6–11 and 12–17 years by food security status ($p \leq 0.0004$, Table 1) as did the prevalence of at-risk-for-overweight and overweight only among children 6–11 years ($p = 0.001$).

3.1. Frequency and Energy Contribution of Broad Food Categories, Sub-Categories, and Foods

The broad food categories, energy contributions and reported frequency of consumption, were compared by food security status for ages 6–11 and 12–17 years in Table 2. Broad food category rankings by frequency and energy contributions were also considered. Ranking revealed broad category "snacks and sweets" as the most frequently consumed items for all children 6–11 years (Table 2). Broad category "beverages" were second or third most frequently consumed but ranked sixth in terms of group contributing to energy. Among those 12–17 years, "snacks and sweets" shared the top ranking with "beverages" and where ranking differed by food security status. "Beverage" contribution to energy ranked third to fifth. "Mixed dishes" ranked lower in frequency compared with contribution to energy ranking among both age groups and all food security categories. "Milk and dairy", "grains", and "protein foods" also had high rankings in both frequency and energy contribution for all ages and food security categories. "Water" and "condiments" added little to energy but ranked higher in terms of frequency.

3.1.1. 6–11 Years

The weighted proportion of the broad category "beverages" ($p = 0.02$, Table 2) and "mixed dishes" ($p = 0.04$) reported by frequency was statistically significantly greater for food insecure compared with secure children 6–11 years (12.7% vs. 11.4%, Table 2). "Mixed dishes" were also more frequently reported among food insecure at 9.3% compared with food secure at 8.0%. In contrast, reported intake of "snacks and sweets" by frequency ($p = 0.02$) and energy contribution ($p = 0.02$) was lower among food insecure compared with secure children of similar age (14.4% vs. 16.1% and 18.3% vs. 21.0%). Additional significant differences resulted among food secure, low and very low food secure groups ($p = 0.02$) for "snacks and sweets" (21.0%, 18.1%, 20.1%).

Food sub-categories contributing to the broad beverage category such as "fruit drinks" captured 3.2%, 4.3%, and 4.1% of reports (Table 3) among food secure, low, and very low food secure children. The pattern was consistent with lower "soft drink" reports for food secure (3.0%) compared with low (3.9%) and very low (3.4%) food secure children. Top items in these sub-categories were "fruit flavored drink from powder", "fruit-flavored caffeine-free soft drink", "cola-type soft drink", "apple juice", "orange juice", "fruit juice drink", and "reduced sugar fruit juice drink" (Supplemental Table S1). The broad "snacks and sweets" category included sub-categories, "cookies and brownies" and "candy without chocolate", with a higher percentage of reports among food secure (both 2.6%) compared with low (1.9%, 1.6%, respectively) and very low (1.5%, 2.2%, respectively) food secure children. "Corn tortilla chips", "hard candy", "chocolate chip cookie", "ice cream" and "snack crackers" were most frequently consumed items in these sub-categories.

Table 3. Top 25 most frequently consumed What We Eat in America food or beverage sub-categories [a], unweighted frequency of reported intake from food or beverage sub-categories, weighted percent and standard error of weighted percent of reported food or beverage sub-categories among all reported sub-categories for food secure, low, and very low food secure U.S. children and adolescents aged 6–11 and 12–17 years using the National Health and Nutrition Examination Survey 2007–2014.

	6–11 Years (n = 4437)									12–17 Years (n = 4696)								
	Food Secure			Low Food Secure			Very Low Food Secure			Food Secure			Low Food Secure			Very Low Food Secure		
Rank	WWEIA Sub-Category [a]	Freq [b]	Wtd % [c,d] (SE)	WWEIA Sub-Category [a]	Freq [b]	Wtd % [c,d] (SE)	WWEIA Sub-Category [a]	Freq [b]	Wtd % [c,d] (SE)	WWEIA Sub-Category [a]	Freq [b]	Wtd % [c,d] (SE)	WWEIA Sub-Category [a]	Freq [b]	Wtd % [c,d] (SE)	WWEIA Sub-Category [a]	Freq [b]	Wtd % [c,d] (SE)
Total		58,077	100		7322	100		1146	100		41,404	100		5187	100		981	100
1	Tap water	3082	5.9 (0.3)	Tap water	350	4.8 (0.4)	Reduced fat milk	53	4.6 (0.4)	Tap water	2166	5.9 (0.3)	Soft drinks	306	6.6 (0.5)	Bottled water	39	5.7 (0.6)
2	Fruit drinks	2747	2.7 (0.1)	Fruit drinks	300	4.3 (0.5)	Tap water	51	4.3 (0.4)	Soft drinks	1957	4.3 (0.2)	Tap water	226	4.5 (0.5)	Soft drinks	63	5.1 (0.4)
3	Yeast breads	1687	3.1 (0.1)	Bottled water	304	4.1 (0.6)	Fruit drinks	46	4.1 (0.9)	Bottled water	1841	4.1 (0.2)	Bottled water	218	4.0 (0.5)	Cheese	35	4.4 (0.5)
4	Cheese	1629	3.1 (0.1)	Soft drinks	296	3.9 (0.5)	Bottled water	41	4.0 (0.6)	Cheese	1295	3.4 (0.2)	Yeast breads	155	3.2 (0.3)	Tea	19	3.6 (0.4)
5	Soft drinks	1925	3.0 (0.2)	Yeast breads	212	3.2 (0.3)	Soft drinks	38	3.4 (0.7)	Yeast breads	1193	2.9 (0.1)	Fruit drinks	179	3.0 (0.4)	Tap water	30	3.5 (0.2)
6	Reduced fat Milk	1681	2.9 (0.2)	Tomato-based condiments	244	3.0 (0.3)	Apples	24	2.2 (0.4)	Tomato-based condiments	1215	2.8 (0.2)	Reduced fat milk	140	3.0 (0.4)	Yeast breads	36	3.3 (0.5)
7	Bottled water	1989	2.9 (0.2)	Cheese	186	2.8 (0.4)	Candy w/o chocolate	22	2.2 (0.8)	Reduced fat milk	1013	2.8 (0.2)	Cheese	145	2.8 (0.3)	Chicken, whole pieces	24	2.8 (0.2)
8	Tomato-based condiments	1523	2.6 (0.1)	Reduced fat milk	200	2.6 (0.3)	Cheese	25	2.2 (0.4)	Fruit drinks	1,189	2.4 (0.1)	Pizza	123	2.2 (0.3)	Fruit drinks	32	2.7 (0.5)
9	Candy w/o chocolate	1415	2.6 (0.2)	Ready-to-eat cereal, higher sugar (≥1.2g/100g)	180	2.3 (0.3)	Rolls and buns	19	2.1 (0.6)	Cookies and brownies	945	2.1 (0.1)	Tomato-based condiments	146	2.1 (0.3)	Lettuce and lettuce salads	20	2.6 (0.2)
10	Cookies and brownies	1398	2.6 (0.1)	Cookies and brownies	153	1.9 (0.2)	Ready-to-eat cereal, higher sugar (≥1.2g/100g)	30	2.1 (0.4)	Rolls and buns	725	1.9 (0.1)	Cookies and brownies	112	2.0 (0.2)	Cold cuts and cured meats	24	2.5 (0.5)
11	Ready-to-eat cereal, higher sugar (≥1.2g/100g)	1333	2.2 (0.1)	Jams, syrups, toppings	112	1.8 (0.2)	Candy w/chocolate	15	2.1 (0.3)	Pizza	856	1.9 (0.1)	Tea	96	2.0 (0.3)	Candy w/chocolate	22	2.4 (0.3)
12	Jams, syrups, toppings	1005	1.8 (0.1)	French fries and fried white potatoes	130	1.8 (0.2)	Pizza	26	2.0 (0.2)	Ready-to-eat cereal, higher sugar (≥1.2g/100g)	776	1.8 (0.1)	Corn tortilla and other chips	108	2.0 (0.2)	Tomato-based condiments	24	2.4 (0.2)

Table 3. Cont.

		6–11 Years (n = 4437)									12–17 Years (n = 3666)								
		Food Secure			Low Food Secure			Very Low Food Secure			Food Secure			Low Food Secure			Very Low Food Secure		
Rank	WWEIA Sub-Category [a]	Freq [b]	Wtd % [c,d] (SE)	WWEIA Sub-Category [a]	Freq [b]	Wtd % [c,d] (SE)	WWEIA Sub-Category [a]	Freq [b]	Wtd % [c,d] (SE)	WWEIA Sub-Category [a]	Freq [b]	Wtd % [c,d] (SE)	WWEIA Sub-Category [a]	Freq [b]	Wtd % [c,d] (SE)	WWEIA Sub-Category [a]	Freq [b]	Wtd % [c,d] (SE)
13	Pizza	1117	1.8 (0.1)	Cold cuts and cured meats	101	1.7 (0.2)	Yeast breads	25	2.0 (0.3)	Candy w/o chocolate	821	1.8 (0.1)	Ice cream and frozen dairy desserts	82	1.8 (0.3)	Rolls and buns	12	2.2 (0.2)
14	Corn tortilla and other chips	978	1.6 (0.1)	Whole milk	127	1.7 (0.3)	Tomato-based condiments	26	1.9 (0.5)	Corn tortilla and other chips	827	1.7 (0.1)	Ready-to-eat cereal, higher sugar (21.2g/100g)	99	1.8 (0.3)	Candy w/o chocolate	19	2.0 (0.1)
15	Rolls and buns	873	1.6 (0.1)	Corn tortilla and other chips	124	1.7 (0.2)	Eggs and omelets	22	1.9 (0.4)	Cold cuts and cured meats	680	1.6 (0.1)	Citrus juice	69	1.6 (0.3)	Reduced fat milk	31	1.9 (0.4)
16	French fries and fried white potatoes	931	1.5 (0.1)	Pizza	147	1.6 (0.2)	Chicken, whole pieces	18	1.9 (0.4)	Tea	589	1.6 (0.1)	Chicken, whole pieces	97	1.6 (0.2)	Ready-to-eat cereal, higher sugar (21.2g/100g)	19	1.8 (0.2)
17	Ice cream and frozen dairy desserts	861	1.5 (0.1)	Candy w/o chocolate	143	1.6 (0.2)	Ice cream and frozen dairy desserts	21	1.9 (0.3)	French fries and fried white potatoes	678	1.5 (0.1)	Lettuce and lettuce salads	77	1.5 (0.2)	Whole milk	12	1.7 (0.1)
18	Apples	838	1.5 (0.1)	Ice cream and frozen dairy desserts	93	1.6 (0.2)	Citrus juice	18	1.6 (0.3)	Chicken, whole pieces	706	1.4 (0.1)	Rolls and buns	95	1.5 (0.2)	Mustard and other condiments	14	1.7 (0.2)
19	Cold cuts and cured meats	775	1.4 (0.1)	Apples	99	1.5 (0.2)	Reduced fat flavored milk	12	1.6 (0.3)	Lettuce and lettuce salads	595	1.4 (0.1)	French fries and fried white potatoes	100	1.5 (0.2)	Bananas	13	1.7 (0.2)
20	Whole milk	911	1.3 (0.1)	Crackers, excludes saltines	62	1.5 (0.3)	Rice	15	1.6 (0.4)	Jams, syrups, toppings	486	1.3 (0.1)	Cold cuts and cured meats	76	1.5 (0.2)	Corn tortilla and other chips	15	1.7 (0.2)
21	Lowfat milk	551	1.3 (0.1)	Chicken, whole pieces	93	1.3 (0.2)	Lettuce and lettuce salads	17	1.6 (0.2)	Ice cream and frozen dairy desserts	501	1.2 (0.1)	Candy w/o chocolate	96	1.5 (0.2)	French fries and fried white potatoes	13	1.6 (0.1)
22	Nuts and seeds	560	1.2 (0.1)	Mayonnaise	65	1.2 (0.2)	Soups	21	1.5 (0.5)	Potato chips	523	1.2 (0.1)	Apples	57	1.3 (0.2)	Pizza	19	1.6 (0.2)
23	Chicken, whole pieces	800	1.2 (0.1)	Rolls and buns	99	1.2 (0.2)	Corn tortilla and other chips	25	1.5 (0.3)	Apples	485	1.2 (0.1)	Candy w/chocolate	60	1.3 (0.2)	Chicken patties, nuggets and tenders	9	1.5 (0.2)
24	Citrus juice	688	1.1 (0.1)	Citrus juice	111	1.1 (0.2)	Beans, peas, legumes	14	1.5 (0.2)	Eggs and omelets	488	1.0 (0.1)	Soups	49	1.2 (0.4)	Doughnuts, sweet rolls, pastries	11	1.5 (0.1)
25	Potato chips	661	1.1 (0.1)	Potato chips	81	1.1 (0.2)	Cookies and brownies	20	1.5 (0.2)	Crackers, excludes saltines	286	1.0 (0.1)	Sugars and honey	46	1.2 (0.2)	Cookies and brownies	21	1.3 (0.2)

[a] The What We Eat in America Food Sub-Categories were applied to categorize all foods and beverages to 150 unique sub-categories. Sub-category was reported without dietary weights. [b] The frequency that a food or beverages sub-category was reported without dietary weights. [c] Survey weights and adjustments for the complex survey design were applied to represent the non-institutionalized U.S. population. [d] Derived from the weighted frequency of the foods or beverages in a sub-category divided by the total weighted frequency of all foods or beverages (n) reported in all sub-categories in a single day, where n = 335,995,769 for food secure 6–11 years, n = 31,155,106 for low food secure 6–11 years, n = 4,126,641 for very low food secure 6–11 years, n = 290,965,789 for food secure 12–17 years, n = 28,444,012 for low food secure 12–17 years, n = 4,749,595 for very low food secure 12–17 years. Estimated weighted percent has been abbreviated by "Wtd %"; SE = Standard Error.

3.1.2. 12–17 Years

Compared with food secure adolescents 12–17 years (12.7%) "beverages" as a broad category were more statistically significantly frequently consumed by low (15.5%) and very low food secure (14.4%) and also combined food insecure groups (15.4%, $p = 0.0001$). A greater contribution of energy from "beverages" ($p = 0.03$) was also determined for food insecure compared with secure (13.0% vs. 11.2%). Alternatively, significantly more frequent intake of "water" was observed among food secure ($p = 0.004$), compared with insecure and low and very low food secure groups (10.3%, 8.7%, 8.6%, 8.8%).

Food secure adolescents reported 4.3% intake frequency of "soft drinks" contrasting with the similar pattern of higher intakes for low food secure at 5.6%, the most frequently consumed sub-category for this group, and 5.1% for very low food secure adolescents as in the younger age group, but with an even greater percentage of reports. Top items were "cola-type soft drink", "fruit-flavored, caffeine free soft drink", "brewed sugar-sweetened iced tea", "orange juice", "fruit flavored drink from powder", "fruit flavored soft drink", "fruit juice drink", and "apple juice". "Tap water" had the reverse pattern as "soft drinks" and comprised the most (5.9%) reports among food secure adolescents while accounting for 4.5% and 3.5% of low and very low food secure reports. "Bottled water", however, was less frequently consumed among food secure and low food secure groups (4.0%, 4.1% respectively) compared with very low (5.2%) food secure reports. "Tap water" and "unsweetened bottled water" were the most frequently consumed items.

4. Discussion

Both the frequency and amount of food and beverage intake are important behavioral exposures characterizing dietary intake. Frequency data permits consideration of the most commonly consumed foods while amount shows the "dose". In this analysis, U.S. children and adolescents had similar frequency of consumption of food categories regardless of food security with the exception of beverage and snack categories. Frequency alone is often overlooked as a component of dietary patterns among children and only two studies are known among adults [23,24]. Traditional dietary assessment, namely food frequency questionnaires, have relied on querying frequency to obtain results focused on contributions to servings of foods, energy and nutrients. Yet, separation of frequency from energy contribution and consideration of frequency as a dietary behavior with potential links to health presents opportunities for behavioral interventions. "Beverages" or "snacks and sweets" were the most frequently consumed broad food groups for all children 6–17 years yet neither ranked as highest contributor to energy, exemplifying their potentially under-recognized importance in children's diets. Their ubiquitous frequency represents potentially impactful targets for intervention to improve overall dietary quality to develop healthy habits for later life [25]. "Beverages" as a broad category represents a spectrum of product types, some without and others with added sugars and key nutrients, respectively [1,14]. However, sub-categories and individual foods ranked by frequency reveal that beverages with a high amount of added sugars are prominent choices [26]. Thus, particular attention to intervention messaging and counseling to improve drink choice among children should be provided. Recommendations for specific beverages and not only broad categories, may be gleaned from these frequency rankings and used to educate healthful patterns. High frequency of snacks and sweets, particularly candy, cookies and brownies, and ice cream, may be targets of interventions more clearly interpreted to broadly limit because of their inherent added sugars [26], yet perhaps more difficult, compared with beverages, to find acceptable substitutions.

Frequency differences in "beverages" and "snacks and sweets" by food security status supports a previous summary of the literature for children 6–11 years for higher added sugar intake [11], sourced from beverages, snacks and sweets among U.S. children [26], and are novel among the sparse evaluation for those 12–17 years [11,27]. "Beverage" intake frequency associated with food insecurity in both age groups may potentially be a manifestation of choices prioritized to satisfy hunger rather than health. Less frequent "water" intake among food insecure adolescents 12–17 years may be related, as a trade-off for higher intake of other beverages [28] or due to lack of potable water supply access among food insecure households [29]. These results support findings showing higher odds of heavy (i.e., more energy) total sweetened beverage intake among low-income compared with high-income children 2–11 years [30]. Older children may be making independent dietary choices and may also be encouraged to obtain food outside the household when also food insecure.

"Soft drinks" were the highest ranking items in the "beverages" category among older food insecure children with caffeinated soft drinks ranking prominently. Older, prevalently low-income children may be working and contributing to family income [31] and using caffeinated beverages to maintain their schedules [32]. Intake frequency and timing of caffeinated beverages may matter more to healthful sleep/wake habits compared with total intake. Previous observational studies have suggested that consumption of caffeinated beverages leads to sleep dysfunction in junior high and high school children [33], and associate with obesity among children 11 years of age [34]. High frequency of caffeinated soft drinks is consistent with these observational results and offers additional evidence supporting dietary interventions to reduce caffeine intake and frequency among all children and especially older food insecure children.

Less frequency and energy contributions of "snacks and sweets" among food insecure compared with secure may represent a relatively more healthful dietary pattern among food insecure 6–11-year-old children. "Snacks and sweets" may be viewed as non-essential foods where budget may be conserved and include high-energy, high-sodium foods [25,35]. As such, the results are unaligned with previous explanations of dietary differences among food insecure groups generalizing a reliance on high energy, low nutrient foods [36].

Frequently consumed foods and beverages among children and adolescents may be used to inform opportunities to promote available and familiar foods that are sources of the nutrients or dietary components that are lacking [11,27], and inform efforts to build on dietary strengths by promoting foods that are already frequently consumed. For example, cow's milk and raw apple were highly reported and may be further promoted in children's food environments. The prominence of "condiments" among frequently consumed foods was apparent. Items like catsup, mustard, mayonnaise, and salsa consumed in relatively small amounts and with little contribution to energy may be used to enhance taste. Their frequent use presents an opportunity to for stealth nutrition interventions to potentially fortify condiments with nutrients most children need more of, and to further reduce components most children need less of (e.g., sodium and sugar).

4.1. Implications

While applications of stealth nutrition may help, the overall poor dietary intake of U.S. children regardless of food security status demand more dramatic changes to improve dietary selection. Primary care contact or public health education among youth provide an ideal environment for education and discussion of dietary habits and suggestions for substitution of soft drinks, for example, with water or low-fat dairy and promotion of fruits and vegetables. Dietary recommendations for food groups and categories may be further translated to specify frequently consumed foods comprising groups recommended for increase or decrease. Federal nutrition assistance programs such as Supplemental Nutrition Assistance Program; Special Supplemental Nutrition Assistance Program for Women, Infants, and Children; and the National School Lunch and Breakfast Programs may similarly apply knowledge of the frequently consumed foods to tailor education and menu components to the 59% of 2016 U.S. food insecure households participating [12]. The National School Lunch and Breakfast Programs play key roles in child nutrition as they represent two main eating occasions of a child's day. Vegetables and fruits may be further promoted through these programs in order to increase their frequency and contributions to total energy. Frequently consumed foods may be key foods for companies to consider nutrient profile improvement to reduce added sugars, sodium and increase calcium, vitamin D, potassium, and fiber [1]. Examination of frequently consumed foods by age group can inform dietary intake questionnaires and be used to populate technology-assisted dietary assessment search tools. Finally, foods listed by frequency may inform monitoring of population dietary intake and potential food environment improvements that enhance safe access to enough foods for healthy, active lifestyles [37].

4.2. Strengths and Limitations

Dietary intake and reporting are reliant on memory and prone to error [38]. Much less is known about the measurement error in children and adolescents self-reported diets compared with adults. Dietary recalls throughout the week allow representation of week and weekend days for U.S. children contributing a strength, yet this analysis is limited as it only represents one day of data for each participant and does not reflect usual intake over time. Aggregation to broad and sub-food categories may highlight food group differences that depend on the groups combined while dis-aggregation may highlight differences that are not meaningful to nutrition such as 'tap water" vs. "bottled water", yet use of broad and sub-food categories aligns with the practical translation of dietary recommendations. Lastly, since food security among household children is reported by a household adult, an individual child's food security may be biased by the perception of the adult and the adult's perception of food security for other children in the household [39]. Older children tend to be under-classified as food insecure while younger children may be over-classified. While imperfect, differences by food security and age were observed in this analysis and add knowledge of the dietary patterns of food insecure children.

5. Conclusions

Among children and adolescents 6–17 years old, similar foods ranked among those frequently consumed. However, frequency-differentiated intake patterns exist for beverages and snack foods by food security across age groups. The main findings reported in this paper may inform dietary recommendations, development of population-specific dietary assessment tools, interventions, menus, and the composition of food packages, and food policy for food insecure children, and adolescents.

Supplementary Materials: The following are available online at http://www.mdpi.com/2072-6643/12/2/304/s1, Table S1: Top 25 most frequently consumed foods or beverages, unweighted frequency of reported foods or beverages, weighted percent of reported foods or beverages, and standard error of weighted percent of reported foods or beverages among all reported foods or beverages for food secure, low, and very low food secure U.S. children and adolescents aged 6–11 and 12–17 years using the National Health and Nutrition Examination Survey 2007–2014.

Author Contributions: Conceptualization, H.A.E.-M.; methodology, H.A.E.-M. and C.J.B.; analysis, H.A.E.-M.; writing—original draft preparation, H.A.E.-M.; writing—review and editing, H.A.E.-M., C.J.B., R.L.B., Y.J.Y. All authors have read and agreed to the published version of the manuscript.

Funding: H.A.E.-M. received support from USDA National Institute of Food and Agriculture, Hatch project IND030489.

Conflicts of Interest: The authors declare no conflict of interest. The funders had no role in the design of the study; in the collection, analyses, or interpretation of data; in the writing of the manuscript, or in the decision to publish the results.

References

1. U.S. Department of Agriculture. Advisory Report to the Secretary of Health and Human Services and the Secretary of Agriculture. Available online: http://www.health.gov/dietaryguidelines/2015-scientific-report/PDFs/Scientific-Report-of-the-2015-Dietary-Guidelines-Advisory-Committee.pdf (accessed on 10 December 2019).
2. Eicher-Miller, H.A.; Park, C.Y.; Bailey, R. Identifying nutritional gaps among Americans. In *Dietary Supplements in Health Promotion*; Wallace, T.C., Ed.; CRN Press: Boca Raton, FL, USA, 2015; pp. 17–54.
3. Anderson, S.A. Core indicators of nutritional state for difficult-to-sample populations. *J. Nutr.* **1990**, *120* (Suppl. 11), 1559–1600. [CrossRef] [PubMed]
4. Alaimo, K.; Olson, C.M.; Frongillo, E.A., Jr. Food insufficiency and American school-aged children's cognitive, academic, and psychosocial development. *Pediatrics* **2001**, *108*, 44–53. [PubMed]

5. Casey, P.H.; Szeto, K.L.; Robbins, J.M.; Stuff, J.E.; Connell, C.; Gossett, J.M.; Simpson, P.M. Child health-related quality of life and household food security. *Arch. Pediatr. Adolesc. Med.* **2005**, *159*, 51–56. [CrossRef] [PubMed]
6. Slopen, N.; Fitzmaurice, G.; Williams, D.R.; Gilman, S.E. Poverty, food insecurity, and the behavior for childhood internalizing and externalizing disorders. *J. Am. Acad. Child. Adolesc. Psychiatry* **2010**, *49*, 444–452. [PubMed]
7. Eicher-Miller, H.A.; Mason, A.C.; Weaver, C.M.; McCabe, G.P.; Boushey, C.J. Food insecurity is associated with iron deficiency anemia in U.S. adolescents. *Am. J. Clin. Nutr.* **2009**, *90*, 1358–1371. [CrossRef]
8. Eicher-Miller, H.A.; Mason, A.C.; Weaver, C.M.; McCabe, G.P.; Boushey, C.J. Food insecurity is associated with diet and bone mass disparities in early adolescent males but not females in the United States. *J. Nutr.* **2011**, *141*, 1738–1751. [CrossRef]
9. Belsky, D.W.; Moffitt, T.E.; Arseneault, L.; Melchior, M.; Caspi, A. Context and sequelae of food insecurity in children's development. *Am. J. Epidemiol.* **2010**, *172*, 809–818. [CrossRef]
10. Gundersen, C.; Ziliak, J.P. Food insecurity and health outcomes. *Health Aff.* **2015**, *34*, 1830–1839. [CrossRef]
11. Eicher-Miller, H.A.; Zhao, Y. Evidence for the age-specific relationship of food insecurity and key dietary outcomes among U.S. children and adolescence. *Nutr. Res. Rev.* **2018**, *31*, 98–113. [CrossRef]
12. Colman-Jensen, A.; Rabbitt, R.P.; Gregory, C.A.; Singh, A. Household Food Security in the United States in 2016. ERR-237. U.S. Department of Agriculture, Economic Research Service. 2017. Available online: https://www.ers.usda.gov/publications/pub-details/?pubid=84972 (accessed on 10 December 2019).
13. Nicklas, T.A.; Baranowski, T.; Cullen, K.W.; Berenson, G. Eating patterns, dietary quality and obesity. *J. Am. Coll. Nutr.* **2001**, *20*, 599–608. [CrossRef]
14. U.S. Department of Agriculture. Agricultural Research Service. What We Eat in America Food Categories. 2016. Available online: https://www.ars.usda.gov/northeast-area/beltsville-md-bhnrc/beltsville-human-nutrition-research-center/food-surveys-research-group/docs/dmr-food-categories (accessed on 10 December 2019).
15. Centers for Disease Control and Prevention (CDC); National Center for Health Statistics (NCHS). National Health and Nutrition Examination Survey Dietary Data. Available online: https://wwwn.cdc.gov/Nchs/Nhanes/Search/DataPage.aspx?Component=Dietary (accessed on 10 December 2019).
16. Centers for Disease Control and Prevention (CDC), National Center for Health Statistics (NCHS). National Health and Nutrition Examination Survey Questionnaire and Examination Protocol. Available online: https://wwwn.cdc.gov/nchs/nhanes/analyticguidelines.aspx (accessed on 10 December 2019).
17. National Center for Health Statistics. NCHS Research Ethics Review Board (ERB) Approval. Available online: https://www.cdc.gov/nchs/nhanes/irba98.htm (accessed on 10 December 2019).
18. Bickel, G.; Nord, M.; Price, C.; Hamilton, W.; Cook, J. Guide to Measuring Household Food Security, Revised 2000. U.S. Department of Agriculture, Food and Nutrition Service. 2000. Available online: https://www.fns.usda.gov/guide-measuring-household-food-security-revised-2000 (accessed on 10 December 2019).
19. Centers for Disease Control and Prevention. A SAS Program for the 2000 CDC Growth Charts. Available online: https://www.cdc.gov/nccdphp/dnpao/growthcharts/resources/sas.htm (accessed on 10 December 2019).
20. Agricultural Research Service USDA. USDA Automated Multiple-Pass Method. Available online: http://www.ars.usda.gov/Services/docs.htm?docid=7710 (accessed on 10 December 2019).
21. Moshfegh, A.J.; Rhodes, D.G.; Baer, D.J.; Murayi, T.; Clemens, J.C.; Rumpler, W.V.; Paul, D.R.; Sebastian, R.S.; Kuczynski, K.J.; Ingwersen, L.A.; et al. The US Department of Agriculture Automated Multiple-Pass Method reduces bias in the collection of energy intakes. *Am. J. Clin. Nutr.* **2008**, *88*, 324–332. [CrossRef] [PubMed]
22. USDA Agricultural Research Service. Food and Nutrient Database for Dietary Studies 2013–2014. Food Surveys Research Group: Beltsville, MD. Available online: http://www.ars.usda.gov/ba/bhnrc/fsrg (accessed on 10 December 2019).
23. Eicher-Miller, H.A.; Boushey, C.J. How often and how much? Differences in dietary intake by frequency and energy contribution vary among U.S. Adults in NHANES 2007–2012. *Nutrients* **2017**, *9*, 86. [CrossRef] [PubMed]
24. Kendall, A.; Olson, C.M.; Frongillo, E.A. Relationship of hunger and food insecurity to food availability and consumption. *J. Am. Diet. Assoc.* **1996**, *96*, 1019–1024. [CrossRef]

25. Fiorito, L.M.; Marini, M.; Mitchell, D.C.; Smiciklas-Wright, H.; Birch, L.L. Girls' early sweetened carbonated beverage intake predicts different patterns of beverage and nutrient intake across childhood and adolescence. *J. Am. Diet. Assoc.* **2010**, *110*, 543–550. [CrossRef]
26. Bailey, R.L.; Fulgoni, V.L.; Cowan, A.E.; Gaine, P.C. Sources of added sugar in young children, adolescents, and adults with low and high intakes of added sugars. *Nutrients* **2018**, *10*, 102. [CrossRef]
27. Hanson, K.L.; Connor L.M. Food insecurity and dietary quality in U.S. adults and children: A systematic review. *Am. J. Clin. Nutr.* **2014**, *100*, 684–692. [CrossRef]
28. Park, S.; Blanck, H.M.; Sherry, B.; Brener, N.; O'Toole, T. Factors associated with low water intake among U.S. High School Students-National Youth Physical Activity and Nutrition Study, 2010. *J. Am. Nutr. Diet.* **2012**, *112*, 1421–1427. [CrossRef]
29. Pinard, C.A.; Kim, S.A.; Story, M.; Yaroch, A.L. The food and water system impacts on obesity. *J. Law Med. Ethics* **2013**, *41*, 52–60. [CrossRef]
30. Han, E.; Powell, L.M. Consumption patterns of sugar-sweetened beverages in the United States. *J. Acad. Nutr. Diet.* **2013**, *113*, 43–53. [CrossRef]
31. Johnson, D.S.; Lino, M. Teenagers: Employment and contributions to family spending. *Mon. Labor. Rev.* **2000**, *123*, 15–25.
32. Miller, K.E.; Dermen, K.H.; Lucke, J.F. Caffeinated energy drink use by U.S. adolescents aged 13–17: A national profile. *Psychol. Addict. Behav.* **2018**, *32*, 647–659. [CrossRef] [PubMed]
33. Orbeta, R.L.; Overpeck, M.D.; Ramcharran, D.; Kogan, M.D.; Ledsky, R. High caffeine intake in adolescents: Associations with difficulty sleeping and feeling tired in the morning. *J. Adolesc. Health* **2006**, *38*, 451–453. [CrossRef] [PubMed]
34. Ludwig, D.S.; Peterson, K.E.; Gortmaker, S.L. Relation between consumption of sugar-sweetened drinks and childhood obesity: A prospective, observational analysis. *Lancet* **2001**, *357*, 505–508. [CrossRef]
35. Dunford, E.K.; Poti, J.M.; Popkin, B.M. Emerging disparities in dietary sodium intake from snacking in the U.S. population. *Nutrients* **2017**, *9*, 610. [CrossRef] [PubMed]
36. Drewnowski, A.; Darmon, N.; Briend, A. Replacing fats and sweets with vegetables and fruits-a question of cost. *Am. J. Public Health* **2004**, *94*, 1555–1559. [CrossRef] [PubMed]
37. Centers for Disease Control and Prevention (CDC) The CDC Guide to Strategies for Reducing the Consumption of Sugar-Sweetened Beverages. Available online: http://www.cdph.ca.gov/SiteCollectionDocuments/StratstoReduce_Sugar_Sweetened_Bevs.pdf (accessed on 10 December 2019).
38. Burrows, T.L.; Martin, R.J.; Collins, C.E. A systematic review of the validity of dietary assessment methods in children when compared with the method of doubly labeled water. *J. Acad. Nutr. Diet.* **2010**, *110*, 1501–1510. [CrossRef]
39. Nord, M.; Bickel, G. Measuring Children's Food Security in U.S. Households, 1995–1999. Food Assistance and Nutrition Research Report No. 25, U.S. Department of Agriculture, Food and Rural Economics Division, Economic Research Service. Available online: https://www.ers.usda.gov/publications/pub-details/?pubid=46624 (accessed on 10 December 2019).

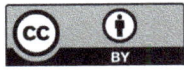

© 2020 by the authors. Licensee MDPI, Basel, Switzerland. This article is an open access article distributed under the terms and conditions of the Creative Commons Attribution (CC BY) license (http://creativecommons.org/licenses/by/4.0/).

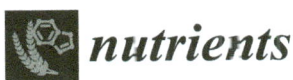 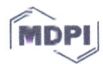

Article

Food Security and Diet Quality in Native Hawaiian, Pacific Islander, and Filipino Infants 3 to 12 Months of Age

Sally Campbell [1,2], John J. Chen [3], Carol J. Boushey [4], Heather Eicher-Miller [5], Fengqing Zhu [3] and Marie K. Fialkowski [3,*]

1. Technological University Dublin, Kevin Street, Saint Peter's, D08X622 Dublin 2, Ireland; campbes7@tcd.ie
2. Trinity College University of Dublin, College Green, Dublin 2, Ireland
3. Department of Human Nutrition, Food and Animal Sciences, College of Tropical Agriculture and Human Resources—University of Hawai'i at Mānoa, Honolulu, HI 96822, USA; jjchen@hawaii.edu
4. Epidemiology Program, University of Hawaii Cancer Center, 701 Ilalo St, Honolulu, HI 96813, USA; cjboushey@cc.hawaii.edu
5. Department Nutrition Science, College of Health and Human Science, Purdue University, West Lafayette, IN 47907, USA; heicherm@purdue.edu (H.E.-M.); zhu0@purdue.edu (F.Z.)
* Correspondence: mariekf@hawaii.edu

Received: 31 May 2020; Accepted: 15 July 2020; Published: 17 July 2020

Abstract: Food insecurity and other nutritional risks in infancy pose a lifelong risk to wellbeing; however, their effect on diet quality in Native Hawaiian, Pacific Islander, and Filipino (NHPIF) infants in Hawai'i is unknown. In this cross-sectional analysis, the association between various indicators of food security and NHPIF infant diet quality were investigated in 70 NHPIF infants aged 3–12 months residing on O'ahu, Hawai'i. The dietary assessments of the infants were collected using a mobile food record^{TM}. Foods consumed across four days were categorized into seven food groups. Indicators for food security were examined through an adapted infant food security index and other indicators. Data were analyzed using chi-square tests, independent sample t-tests, multinomial logistic regression, and linear regression models. In models adjusting for age and sex, infants defined as food insecure by the adapted index were found to consume foods from more food groups and consume flesh foods on a greater proportion of days. Of the indicators examined, the adapted index was shown to be the best indicator for food group consumption. Further work is needed on a more representative sample of NHPIF infants to determine the impact that food security has on nutritional status and other indicators of health.

Keywords: infants; minority; food security; diet diversity; diet quality

1. Introduction

Food insecurity is defined as limited or uncertain availability of nutritionally adequate foods. It is considered a high priority for public health stakeholders given its economic and health impacts and the associated nutritional risks [1]. These impacts include worse developmental outcomes and chronic illness among children [2], and poorer health outcomes in infants [3]. Situations of food insecurity are linked with disrupted eating patterns, poor diet quality and nutritional inadequacy across age groups and demographics [4]. Infants aged 0–12 months are more susceptible to the adverse effects of food insecurity given their high nutritional requirements for growth and dependence on others for nutrition [3]. Optimal nutrition during infancy protects against morbidity and mortality, reduces the risk of chronic disease, and promotes better overall development, and thus efforts to understand and mitigate nutritional risks such as infant food insecurity and improved nutrition in early life may have far-reaching implications [5].

An eighteen-item survey known as the U.S. Household Food Security Survey Module (USHFSSM) was developed by the United States Department of Agriculture (USDA) to assess household food security; a portion of the survey questions may be used to determine the food security of a child or children within the household [6]. In contrast to this method, Schlichting D. et al. devised a food security index which aims to assess the food security of an infant at an individual level within a household [3]. In addition to food security status, another indicator of nutritional risk is household income as it is theorized that some low-income households lack economic access to healthy foods [7,8]. Similarly, eligibility to food assistance programs, such as the Special Supplemental Nutrition Program for Women, Infants and Children (WIC) and the Supplemental Nutrition Assistance Program (SNAP), are based on household income criteria and may also indicate nutritional risk [8–10]. The separate associations between each of these indicators of nutritional risk: food insecurity, household income, and food assistance program participation, with overall dietary quality, reveals disagreement across the literature. These nutritional risks may have contrasting influences on the diet quality of different demographics, namely by age and ethnic group.

Food insecurity disproportionately influences households headed by individuals of minority race/ethnicity [4]. For example, the odds of food insecurity were higher among ethnic minority infants including Maori, Pacific Islander, and Asian infants when compared to all other infants, in a representative sample of the New Zealand infant population [3]. This race/ethnicity disparity in food insecurity extends to associations with poor dietary intake among food-insecure minority groups. Leung C et al. studied a population of 4393 adults from the National Nutrition and Health Examination Survey (NHANES) and found food insecurity was associated with a lower diet quality indicated by Healthy Eating Index (HEI) score, and this association was most pronounced among those who identify as American Indian or Alaska Native, Native Hawaiian or Pacific Islander or as multiracial [4]. Despite their inclusion in this sample, the Native Hawaiian or Pacific Islander population represents a unique group within the US at risk of poorer health outcomes than the overall population [11]. Heinrich K. and colleagues found that a combination of high living costs and low-income negatively impacts some low-income residents in Hawai'i, contributing to food insecurity [12].

Minority groups such as Native Hawaiian, Pacific Islander or Filipinos (NHPIF) in Hawai'i report higher levels of food insecurity than other ethnicities [13]. Yet the relationship between food insecurity and other indicators of nutritional risk, household income and food assistance participation, to diet quality among NHPIF infants in Hawai'i is not known, nor is which indicator has a stronger relationship to dietary quality. Therefore, the objective of this study was to determine which indicator of nutritional risk would have the strongest association with the diet quality of NHPIF infants 3–12 months of age. This was assessed using responses to two questions modified from the USHFSSM relating to money running out for food and utilities, participation in food assistance programs, annual household income, or an adapted infant food security index. A Minimum Dietary Diversity (MDD) score is used when evaluating the diet quality of infants aged 6–12 months, and thus MDD was used for this analysis. The diet quality of infants aged 3–12 months was examined by food group consumption. Authors hypothesized that an adapted infant food security index, which takes into account multiple indicators of food insecurity, would have the strongest association with diet quality assessed using the MDD and food group consumption [14].

2. Materials and Methods

2.1. Study Sample

The target population for this cross-sectional study was NHPIF infants between 3–12 months of age residing on O'ahu, Hawai'i. To be eligible to participate in the study, the infant's caregiver(s) had to be 18 years of age or older, have an iOS mobile device, and have reliable access to the Internet. The infant participants had to have commenced complementary feeding prior to study onset and be reported by the caregiver as at least part Native Hawaiian, Pacific Islander or Filipino. A convenient sample of NHPIF infants was primarily recruited through community-based events (e.g., Baby Expo), programs (e.g., WIC), and networking. Seventy infants and their caregivers completed the study, of which 56 of the infants were aged 6–12 months. Institutional Review Board (IRB) exemption from the University of Hawai'i was received prior to the collection of data (IRB reference number: 2017-00845). Consent was obtained in writing from the caregivers for both their participation and their infant's participation prior to collecting any data. Data was collected between March 2018–February 2019.

2.2. Participant Characteristics

At study onset, caregivers completed a questionnaire using a secure on-line web application. Topics included feeding practices followed prior to enrolment in the study. Demographic information included annual household income, information relating to household food security status including household participation in food assistance programs such as WIC, SNAP, free or reduced cost school meals, food banks since the child was born and two questions informed from the USHFSSM [6]. The two questions modified from the USHFSSM were:

1. *In the past 12 months, how often did your money for food run out before the end of the month? (Never, Seldom, Sometimes, Most times, Always, Do not know, No response)*
2. *In the past 12 months, how often did your money for household utilities (e.g., water, fuel, oil, electricity) run out before the end of the month? (Never, Seldom, Sometimes, Most times, Always, Do not know, No response)*

2.3. Dietary Assessment

Infant dietary assessment was completed through surrogate reporting via the caregiver with the mobile food record^{TM} (mFR^{TM}) [15]. The mFR^{TM} is an application designed specifically for the assessment of dietary intake from the Technology Assisted Dietary Assessment^{TM} project (http://tadaproject.org/) which uses the camera on a mobile device to capture food and beverage intake, which is then used to estimate energy, nutrients, food and beverage intakes [15–18]. The mFR^{TM} was loaded on to the caregiver's mobile device and training on the mFR^{TM} application was completed prior to data collection. Caregivers were instructed to take before and after images of all foods and beverages the participant consumed over a 4-day collection period (Thursday–Sunday). After the collection period concluded, a member of the research team reviewed the images with caregivers to verify content, as needed, and to probe for any forgotten foods or beverages. At the end of the data collection period, caregivers were compensated with a $40 gift card.

2.4. Dietary Diversity Score

The global metric Minimum Dietary Diversity (MDD) score from the World Health Organisation's (WHO) indicators for assessing infant and young child feeding practices (IYCF, 2007) [14] was used to examine infant diet quality. Consuming a wide range of foods to meet one's nutrient needs is one tenet of a healthy diet and, in infancy, the number of food groups consumed can predict the nutrient density of the diet [19]. Given the absence of an HEI for children aged below 2 years [20] and the limited selection of infant diet quality scoring metrics in the US, MDD was implemented as an indicator of the micronutrient adequacy of NHPIF infants. The WHO recommends the initiation of complementary feeding from 6 months onward [21]; thus, this assessment is appropriate only for infants aged 6 months and older. Solid foods and liquids consumed in any amount more than a condiment were enumerated over the 4 days using the mFR^{TM} images. Using the MDD metric, solids and liquids consumed in a day were categorized into seven food groups: (1) grains, roots, and tubers; (2) legumes and nuts; (3) dairy products (milk, including formula, yogurt, cheese); (4) flesh foods (meat, fish, poultry, liver/organ meats); (5) eggs; (6) vitamin A-rich fruits and vegetables; and (7) other fruits and vegetables. Particular attention is given by the WHO to assess vitamin A intake in children aged 6–59 months. This is because vitamin A deficiency in infancy is a public health problem in many developing countries. Furthermore, vitamin A deficiency can cause visual impairment and may increase the risk of illness and death from childhood infections [22]. MDD was considered met if the infant consumed four or more of the seven food groups, on average, each day and unmet if less than four food groups had been consumed, on average, each day. Human milk is not counted in a food group in the version of the WHO MDD metric used [14].

2.5. Adapted Food Security Index

A food security index was adapted from an index developed by Schlichting D. et al. and is outlined in Table 1 [3]. The adapted index estimates the degree of infant food security as a weighted sum of scores from two of the modified USHFSSM questions, i.e., use of defined methods to cope with food insecurity such as using food banks, and infant breastfeeding status at 3 months. Breastfeeding status at this age was chosen as each participant had commenced complementary feeding prior to study onset and the minimum participant age was 3 months. Positive points were awarded for breastfeeding to 3 months and never running out of money for food or utilities, while scoring was reversed and points deducted for the use of coping methods such as using food assistance programs. The range of scores was −14 to 4. For ease of discussion, a constant equal to the lowest value (−14) was added to all scores, shifting the range upward to 0–18 where 0 represents the lowest status of food security and 18 the highest. A cutoff for infant food insecurity was set at half a standard deviation below the mean (12.76). This cutoff point is consistent with other authors who claim it represents the minimum socially acceptable level of food insecurity prevalence. Infants were classified by this index into either extremely, highly or moderately food insecure or extremely, highly or moderately food secure (see Table 1 and Table 5) [3].

Table 1. The adapted infant food security index [a] components, weights, scores, and ranges applied to this study.

	Adapted Infant Food Security Index Used in this Study			
	Component	Weight	Min	Max
Coping	Money for food runs out by the end of the month	Never = 1 Seldom = 0 Sometimes = −1 Most times = −2 Always = −3	−3	1
	Money for utilities runs out by the end of the month	Never = 1 Seldom = 0 Sometimes = −1 Most times = −2 Always = −3	−3	1
	Participation in WIC	Yes = −2 No = 0	−2	0
	Participation in SNAP	Yes = −2 No = 0	−2	0
	Receives reduced cost/free school meals	Yes = −2 No = 0	−2	0
	Receives other food assistance	Yes = −2 No = 0	−2	0

Table 1. *Cont.*

Adapted Infant Food Security Index Used in this Study				
	Component	Weight	Min	Max
BF	Breastfeeding to 3 months	Exclusive = +2 BF and Formula Feeding = +1 Formula only or BF < 3 month = 0	0	2
	Total Score		−14	4
	Add constant of 14		0	18

[a] Adapted from Schlichting D. et al. [3].

2.6. Analysis

Descriptive statistics were used to categorize the sample. Mean and standard deviations (SD) were used to describe age and food group consumption. Frequencies and percentages were used to describe food security prevalence by the various indicators. Participation in food assistance programs was examined from the dichotomous responses: yes or no. Responses to the modified USHFSSM questions on running out of money for food or utilities were collapsed into dichotomous variables (yes or no). The responses never or seldom to either question was reported as not experiencing (no) while the responses sometimes, most times or always were reported as experiencing it (yes). The mean daily consumption of the 7 food groups was calculated as a mean of all four mFR^{TM} days, a method commonly used [3,23]. The frequency of consumption of each food group with the average number of food groups consumed was examined in all participants (i.e., 3–12 months). Quantitative variables were compared between food-secure and food-insecure subgroups using both independent samples t-test methods and the non-parametric Mann–Whitney U tests. Independent sample t-test p-value results were presented when the results from the two approaches were similar. Categorical variables were compared using Chi-squared tests or Fisher's exact tests [23]. Spearman's rho correlation coefficient was used in examining correlation between food security indicators and food groups consumed [24]. The proportion meeting/not meeting the MDD ($\geq$4 food groups) was determined in the participants 6–12 months of age subgroup only, across all four days of the mFR^{TM}. A sequence of multivariable logistic regression and linear regression models were developed to investigate the relationships between MDD and individual and total food group intake, and those variables that yielded significant results in the bivariate analysis. In logistic regression analysis, MDD was met or not, on average, across the four days (yes or no) was used as the dependent variable to investigate its associations with the adapted food security index score, household income or the response to running out of money for food, adjusting for age and sex. In the linear regression analysis, total and individual food group consumption was used as the dependent variable to study its relationships with the adapted food security index score, household income, responses to running out of money for food and utilities or WIC and SNAP participation status, adjusting for age and sex as considered in similar studies [23]. Statistical significance was set at p-value < 0.05. All statistical analyses were performed using SPSS version 26 (Armonk, NY, USA). As this was a secondary analysis, a power calculation was not conducted to identify the sample size.

3. Results

3.1. Food Security Classification Using the Adapted Food Security Index

Of the 70 infants, approximately one quarter were classified as food insecure, with over 20% being classified as moderately or highly or extremely food insecure. Over 40% were highly food secure, while no infant was classified as extremely food secure (see Table 2).

Table 2. Food security classifications using an adapted food security index among infants aged 3–12 months in the cross-sectional study ($n = 70$) [a].

SD Cut Point	Score Range	Definition	Prevalence, n (%)
<−2 SD	<7.12	Extremely food insecure	4 (5.7)
−2 SD ≤ • < −1 SD	7.13–10.88	Highly food insecure	5 (7.1)
−1 SD ≤ • < −0.5 SD	10.89–12.76	Moderately food insecure	9 (12.9)
−0.5 SD ≤ • < +0.5 SD	12.77–16.52	Moderately food secure	16 (22.9)
+0.5 SD ≤ • < +1 SD	16.53–18.40	Highly food secure	31 (44.3)
≥+1 SD	≥18.41	Extremely food secure	0 (0)

SD = standard deviation. [a] Total number of responses = 65 as there were 5 (7.1%) incomplete responses.

3.2. Other Characteristics of Participants

Approximately half of the infants were girls and the mean age was 7.4 months. A greater proportion of food-secure infant caregivers were married and earning higher incomes. Likewise, a greater proportion of food-secure infant caregivers attended college (see Table 3).

Table 3. Characteristics of food-secure and food-insecure infants and their caregivers included in this cross-sectional study examining food security and Native Hawaiian, Pacific Islander, and Filipino (NHPIF) [a] infant diet ($n = 70$).

Characteristics		Total Sample	Food-[b] Secure Subsample	Food-Insecure Subsample	p-Value [c]
Age	Months (mean ± SD)	7.4 ± 2.1	7.2 ± 2.1	8 ± 2.2	
	3–6 months, n (%)	14 (20.1)	10 (21.4)	4 (27.9)	0.2
	6–12 months, n (%)	56 (79.9)	37 (78.7)	14 (72.1)	
Sex	Boy, n (%)	38 (54.3)	27 (57.4)	8 (44.4)	0.4
	Girl, n (%)	32 (45.7)	20 (42.6)	10 (55.6)	
Marital Status	Married, n (%)	46 (61.3)	36 (76.6)	10 (55.6)	0.02
	Single/divorced/widowed, n (%)	24 (31.9)	11 (23.4)	8 (44.4)	
Highest Level of Education Attended	College, n (%)	50 (66.6)	37 (78.7)	9 (50)	0.03
	Grade School (Elementary–High School), n (%)	20 (26.6)	10 (21.3)	9 (50)	
Employed for Wages	Yes, n (%)	42 (60)	28 (59.6)	10 (55.6)	0.8
	No, n (%)	28 (40)	19 (40.4)	8 (44.4)	
Annual Household Income	>$35,000	48 (81.4)	38 (90.5)	10 (58.8)	0.01
	<$35,000	11 (18.6)	4 (9.5)	7 (41.2)	

[a] Native Hawaiian, Pacific Islander or Filipino ethnicity. [b] As categorized by the adapted infant food security index used in this study. [c] p-values comparing food-secure and food-insecure subsamples.

Table 4 displays the proportion of infants classified as food secure or insecure by component on the food security index adapted from Schlichting D. et al. [3]. Most infants classified as food insecure were part of households who experienced running out of money for food or utilities by the end of the month. Additionally, over 80% of food-insecure infants' households participated in WIC and over 50% participated in SNAP.

Table 4. Proportion of infants aged 3–12 months enrolled in the cross-sectional study classified as food secure or insecure by each component of the adapted infant food security index used in this study ($n = 70$) [a,b].

Component			Food Security Status		Chi-Squared p-Value
			Food Secure n (%)	Food Insecure n (%)	
Coping	Money for food runs out by the end of the month	Yes No	3 (6.4) 44 (93.6)	15 (83.3) 3 (16.7)	0.001
	Money for utilities runs out by the end of the month	Yes No	6 (11.5) 46 (88.5)	12 (92.3) 1 (7.7)	<0.0001
	Participation in Special Supplemental Nutrition Program for Women (WIC)	Yes No	7 (14.9) 40 (85.1)	15 (83.3) 3 (16.7)	<0.0001
	Participation in Supplemental Nutrition Assistance Program (SNAP)	Yes No	3 (6.4) 44 (93.6)	10 (55.6) 8 (44.4)	<0.0001
	Receives reduced cost/free school meals	Yes No	0 (0) 47 (100)	7 (38.9) 11 (61.1)	0.001
	Receives food assistance (Food Bank/Food Pantries or Commodity Foods)	Yes No	0 (0) 47 (100)	2 (11.1) 16 (88.9)	0.07
Breastfeeding	Exclusive breastfeeding to 3 months		30 (63.8)	14 (77.8)	0.7
	Breast and formula feeding to 3 months		13 (28.7)	2 (11.1)	0.2
	Formula only or breastfeeding <3 months		4 (8.5)	2 (11.1)	0.1

[a] Adapted from Schlichting D. et al. [3]. [b] Total number of responses were 65. 5 (7.1%) incomplete responses.

3.3. Average Percentage Daily Food Group Consumption by Food Security Status

The seven food groups used to classify the infants' dietary characteristics are shown in Table 5. Grains, roots or tubers were the most commonly consumed foods followed by other fruits and vegetables and dairy products. The mean total number of food groups consumed daily was a little over 3.0 food groups with a range between 1.0–5.3. The mean consumption of food groups by infants, 3–12 months, from households who experience running out of money for food or utilities at the end of the month was almost four food groups each day, while infants from households who do not experience running out of money for food or utilities at the end of the month had, on average, three food groups each day. Infants, 3–12 months, from households not experiencing running out of money for food or utilities at the end of the month consumed a flesh food more than half of the time, while those who did not experience running out of money for food or utilities by the end of the month consumed a flesh food approximately 20% of the time. A marginal but statistically significant difference in the consumption of grains, roots and tubers, between those who do and do not experience running out of money for food, was also identified. Infants, 3–12 months, from households who do experience running out of money for food at the end of the month consumed a grain root or tuber almost 100% of the time, while those who do not experience running out of money for food by the end of the month consumed a grain, root or tuber approximately 80% of the time.

Table 5. Mean percent daily food group consumption by various indicators of food security applied in this analysis for infants aged 3–12 months enrolled in the cross-sectional study ($n = 70$).

Food Group	Infants Total (%)	FSSS Q1 [a]			FSSS Q2 [b]			WIC			SNAP			FIS (%)	FS (%)	Index Score [c]			Income		
		Yes (%)	No (%)	p	Yes (%)	No (%)	p	Yes (%)	No (%)	p	Yes (%)	No (%)	p			p	Corr	p	Low Income (%)	High Income (%)	p	Corr	p
Grains, roots and tubers	85	96	79	0.001	96	82	0.089	93	80	0.023	95	82	0.173 Y	96	80	0.002	−0.359	0.003	94	82	0.030	−0.227	0.058
Legumes and nuts	8	4	9	0.505 Y	6	8	0.948 Y	6	9	0.973 Y	11	7	0.085 Y	6	9	0.935 Y	−0.042	0.742	13	7	0.251	−0.132	0.275
Dairy products	61	65	60	0.659	48	63	0.283	69	56	0.252	68	59	0.621 Y	58	62	0.802	−0.016	0.902	77	59	0.224	−0.177	0.143
Flesh foods	28	57	17	0.000	63	20	0.000	33	24	0.338	40	25	0.203	61	16	0.000	−0.362	0.003	50	24	0.085	−0.187	0.122
Eggs	8	10	7	0.469	6	8	0.767	9	7	0.628	17	6	0.116	12	6	0.146 Y	−0.002	0.987	20	5	0.067	−0.141	0.247
Vitamin A-rich fruits and vegetables	56	65	54	0.192	71	53	0.071	61	54	0.398	63	55	0.570 Y	63	54	0.361	−0.220	0.078	67	54	0.171	−0.095	0.432
Other fruits and vegetables	73	78	71	0.487	85	71	0.186	74	72	0.680 Y	75	72	0.944 Y	78	71	0.450	−0.138	0.274	77	72	0.666	−0.056	0.643
Total food groups (n)	3.2	3.8	3.0	0.005	3.8	3.0	0.018	3.5	3.0	0.110	3.7	3.1	0.055	3.8	3.0	0.008	−0.317	0.010	4.0	3.0	0.003	−0.294	0.014

Y indicates Mann–Whitney U test result. Special Supplemental Nutrition Program for Women, Infants and Children (WIC), The Supplemental Nutrition Assistance Program (SNAP), p value (p), correlation (Corr, Spearman's rho), grains, roots and tubers (Grains), legumes and nuts (Legumes), vitamin A-rich fruits and vegetables (Vitamin A), other fruits and vegetables (Other). [a] Adapted USDA Food Security Survey Scale Question. Money for food runs out by the end of the month. No = Never/seldom. Yes = Sometimes/most times/always. [b] Adapted USDA Food Security Survey Scale Question. Money for utilities runs out by the end of the month. No = Never/seldom. Yes = Sometimes/most times/always. [c] Adapted Infant Food Security Index used in this study. Classified as food secure (FS). Classified as food insecure (FIS).

Only one marginal, but statistically significant, difference in infant daily food group consumption was identified between households who do and do not participate in WIC and SNAP. Infants in households who participate in WIC or SNAP consumed a grain, root or tuber over 90% of the time, while those who do not participate in WIC or SNAP consumed a grain, root or tuber approximately 80% of the time. On average, infants in households who participate in WIC or SNAP consumed foods from approximately 3.5 food groups each day, while infants in households who do not participate in WIC or SNAP consumed foods from approximately 3.0 food groups each day (see Table 5).

There was a significant difference in the intake of flesh foods between those infants who were and were not defined as food insecure by the adapted food security index. Those defined as food insecure had a flesh food intake over 60% of the time, while those defined as food secure had a flesh food intake more than 15% of the time. Likewise, infants defined as food insecure had a grain, root or tuber group over 95% of the time versus approximately 80% of the time by those defined as food secure. Furthermore, infants defined as food insecure had, on average, 3.76 out of seven food groups a day, while those defined as food secure had, on average, almost 3.0 food groups (see Table 5).

Weak to moderate, but statistically significant negative spearman correlations were observed between infant food security by the adapted index and total food group, the grain, root, and tuber food group and the flesh food group consumption. Likewise, weak, but significant negative spearman correlations were found between household income and total food group consumption (see Table 5).

3.4. Proportion of Infants Aged 6–12 Months Meeting the MDD by Food Security Indicators

Table 6 presents the proportion of infants 6–12 months who did and did not meet the MDD by the various indicators of food security examined in this study. The highest proportion of infants to meet the MDD were those classified as moderately food insecure by the adapted infant food security index, of whom over 70% met the MDD. Significantly more food-insecure infants met the MDD in comparison to food-secure infants. In addition, over two-thirds of infants from households with an annual income of <$35,000, met the MDD whereas a little less than 30% of infants from households with an annual income of >$35,000 met the MDD. Similarly, the income bracket with the highest proportion of infants (approximately 80%) meeting the MDD was <$10,000 while the lowest proportion of infants (over 15%) meeting the MDD were from the $60,000–75,000 bracket followed by the >$75,000 bracket with over 25%.

Table 6. Proportion of infants aged 6–12 months enrolled in the cross-sectional study meeting the Minimum Dietary Diversity (MDD) score [a] by the various indicators of food security examined in this study (n = 70) [b].

		Met MDD n (%)	Did not Meet MDD n (%)	Chi Square p Values
Total		20 (35.7)	36 (64.3)	-
Money for food running out by the end of the month [c]	No	10 (26.3)	28 (73.7)	0.052
	Yes	8 (57.1)	6 (42.9)	
Money for utilities running out by the end of the month [d]	No	13 (31)	29 (69)	0.173
	Yes	6 (54.5)	5 (45.5)	
Participation in WIC	No	10 (28.6)	25 (71.4)	0.165
	Yes	10 (47.6)	11 (52.4)	
Participation in SNAP	No	13 (29.5)	31 (70.5)	0.092
	Yes	7 (58.3)	5 (41.7)	

Table 6. Cont.

		Met MDD n (%)	Did not Meet MDD n (%)	Chi Square p Values
Food Security Index Status [e]	Extremely food insecure	2 (66.7)	1 (33.3)	0.046
	Highly food insecure	2 (50)	2 (50)	
	Moderately food insecure	5 (71.4)	2 (28.6)	
	Moderately food secure	2 (16.7)	10 (83.3)	
	Highly food secure	7 (28)	18 (72)	
	Extremely food secure	0 (0)	0 (0)	
Food Security Index Classification [e]	Food insecure	9 (24.3)	28 (75.7)	0.019
	Food secure	9 (64.3)	5 (35.7)	
Annual Household Income ($)	<10,000	4 (80)	1 (20)	0.008
	10,000–20,000	1 (50)	1 (50)	
	20,000–35,000	3 (60)	2 (40)	
	35,000–60,000	3 (42.9)	4 (57.1)	
	60,000–75,000	1 (16.7)	5 (83.3)	
	>75,000	7 (28)	18 (72)	
	<35,000	8 (66.7)	4 (33.3)	0.038
	>35,000	11 (28.9)	27 (71.1)	

Special Supplemental Nutrition Program for Women, Infants and Children (WIC), The Supplemental Nutrition Assistance Program (SNAP). [a] Minimum Dietary Diversity Score. [b] Total number of responses 65. 5 (7.1%) incomplete responses. [c] No = Never/seldom. Yes = Sometimes/most times/always. [d] No = Never/seldom. Yes = Sometimes/most times/always. [e] Based on the adapted Infant Food Security Index used in this study.

3.5. Infant Food Security Indicators and Food Group Consumption Examined Using Linear Regression Analysis

Presented in Table 7 are the statistically significant results of linear regression analysis between food security indicators and total food group consumption, grain, root, and tuber food group consumption, and flesh group consumption. The regression findings indicate a statistically significant association between food security score and grain, root, and tuber consumption. For each unit increase in food security classification from extremely food insecure to extremely food secure by the adapted food security index, the frequency of daily grain, root, and tuber consumption decreases by approximately 6% after controlling for age and sex. A similar trend is observed across the models whereby running out of money for food or utilities by the end of the month and lower food security score results in a higher percentage increase in either of total food group, grain, root, and tuber food group consumption, and flesh group consumption.

3.6. Infant Food Security Indicators and Meeting the MDD Examined Using Multivariable Logistic Regression Analysis

Multivariable logistic regression results, which adjusted for age and sex, did not find significant associations between meeting the MDD and running out of money for food by the end of the month, being defined as food insecure by the adapted infant food security index and having a low household income (see Table A1).

Table 7. The association between infant food security indicators and total and individual food group consumption in infants 3–12 months examined using linear regression ($n = 70$) [a].

Total Food Group Consumption

	Model 1			Model 2			Model 3		
	B	SE	p-value	B	SE	p-value	B	SE	p-value
Running out of money for food by the end of the month	2.961	0.749	<0.0001						
Constant	0.831	0.285	0.01	0.411		0.01	0.957	0.503	0.1
Age				0.251	0.434	0.01	0.689	0.256	0.01
Sex				0.053	0.296	<0.0001	0.238	0.054	<0.0001
					0.057		0.190	0.229	0.4
R-Squared	0.117			0.333			0.341		
Adjusted R-Squared	0.103			0.312			0.309		

	Model 4			Model 5			Model 6		
	B	SE	p-value	B	SE	p-value	B	SE	p-value
Running out of money for utilities by the end of the month	3.044	0.146	<0.0001						
Constant	0.802	0.332	0.02	1.235	0.434	0.01	0.795	0.528	0.1
Running out of money for utilities by the end of the month				0.653	0.296	0.03	0.664	0.293	0.03
Age				0.247	0.057	<0.0001	0.240	0.056	<0.0001
Sex							0.333	0.231	0.2
R-Squared	0.082			0.293			0.316		
Adjusted R-Squared	0.068			0.271			0.283		

	Model 7			Model 8			Model 9		
	B	SE	p-value	B	SE	p-value	B	SE	p-value
Food Security Score [b]	4.307	0.449	<0.0001						
Constant	−0.279	0.107	0.01	2.350	0.586	<0.0001	1.970	0.676	0.01
Food Security Score				−0.247	0.094	0.01	−0.237	0.094	0.02
Age				0.246	0.055	<0.0001	0.241	0.055	<0.0001
Sex							0.258	0.230	0.3
R-Squared	0.097			0.319			0.333		
Adjusted R-Squared	0.083			0.297			0.300		

Grain, root and tuber consumption

	Model 10			Model 11			Model 12		
	B	SE	p-value	B	SE	p-value	B	SE	p-value
Food security score [b]	1.117	0.108	<0.0001						
Constant	−0.068	0.026	0.01	0.907	0.158	<0.0001	0.842	0.184	<0.0001
Food Security Score				−0.064	0.025	0.01	−0.062	0.026	0.03
Age				0.026	0.015	0.1	0.026	0.015	0.1
Sex							0.044	0.063	0.5
R-Squared	0.099			0.143			0.150		
Adjusted R-Squared	0.084			0.115			0.108		

Table 7. Cont.

Flesh food consumption

	Model 13			Model 14			Model 15		
	B	SE	p-value	B	SE	p-value	B	SE	p-value
Running out of money for food by the end of the month									
Constant	0.172	0.050	0.001	-0.413	0.139	0.004	-0.416	0.171	0.02
Running out of money for food by the end of the month	0.398	0.096	<0.0001	0.364	0.085	<0.0001	0.363	0.087	<0.0001
Age				0.080	0.018	<0.0001	0.080	0.018	<0.0001
Sex							0.002	0.078	0.98
R-Squared	0.211			0.398			0.398		
Adjusted R-Squared	0.198			0.379			0.369		

	Model 16			Model 17			Model 18		
	B	SE	p-value	B	SE	p-value	B	SE	p-value
Running out of money for utilities by the end of the month									
Constant	0.204	0.048	<0.0001	-0.376	0.143	0.01	-0.468	0.176	0.01
Running out of money for utilities by the end of the month	0.431	0.109	<0.0001	0.383	0.098	<0.0001	0.386	0.098	<0.0001
Age				0.079	0.019	<0.0001	0.078	0.019	<0.0001
Sex							0.070	0.077	0.4
R-Squared	0.194			0.370			0.378		
Adjusted R-Squared	0.182			0.351			0.349		

	Model 19			Model 20			Model 21		
	B	SE	p-value	B	SE	p-value	B	SE	p-value
Food security score [a]									
Constant	0.753	0.156	<0.0001	0.103	0.206	0.6	0.052	0.240	0.8
Food Security Score	-0.117	0.037	0.003	-0.106	0.033	0.002	-0.105	0.034	0.003
Age				0.082	0.019	<0.0001	0.081	0.019	<0.0001
Sex							0.035	0.082	0.7
R-Squared	0.135			0.330			0.332		
Adjusted R-Squared	0.122			0.309			0.299		

Special Supplemental Nutrition Program for Women, Infants and Children (WIC), The Supplemental Nutrition Assistance Program (SNAP). Model 1 + 13: Running out of money for food by the end of the month. Model 2 + 14: Running out of money for food by the end of the month + age. Model 3 + 15: Running out of money for food by the end of the month + age + sex. Model 4 + 16: Running out of money for utilities by the end of the month. Model 5 + 17: Running out of money for utilities by the end of the month + age. Model 6 + 18: Running out of money for utilities by the end of the month + age + sex. Model 7, 10 + 19: Food Security Score. Model 8, 11 + 20: Food Security Score + age. Model 9, 12 + 21: Food Security Score + age + sex. [a] Total number of responses 65. 5 (7.1%) incomplete responses. [b] Based on the adapted Infant Food Security Index used in this study.

4. Discussion

As hypothesized, the indicator of nutritional risk which had the strongest association with the diet quality of NHPIF infants 3–12 months was the adapted infant food security index, which takes into account multiple indicators of food insecurity. Significant associations after adjusting for infant age and sex were only found with the adapted infant food security index and the two modified USHFSSM questions regarding food group consumption as an indicator of dietary quality. Food-insecure NHPIF infants classified by the adapted infant food security index used in this study consumed a greater number of food groups on average each day, had a greater intake of flesh foods and a greater intake of grains, roots and tubers compared to those classified as food secure by the index. Households who experienced running out of money for food or utilities by the end of the month were significantly associated with greater total food group and more frequent daily flesh food consumption compared to those who did not experience running out of money for food or utilities by the end of the month. However, significant differences in the intake of legumes and nuts, dairy products, eggs, vitamin A-rich fruit or vegetables or other fruit and vegetables were not apparent between infants defined as food secure or insecure by any of the nutritional risk indicators. Based on these findings, the adapted infant food security index may be the better indicator to use to assess the association between food security and food group consumption within this sample of NHPIF infants compared with the two questions modified from the USHFSSM, participation in food assistance programs, annual household income.

Of the infants in this study, 36% met the MDD, on average, each day. This is higher than what has been reported in a cohort of infants aged 8–12 months in Cincinnati, Ohio, where only 28% of infants were found to meet the MDD, on average, each day [25]. In the present study, none of the associations between MDD and any indicators of nutritional risk remained significant in multivariable logistic regression models adjusting for infant age and sex. These findings may be attributed to the small sample size available in this study for infants 6–12 months.

The association between total food group consumption and infant food insecurity by the adapted food security index found in this study was interesting but not unique among the literature. In a study conducted in South Africa, where socioeconomic status (SES) was measured using a composite score of assets and market access, household income, employment status, and educational attainment, MDD was higher among lower SES 6–12-month-old infants. The authors report that their results may have been reflective of the small sample size when stratified by SES and age [23]. A similar justification could be considered for this study whereby infants classified as food insecure by the index used in this study made up only 25.7% ($n = 18$) of the sample. In addition, this study was a secondary analysis and was not sampled to be representative of NHPIF food-insecure infants in Hawai'i. Thus, the food group consumption identified in this study may not be generalized for the population. These results are suggestive, however, that NHPIF food-insecure infants in Hawai'i are not at nutritional disadvantage compared to those that are food secure. Rossen L.M et al. similarly reported that food insecurity was largely not associated with dietary intake in a representative sample of 5136 US children aged 2–15 years from NHANES [26]. Likewise, Shinyoung J. et al. did not find a substantial difference in diet quality by household food security or food security among a sample of 5540 children from NHANES 2011–2014 [27]. Other research from a representative sample of New Zealand infants found that food-secure infants had a more diverse diet compared to those who were food insecure [3]. Infants defined as food insecure by the adapted index applied in this study may be employing coping mechanisms such as participation in food assistant programs such as WIC and SNAP. Furthermore, the nutrition of these infants may be prioritized by their caregiver, providing protection against the lack of food resources in the household, as seen in other studies [27].

Similar patterns of higher flesh food intake were identified among lower SES infants in South Africa, as in the results of this study, where the most common type of flesh food consumed daily by low SES infants was processed meat followed by red meat [23]. Processed meats are high in sodium and fat and their intake during infancy has been associated with hypertension and coronary artery disease during adulthood [23,28]. While studies have shown the benefits of flesh foods on infant growth and cognitive development [28,29], the effect of high flesh food consumption in food-insecure infants found in this study was not clear, nor was the type of flesh foods consumed. Meat as a complementary food in infancy is a key source of the micronutrients zinc, iron and vitamin B12 [30]. The pattern of high flesh food intake may contribute to the intake of these micronutrients; however, as this study does not address the type and quantity of foods consumed in each food group, micronutrient intake remains unclear. Factors such as poor maternal nutrition knowledge, delayed introduction of flesh foods, or concerns about potentially allergenic foods [23,31] may influence flesh food consumption patterns during this stage of life.

While authors suggest that dietary diversity is generally associated with child nutritional status and that the associations remain when controlling for household wealth and welfare factors [32], there are drawbacks of assessing infant diet using the global MDD score from the WHO for assessing infant and young child feeding practices. Firstly, food is enumerated when consumed; however, there is no amount recorded. This decision by the creators of the MDD, may be a result of infant portion sizes being small and overall differences in portion sizes having a minimal impact. Secondly, the MDD does not adjust for total energy (kcal). Higher energy intakes could contribute to being overweight during infancy, which is consistently associated with a risk of obesity in childhood and adult life. This association is especially important in populations where the obesity risk is higher such as those of NHPIF ancestry [11]. Thirdly, the designated food groups do not completely distinguish added sugars, sodium and saturated fats. As an example, guidelines for the grains, roots and tubers group does not distinguish a French fry from a boiled wholefood sweet potato. Thus, we identified a greater diversity of foods being eaten by food-insecure infants, however, the quality and quantity of these foods were not assessed using the MDD score. This issue was addressed by Schlichting et al., who added an additional grouping of energy dense nutrient poor foods, which gave an indication of the unhealthy foods consumed [3]. Importantly, the outcome of diet diversity is a concept unique from more traditional dietary quality indices. Furthermore, this dietary assessment method did not incorporate a breastfeeding assessment element. The WHO updated the MDD in 2017 to reflect inclusion of breast milk as the eighth food group [33]. In the present study, breastfeeding status was only considered within the adapted infant food security index.

WIC and SNAP are two important food and nutrition assistance programs conducted by USDA to improve the nutritional well-being of low-income individuals, and there is ongoing interest in investigating the roles of these programs in accomplishing these intentions. One study reported, from a NHANES sample of 1197 children aged 2 to 4 years from low-income households, that WIC food packages are associated with higher diet quality for low-income children [34]. Another study, which addressed the participation and effectiveness of SNAP and WIC in a multi-equation framework for nutrient intakes for young children in the US, found that WIC participation increases the intakes of iron, potassium, and fiber; however, no nutritional effects were found with SNAP participation [35]. The results of this study demonstrate that despite residing in lower income WIC- and SNAP-participating households, these infants may not be at a disadvantage nutritionally compared to those who do not participate in these programs and who are assumed to be of higher income. These results suggest that participation in WIC and SNAP supports more healthful food group consumption. However, further investigation on how these programs mitigate food insecurity and diet quality are needed to inform program implementation in the NHPIF population.

The strengths of this study include the application of an adapted infant food security index which classified food security at the level of the infant and incorporated various indicators of food security. However, this adapted index did not undergo any tests for validity and it did not include the complete 18-item USHFSSM, nor the eight items specific to determining child food security, which would have provided another indicator of food security status. Another strength of the study is that it is the first known examination of food security in this particular population, which acts to fill the relative deficit of such data and provides a base of work for further research. This collection of infant dietary intake by an image-based mFR^{TM} served to reduce the confounding of results, which can occur due to misreporting dietary intake [16]. The mFR^{TM} images enabled a more accurate distinction of foods into appropriate food groups, giving more confidence to the assessment of diet by diversity. Given the cross-sectional nature of this study, only associations can be estimated. In addition, this study was unable to indicate portion size, report on the types of foods consumed within each food group or assess the nutrient quality of foods consumed. This study was only able to report on whether different types of food were consumed. Additionally, the small sample size in this secondary data analysis may have limited the statistical power, and may not be representative of NHPIF infants residing on O'ahu, Hawai'i.

5. Conclusions

This study investigated various nutritional risk indicators and examined their association with MDD and individual and total food group intake in NHPIF infants. Infants defined as food secure based on the adapted infant food security index had greater overall, flesh food, and grain, tuber and root consumption compared to those defined as food secure. The caregivers of these infants may be employing coping mechanisms such as participation in food assistance programs such as WIC and SNAP. Likewise, these infants may be protected from the effects of food insecurity as their nutrition is prioritized by their caregivers. Of the nutritional risk indicators examined, two questions modified from the USHFSSS, participation in food assistance programs, an adapted infant food security index, and household income, the adapted infant food security index was shown to be the best indicator for consuming more food groups. Further research is needed on a more representative sample of NHPIF infants to determine the most appropriate indicator for food security risk and MDD.

Author Contributions: Conceptualization, S.C., H.E.-M., M.K.F.; methodology, M.K.F., C.J.B. and, F.Z.; formal Analysis, S.C., J.J.C., C.J.B., M.K.F.; writing—original draft preparation, S.C.; writing—review & editing, M.K.F., S.C., H.E.-M., C.J.B., and F.Z. supervision, M.K.F. All authors have read and agreed to the published version of the manuscript.

Funding: The project was supported by award number U54MD007601 by the National Institute on Minority Health and Health Disparities of the National Institutes of Health, the HMSA Foundation Community Fund grant #CF-021803, and the University of Hawai'i at Mānoa Native Hawaiian Student Services 'Ōiwi Undergraduate Research Fellowship Program.

Acknowledgments: The authors would like to thank Sheila Sugrue, Jessie Kai, Gemady Langfelder and Christina Gar Lai Young for their research contributions. The authors would also like to thank the study participants and community partners.

Conflicts of Interest: The authors declare no conflict of interest.

Appendix A

Table A1. Multinomial logistic regression results examining the association between food security indicators and meeting the MDD in infants 6–12 Months ($n = 56$).

	B	SE	p-Value	OR	95% CI
Model 1					
Intercept	−0.693	0.612	0.258	-	
Household income <$35,000	1.591	0.709	0.025	4.909	1.223–19.709
Model 2					
Intercept	7.650	2.543	0.003	-	
Age	−1.006	0.304	0.001	0.366	0.202–0.663
Household income <$35,000	1.736	0.896	0.053	5.672	0.979–32.855
Model 3					
Intercept	8.842	2.905	0.002	-	
Age	−0.994	0.305	0.001	0.370	0.204–0.673
Sex	−0.800	0.778	0.304	0.449	0.098–2.065
Household income <$35,000	1.647	0.908	0.070	5.191	0.875–30.779

Table A1. *Cont.*

	β	SE	p	OR	95% CI
Model 4					
Intercept	−0.288	0.540	0.594	-	
Running out of money for food by the end of the month	1.317	0.654	0.044	3.733	1.037–13.445
Model 5					
Intercept	7.751	2.585	0.003	-	
Age	−0.923	0.290	0.001	0.397	0.225–0.701
Running out of money for food by the end of the month	1.037	0.755	0.170	2.820	0.642–12.392
Model 6					
Intercept	8.810	2.905	0.002	-	
Age	−0.908	0.289	0.002	0.404	0.229–0.711
Sex	−0.714	0.750	0.341	0.489	0.113–2.127
Running out of money for food by the end of the month	0.842	0.785	0.283	2.321	0.499–10.803
Model 7					
Intercept	−0.588	0.558	0.292	-	
Food security index score	1.723	0.677	0.011	5.600	1.487–21.096
Model 8					
Intercept	7.081	2.587	0.006	-	
Age	−0.873	0.288	0.002	0.418	0.238–0.734
Food security index score	1.387	0.775	0.073	4.003	0.877–18.271
Model 9					
Intercept	8.039	2.898	0.006	-	
Age	−0.862	0.288	0.003	0.422	0.240–0.743
Sex	−0.641	0.757	0.397	0.527	0.120–2.323
Food security index score	1.229	0.799	0.124	3.419	0.715–16.356

Model 1–3: food security indicator: Household income <$35,000. Model 4–6: food security indicator: Running out of money for food by the end of the month. Model 6–8: food security indicator: Food security index score. Model 1, 4, 7: Food security indicator. Model 2, 5, 8: Food security indicator + age. Model 3, 6, 9: Food security indicator + age + sex.

References

1. Zaslow, M.; Bronte-Tinkew, J.; Capps, R.; Horowitz, A.; Moore, K.A.; Weinstein, D. Food Security During Infancy: Implications for Attachment and Mental Proficiency in Toddlerhood. *Matern. Child Health* **2009**, *13*, 66–80. [CrossRef] [PubMed]
2. Gundersen, C.; Kreider, B. Bounding the effects of food insecurity on children's health outcomes. *J. Health Econ.* **2009**, *28*, 971–983. [CrossRef]
3. Schlichting, D.; Hashemi, L.; Grant, C. Infant Food Security in New Zealand: A Multidimensional Index Developed from Cohort Data. *Int. J. Environ. Res. Public Health* **2019**, *16*, 283. [CrossRef] [PubMed]
4. Leung, C.W.; Tester, J.M. The Association between Food Insecurity and Diet Quality Varies by Race/Ethnicity: An Analysis of National Health and Nutrition Examination Survey 2011–2014 Results. *J. Acad. Nutr. Diet.* **2019**, *119*, 1676–1686. [CrossRef] [PubMed]
5. McGuire, S. World Health Organization. Comprehensive Implementation Plan on Maternal, Infant, and Young Child Nutrition. Geneva, Switzerland, 2014. *Adv. Nutr.* **2015**, *6*, 134–135. [CrossRef] [PubMed]
6. Bickel, G.; Mark, N.; Cristofer, P.; William, H.; John, C. *Guide to Measuring Household Food Security, Revised 2000*; U.S. Department of Agriculture, Food and Nutrition Service: Alexandria, VA, USA, 2000.
7. Butcher, L.M.; O'Sullivan, T.A.; Ryan, M.M.; Lo, J.; Devine, A. Utilising a multi-item questionnaire to assess household food security in Australia. *Health Promot. J. Aust.* **2019**, *30*, 9–17. [CrossRef]
8. Jones, A.D.; Ngure, F.M.; Pelto, G.; Young, S.L. What Are We Assessing When We Measure Food Security? A Compendium and Review of Current Metrics. *Adv. Nutr.* **2013**, *4*, 481–505. [CrossRef]
9. Oberholser, C.A.; Tuttle, C.R. Assessment of Household Food Security among Food Stamp Recipient Families in Maryland. *Am. J. Public Health* **2004**, *94*, 790–795. [CrossRef]
10. Tomayko, E.J.; Mosso, K.L.; Cronin, K.A.; Carmichael, L.; Kim, K.; Parker, T.; Yaroch, A.L.; Adams, A.K. Household food insecurity and dietary patterns in rural and urban American Indian families with young children. *BMC Public Health* **2017**, *17*, 611. [CrossRef]

11. Galinsky, A.M.; Zelaya, C.E.; Simile, C.; Barnes, P.M. Health Conditions and Behaviors of Native Hawaiian and Pacific Islander Persons in the United States, 2014. *Vital Health Stat.* **2017**, *40*, 1–99.
12. Katie, M.H.; Laura, J.Y.H.; Courtney, B.J.; Yuka, J.; Martha, R.; Jay, E.M. Food security issues for low-income Hawaii residents. *Asia Pac. J. Public Health* **2008**, *20*, 64–69.
13. Stupplebeen, D.A. Housing and Food Insecurity and Chronic Disease among Three Racial Groups in Hawai'i. *Prev. Chronic Dis.* **2019**, *16*, E13. [CrossRef]
14. World Health Organisation. *Indicators for Assessing Infant and Young Child Feeding Practices*; World Health Organisation: Washington, DC, USA, 2008.
15. Ahmad, Z.; Bosch, M.; Khanna, N.; Kerr, D.A.; Boushey, C.J.; Zhu, F.Q.; Delp, E.J. A Mobile Food Record for Integrated Dietary Assessment. In Proceedings of the 2nd International Workshop on Multimedia Assisted Dietary Management, MADiMa16 (2016), Amsterdam, The Netherlands, 16 October 2016; pp. 53–62. [CrossRef]
16. Zhu, F.; Bosch, M.; Woo, I.; Kim, S.; Boushey, C.J.; Ebert, D.S.; Delp, E.J. The Use of Mobile Devices in Aiding Dietary Assessment and Evaluation. *IEEE J. Sel. Top. Signal Process.* **2010**, *4*, 756–766. [CrossRef]
17. Zhu, F.; Bosch, M.; Khanna, N.; Boushey, C.J.; Delp, E.J. Multiple hypotheses image segmentation and classification with application to dietary assessment. *IEEE J. Biomed. Health Inf.* **2015**, *19*, 377–388. [CrossRef] [PubMed]
18. Fang, S.; Shao, Z.; Kerr, D.A.; Boushey, C.J.; Zhu, F. An End-to-End Image-Based Automatic Food Energy Estimation Technique Based on Learned Energy Distribution Images: Protocol and Methodology. *Nutrients* **2019**, *11*, 877. [CrossRef] [PubMed]
19. Steyn, N.; Nel, J.; Nantel, G.; Kennedy, G.; Labadarios, D. Food variety and dietary diversity scores in children: Are they good indicators of dietary adequacy? *Public Health Nutr.* **2006**, *9*, 644–650. [CrossRef] [PubMed]
20. Pérez-Escamilla, R.S.-P.S.; Lott, M. *Feeding Guidelines for Infants and Young Toddlers: A Responsive Parenting Approach*; Healthy Eating Research: Durham, NC, USA, 2017.
21. World Health Organization. Complementary Feeding. Available online: https://www.who.int/nutrition/topics/complementary_feeding/en/ (accessed on 17 February 2020).
22. WHO. *Guideline: Vitamin A supplementation in Infants 1–5 Months of Age*; World Health Organization: Geneva, Switzerland, 2011.
23. Budree, S.; Goddard, E.; Brittain, K.; Cader, S.; Myer, L.; Zar, H.J. Infant feeding practices in a South African birth cohort-A longitudinal study. *Matern. Child Nutr.* **2017**, *13*, e12371. [CrossRef]
24. Peat, J.K.; Belind, B. *Medical Statistics: A Guide to SPSS, Data Analysis and Critical Appraisal*, 2nd ed.; BMJ Books: Chichester, UK, 2014.
25. Woo, J.G.; Herbers, P.M.; McMahon, R.J.; Davidson, B.S.; Ruiz-Palacios, G.M.; Peng, Y.-M.; Morrow, A.L. Longitudinal Development of Infant Complementary Diet Diversity in 3 International Cohorts. *J. Pediatr.* **2015**, *167*, 969–974.e1. [CrossRef]
26. Rossen, L.M.; Kobernik, E.K. Food insecurity and dietary intake among US youth, 2007–2010. *Pediatr. Obes.* **2016**, *11*, 187–193. [CrossRef]
27. Jun, S.; Zeh, M.J.; Eicher-Miller, H.A.; Bailey, R.L. Children's Dietary Quality and Micronutrient Adequacy by Food Security in the Household and among Household Children. *Nutrients* **2019**, *11*, 965. [CrossRef] [PubMed]
28. Mauch, C.E.; Perry, R.A.; Magarey, A.M.; Daniels, L.A. Dietary intake in Australian children aged 4–24 months: Consumption of meat and meat alternatives. *Br. J. Nutr.* **2015**, *113*, 1761–1772. [CrossRef]
29. Allen, L.H. Global dietary patterns and diets in childhood: Implications for health outcomes. *Ann. Nutr. Metab.* **2012**, *61* (Suppl. 1), 29–37. [CrossRef] [PubMed]
30. Hambidge, K.M.; Sheng, X.; Mazariegos, M.; Jiang, T.; Garces, A.; Li, D.; Westcott, J.; Tshefu, A.; Sami, N.; Pasha, O.; et al. Evaluation of meat as a first complementary food for breastfed infants: Impact on iron intake. *Nutr. Rev.* **2011**, *59*, S57–S63. [CrossRef] [PubMed]
31. Woo, J.G.; Guerrero, M.L.; Ruiz-Palacios, G.M.; Peng, Y.-m.; Herbers, P.M.; Yao, W.; Ortega, H.; Davidson, B.S.; McMahon, R.J.; Morrow, A.L. Specific infant feeding practices do not consistently explain variation in anthropometry at age 1 year in urban United States, Mexico, and China cohorts. *J. Nutr.* **2013**, *143*, 166–174. [CrossRef] [PubMed]

32. Arimond, M.; Ruel, M.T. Dietary Diversity Is Associated with Child Nutritional Status: Evidence from 11 Demographic and Health Surveys. *J. Nutr.* **2004**, *134*, 2579–2585. [CrossRef] [PubMed]
33. World Health Organisation. *Global Nutrition Monitoring Framework: Operational Guidance for Tracking Progress in Meeting Targets for 2025*; World Health Organization: Geneva, Switzerland, 2017.
34. Tester, J.M.; Leung, C.W.; Crawford, P.B. Revised WIC Food Package and Childrens Diet Quality. *Pediatrics* **2016**, *137*, e20153557. [CrossRef] [PubMed]
35. Yen, S.T. The effects of SNAP and WIC programs on nutrient intakes of children. *Food Policy* **2010**, *35*, 576–583. [CrossRef]

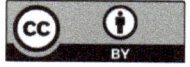

© 2020 by the authors. Licensee MDPI, Basel, Switzerland. This article is an open access article distributed under the terms and conditions of the Creative Commons Attribution (CC BY) license (http://creativecommons.org/licenses/by/4.0/).

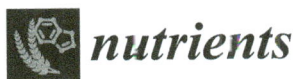

Article

Prevalence and Predictors of Overweight and Obesity among Young Children in the Children's Healthy Living Study on Guam

Rachael T. Leon Guerrero [1,*], L. Robert Barber [1], Tanisha F. Aflague [1], Yvette C. Paulino [1], Margaret P. Hattori-Uchima [1], Mark Acosta [1], Lynne R. Wilkens [2] and Rachel Novotny [3]

1. Office of Research & Sponsored Programs, University of Guam, Mangilao, Guam 96923, USA; bbarber@triton.uog.edu (L.R.B.); taflague@triton.uog.edu (T.F.A.); paulinoy@triton.uog.edu (Y.C.P.); muchima@triton.uog.edu (M.P.H.-U.); macosta@triton.uog.edu (M.A.)
2. University of Hawaii Cancer Center, Honolulu, HI 96813, USA; lynne@cc.hawaii.edu
3. College of Tropical Agriculture and Human Resources, University of Hawaii At Manoa, Honolulu, HI 96822, USA; novotny@hawaii.edu
* Correspondence: rachaeltlg@triton.uog.edu; Tel.: +1-671-735-2170

Received: 12 July 2020; Accepted: 12 August 2020; Published: 20 August 2020

Abstract: This study is part of the Children's Healthy Living program in U.S. Affiliated Pacific region. The objectives were to estimate overweight and obesity (OWOB) prevalence and identify possible related risk factors among ethnic groups in Guam. In 2013, 865 children (2–8 years) were recruited via community-based sampling from select communities in Guam. Children's demographic and health behavior information; dietary intake; and anthropometric measurements were collected. Logistic regression, odds ratio, t-tests, and chi-square tests were used to determine differences and assess covariates of OWOB. The results indicate that 58% of children were living below the poverty level, 80% were receiving food assistance, and 51% experienced food insecurity. The majority of children surveyed did not meet recommendations for: sleep duration (59.6%), sedentary screen-time (83.11%), or fruit (58.7%) and vegetable (99.1%) intake, and consumed sugar sweetened beverages (SSB) (73.7%). OWOB affected 27.4% of children. Children affected by OWOB in this study were statistically more likely ($p = 0.042$) to suffer from sleep disturbances ($p = 0.042$) and consume marginally higher amounts (p value = 0.07) of SSB compared to children with healthy weight. Among Other Micronesians, children from families who considered themselves 'integrated' into the culture were 2.05 (CI 0.81–5.20) times more likely to be affected by OWOB. In conclusion, the OWOB prevalence among 2–8-year-olds in Guam was 27.4%; and compared with healthy weight children, children with OWOB were more likely to have educated caregivers and consume more SSBs. Results provide a basis for health promotion and obesity prevention guidance for children in Guam.

Keywords: child obesity; Guam; Children's Healthy Living (CHL); islander; Pacific; Micronesia

1. Introduction

Childhood overweight and obesity (OWOB) is a global epidemic affecting many countries [1–5], including the United States (US) and the US Affiliated Pacific region (USAP). In the US a high prevalence of CWOB among racial/ethnic minority groups for children 2–19 years is reported, specifically Non-Hispanic black (19.5%) and Hispanic (21.9%), yet Native Hawaiian or Other Pacific Islanders are not included [1,2]. Novotny and colleagues conducted a systematic review of childhood OWOB in the USAP region and estimated that the prevalence of OWOB for children 2–8 years was 21%, and that the prevalence increased to 39% by age 8 [6]. Similarly, the proportion of obese children increased from 10% at age 2 years to 23% at age 8 years, with the highest prevalence of obesity in both Guam and American Samoa [6]. The systematic review found that in Guam, OWOB prevalence (39%) among children ages 3 to 5 years [6] exceeded the US national average (23%) for children aged 2 to 5 years [1,2].

Guam is a U.S. Territory located in the northwestern Pacific Ocean, approximately 3700 miles west of Hawaii, 6000 miles west of California, and 1300 miles southeast of Japan. CHamorus are the original inhabitants of Guam [7,8], and are typically grouped with other Pacific Islanders. However, the current population of Guam is characterized by substantial ethnic variation [9]: 37% CHamoru, 26% Filipino, 12% other Pacific Islander, 11% other ethnicity, 7% White, and 7% other Asian. This ethnic diversity evolved through centuries of colonization and migration that continues today [10] and may modify the burden and predictors of OWOB among CHamorus. Factors related to OWOB are sleep, physical activity, psychosocial, life course exposure, SES, and diet [11,12] that for many racial/ethnic groups in Guam is influenced by this history [12,13]. OWOB prevalence among adults is higher among CHamorus compared to other ethnic groups on Guam [11]. In a study among adults in the two largest ethnic populations in Guam then (2008) and now, CHamorus and Filipinos, there was a significant difference in energy density of diets between the two groups, where CHamorus had a higher energy and added sugar intake [11]. In 2009 and 2010, prevalence of OWOB was highest among CHamorus followed by Other Micronesians reported in one of the first reports to disaggregate BRFSS data by ethnicity [14].

Children who are overweight or obese have a higher risk of being overweight or obese adults [15] with an increased risk of chronic diseases later in life [16]. However, there is limited information about young children in Guam, and data are needed to understand the burden of and determine the appropriate intervention for childhood OWOB. Therefore, the purpose of this study is to estimate the prevalence of OWOB among children in Guam and identify demographic or other risk factors targeted by the Children's Healthy Living (CHL) program for overweight and obesity in CHamoru children.

2. Methods

The Children's Healthy Living Program for Remote Underserved Minority Populations in the Pacific Region (CHL) program is a partnership of universities and local organizations across the remote USAP (Alaska, American Samoa, Commonwealth of the Northern Marianas, Federated States of Micronesia, Republic of Marshall Islands, Republic of Palau, Hawaii, and Guam) working to prevent childhood obesity in the Pacific. Detailed information on the study design of the CHL program can be found elsewhere [17,18]. Briefly, approximately 900 children (2–8 years) and their parents/caregivers from each participating USAP jurisdiction were recruited to participate in the study at both baseline and 24-month follow-up. On Guam, a total of 865 children were recruited at baseline (2013) and 696 children were recruited from the same communities at 24-month follow-up. This paper will focus on baseline data of the 865 children on Guam recruited from communities (Agana Heights, Sinajana, Agat, Santa Rita, Yigo, Yona, Talafofo, and Dededo) selected due to their size, representation of indigenous (CHamoru) residents, and isolation and cohesiveness (for purpose of intervention) [17]. Behavioral targets of the CHL program were increasing sleep, water intake, fruit and vegetable intake, physical activity and decreasing sugar sweetened beverage intake and sedentary behavior [17].

Child participants were recruited primarily at early childhood education centers (e.g., Guam Head Start program, daycares, and public elementary schools) and community-based settings (e.g., municipal centers and public housing areas) on Guam. Data collection occurred over a minimum of two visits at these recruitment sites. Further details on recruitment is described elsewhere [17,18]. Child participants with parents' consent and who provided assent were assessed.

At the first visit, parents/caregivers completed surveys on demographic information (i.e., child age, place of birth, race/ethnicity, and sex; household composition and food security; parent/caregiver educational level and income); cultural identity of the parent/caregiver; and general health status, early life feeding behaviors, and sedentary screen-time and sleep behavior germane to the child. They also received instructions for completing a two-day food and activity log at home during the week. Sleep quality was measured with the Tayside Children's Sleep Questionnaire (TCSQ) [19] and sleep duration [20] was reported by the parent/caregiver as hours asleep at night and during naps. Other surveys were adapted from previous studies [17] with some local terminology added for participant clarity.

Detailed information was collected in CHL on race/ethnic groups, allowing for multiple groups to be selected; classification prioritized ethnic groups indigenous to the jurisdiction. On Guam, the indigenous ethnic group is CHamoru [7,8]. If more than one race/ethnicity was indicated for the child and CHamoru was selected, the child was categorized as CHamoru. If a child identified as not CHamoru and as one of the other Micronesian Pacific Island ethnic groups, such as Chuukese, Palauan, Yapese, Carolinian, Marshallese, or Kosraean, that child was categorized as 'Other Micronesian', because the only other Pacific Island ethnic groups identified in the Guam sample were from Micronesia and not Polynesia (e.g., Native Hawaiians or Samoans). These other Micronesian Pacific Islander groups were grouped together as their numbers were small and they were all from neighboring Micronesian islands.

Food insecurity was determined by asking one question from the US Department of Agriculture's Core Food Security Module: "In the past 12 months how often does money for food run out by the end of the month?" (never, seldom, sometimes, most times, always, don't know, or no response [21]. In this study, options of don't know or no response were treated as missing values. Household food insecurity was considered present if the respondent chose sometimes, most times, or always. Parent's cultural identity, or "acculturation," was determined using their responses reported on a cultural affiliation questionnaire, which assesses one of four modes of acculturation, from two cultural identity subscales (i.e., respondent's ethnic group and the US): traditional (high ethnic and low US subscale scores), integrated (high ethnic and high US subscale scores), assimilated (low ethnic and high US subscale scores), or marginalized (low ethnic and low US scores) [22]. The same scoring system was used as described by Kaholokula and others [22].

After providing assent, each child was measured for weight, height, and waist circumference (WC) by trained and standardized research staff [23] and described in detail elsewhere [17]. These measures were used to compute Body Mass Index (BMI) [weight (kg)/height(m)^2], WC (cm) to height (cm) ratios, and subsequent BMI z-score, BMI-for-age-percentiles, and waist circumference- for-age percentiles [24,25]. BMI percentiles and z-scores were calculated according to CDC reference data [26] and BMI categories were assigned accordingly: underweight (<5th percentile), healthy weight (5th–84th percentile), overweight (85th–94th percentile), and obese (≥95th percentile). Children were considered to have OWOB if their BMI percentile was greater than the 85th percentile for age and sex. Cutoff values for biologically implausible values defined as <−5 or >4 standard deviations (SD) for height-for-age z-score and <−4 or >8 SD for BMI z-score (according to CDC reference data) were removed from the analysis. Child participants were considered to have abdominal obesity if their WC was greater than the International Diabetes Federation [27] cut-point.

Fruit, vegetable, and beverage intake were estimated using data recorded in the child's two-day food logs reported by the child's parent/caregiver and data collection methods are described in detail elsewhere [17]. Parents/caregivers were asked to complete the food log of everything their children ate or drank for two randomly assigned non-consecutive days, which included weekdays and weekend days, between visit one and two, approximately 6 days apart. Assignment of recording days was based on the day of the child's first visit (Monday–Saturday). Parents/caregivers were instructed in record keeping techniques with the aid of food models, service ware, and measuring utensils. During visit two, research staff reviewed the food log with the parents/caregivers (e.g., for completeness of food entries, portion size estimation, food preparation methods, and/or accuracy of recording data). Trained staff entered the food log data into the Pacific Tracker3 (PacTrac3), which includes a food composition database developed in collaboration with the University of Hawaii Cancer Center for use in the Pacific region [28–30]. For this study, PacTrac3 data were used to classify beverage type (i.e., sugar-sweetened beverages (SSB), milk, or water), fruit, and vegetable, as well as, calculate intake (e.g., cups/day, grams/day). All soft drinks, fruit drinks (fruit flavored or containing less than 100% juice), sports drinks, energy drinks, sweetened tea, and sweetened coffee reported were classified as SSB. Milk intake in cups was calculated for food log entries and included all fluid milk (cow and/or goat), chocolate milk, lactose-reduced milk, lactose-free milk, filled milk, dry milk, and evaporated milk. Fruit, vegetable, milk, water, and SSB intake per day was adjusted for within person variance and then averaged over the two days of records, weighted for weekday and weekend days.

Compensation for study participation was provided at visits one and two [17]. The CHL program was funded by the United States Department of Agriculture (USDA), Agriculture and Food Research Initiative. Ethical approval for this project was granted by both the University of Guam Committee on Human Research Subjects (IRB) (CHRS#12-74) and the University of Hawaii Institutional Review Board (CHS#18915); written consent was given by all parents and oral assent was given by all child participants prior to their inclusion, in accordance with the Declaration of Helsinki.

Statistical analyses were performed using IBM SPSS Statistics version 26 (IBM Corporation, Armonk, NY, USA). Data analysis included the calculation of percentages for ordinal and nominal data, and means and standard errors for the interval and continuous data. t-tests and chi-square tests were used to test for differences in continuous and categorical variables, respectively, between BMI groups and ethnic groups. Binary logistic regression models of OWOB assessed its relationship with several potential covariates, adjusted for sex, age, and ethnicity and with the variance corrected for clustering of children within communities. Odds ratios and 95% CI were the primary statistics reported from the models. ORs were calculated for each of the following child factors from all ethnic groups combined and in CHamoru and Other Micronesian children separately: child age, sex, ever breastfed, sleep, sedentary screen-time, vegetable intake, fruit intake, water intake, and SSB intake; and parent/caregiver education, acculturation and marital status; and household income, food insecurity, food assistance, and household size. Does-response was assessed using a trend variable assigned consecutive integers (1, 2, ...) to each ordered category. These factors were selected among demographic and lifestyle-related variables because they have been reported to be risk factors for OWOB among children [17,25,31,32] and/or were behaviors of interest for the CHL Program. p values < 0.05 were considered statistically significant, whereas p values of 0.05 to 0.10 were described as borderline significant.

3. Results

3.1. Demographics

The descriptive characteristics of child participants at baseline are summarized by ethnicity in Table 1. The average age of child participants was 5.79 years (sem 0.062). The majority of child participants were male (51.7%), 2–5 years old (53.8%), CHamoru ethnicity (64.8%), born on Guam (84.5%), from households where parents were not married (60.7%) or there were 3 or more children (76.2%), and considered as being 'integrated' (79.9%) as reported by parent/caregiver.

Overall, more than half of participating children (57.9%) came from families whose annual income was less than $20,000, which was slightly below the poverty level for a 3-person household in 2015 [33]. A significantly higher ($p < 0.001$) proportion of Other Micronesian children (82.9%) came from families whose annual income was less than $20,000 compared to CHamoru (54.2%), Filipino (43.24%) and Other (40%) children. Parents of Filipino children reported significantly higher ($p < 0.001$) education attainment levels compared to both CHamoru and Other Micronesians.

3.2. OWOB Prevalence

OWOB prevalence among child participants in this study is 27.4%. A significantly ($p = 0.03$) higher proportion of Other Micronesian children were affected by obesity (BMI ≥ 95th percentile) compared to CHamoru children (18.3% versus 11.0%) (Table 1).

Table 1. Characteristics * of child participants from Guam in the Children's Healthy Living (CHL) Program by ethnicity.

	Total	CHamoru (n = 561)	Other Micronesians (n = 223)	Filipino (n = 81)	Other (n = 10)	p Value
Child Participant						
Age, years	5.79 ± 0.062	5.80 ± 0.070	5.66 ± 0.123	5.99 ± 0.062	6.24 ± 0.070	0.418
2–5 years old	465 (53.76%)	296 (52.76%)	123 (57.76%)	42 (51.85%)	4 (40%)	
6–8 years old	400 (46.24%)	265 (47.23%)	90 (42.25%)	39 (48.14%)	6 (60%)	
Birthplace						0.0001
Guam	723 (84.46%)	488 (88.09%)	170 (80.19%)	62 (76.54%)	3 (33.33%)	
U.S. Mainland	52 (6.08%)	36 (6.50%)	9 (1.25%)	3 (3.70%)	4 (44.44%)	
Saipan, CNMI	34 (3.97%)	28 (5.05%)	5 (2.36%)	1 (1.24%)	0 (0%)	
Other Islands in Micronesia	28 (3.27%)	0 (0%)	28 (13.21%)	0 (0%)	0 (0%)	
Philippines	15 (1.75%)	0 (0%)	0 (0%)	15 (18.52%)	0 (0%)	
Other	4 (0.47%)	2 (0.36%)	0 (0%)	0 (0%)	2 (22.22%)	
Ever Breastfed?						0.0006
Yes	557 (67.19%)	341 (62.80%)	155 (78.68%)	53 (67.09%)	8 (80%)	
No	272 (32.81%)	202 (37.20%)	42 (21.32%)	26 (32.91%)	2 (20%)	
Child fed both breastmilk & infant formula						0.8223
Yes	443 (54.23%)	291 (54.09%)	102 (53.40%)	46 (58.23%)	4 (44.45%)	
No	374 (45.77%)	247 (45.91%)	89 (46.60%)	33 (41.77%)	5 (55.55%)	
Child age (months) when weaned from breastmilk	9.76 ± 0.438	8.63 ± 0.519	12.48 ± 0.958	8.511 ± 1.165	18.0 ± 3.928	0.0001
Average Sleep Duration (h/d)	8.61 ± 0.078	8.86 ± 0.086 [†]	7.75 ± 0.200	8.99 ± 0.206 [†]	9.05 ± 0.273	
TCSQ Sleep Score	6.34 ± 0.205	6.583 ± 0.246	6.011 ± 0.4621	5.231 ± 0.554	8.00 ± 3.386	0.0136
Met Sleep Recommendations [F]						
Yes	343 (40.35%)	240 (43.09%)	63 (30.58%)	35 (43.75%)	5 (50%)	
No	507 (59.65%)	317 (56.91%)	143 (69.42%)	45 (65.25%)	5 (50%)	
Average Screen-time (hr/d)	5.29 ± 0.132	5.13 ± 0.154 [§]	5.45 ± 0.308	6.24 ± 0.425	3.59 ± 0.550	
Met Screen-time Recommendations [Ω]						0.0069
Yes	124 (16.89%)	82 (16.73%)	39 (22.54%)	3 (4.61%)	0 (0%)	
No	610 (83.11%)	408 (83.27%)	134 (77.46%)	62 (95.39%)	6 (100%)	
Height (cm)	110.56 ± 0.46	109.07 ± 0.59	111.31 ± 1.71	112.98 ± 1.22	114.75 ± 5.03	
Weight (kg)	21.05 ± 0.25	20.78 ± 0.31	21.50 ± 0.54	21.55 ± 0.72	22.4 ± 2.44	
Body Mass Index (kg/m²)	16.84 ± 0.11	16.77 ± 0.14	17.09 ± 0.43	16.65 ± 0.27	16.42 ± 0.61	
BMI z-score	0.402 ± 0.039	0.352 ± 0.048 [†]	0.544 ± 0.08	0.395 ± 0.132	0.189 ± 0.284	0.0397
BMI Categories [§]						
Underweight	25 (2.96%)	18 (32.91%)	4 (1.93%)	3 (3.75%)	0 (0%)	0.6945
Healthy weight	595 (70.49%)	392 (71.66%)	144 (69.56%)	51 (63.75%)	8 (80%)	0.4523
Overweight, % (≥85th%ile)	113 (13.39%)	77 (14.08%)	21 (10.14%)	14 (17.50%)	1 (10%)	0.3385
Obesity, % (≥95th%ile)	111 (13.15%)	60 (10.97%)	38 (18.36%)	12 (15.0%)	1 (10%)	0.0314
OWOB by Age						
2–5 years old	107 (23.94%)	59 (20.85%)	32 (26.89%)	16 (39.02%)	0 (0%)	0.0378
6–8 years old	117 (29.47%)	78 (29.54%)	27 (30.68%)	10 (25.64%)	2 (33.33%)	0.9441
Waist Circumference (cm)	55.07 ± 0.30	54.76 ± 0.38	55.44 ± 0.58	56.104 ± 0.95	55.64 ± 2.50	

Table 1. Cont.

	Total	CHamoru (n = 561)	Other Micronesians (n = 223)	Filipino (n = 81)	Other (n = 10)	p Value
Child Participant						
Abdominal Obesity €						0.6782
Yes	76 (8.94%)	48 (8.77%)	17 (7.98%)	10 (12.50%)	1 (10%)	
No	774 (91.06%)	499 (91.23%)	196 (92.02%)	70 (87.5%)	9 (90%)	
Consumed SSB?						0.0001
Yes	497 (74.74%)	361 (81.49%)	95 (61.29%)	36 (59.01%)	5 (50%)	
No	168 (25.26%)	82 (18.51%)	60 (38.71%)	25 (40.99%)	5 (50%)	
Beverage Consumption ‡¶						
Water (c/d)	1.47 ± 0.048	1.306 ± 0.45	1.298 ± 0.66	1.401 ± 0.105	1.522 ± 0.429	
Milk (c/d)	1.241 ± 0.024	1.280 ± 0.029 †§	1.028 ± 0.045 †	1.454 ± 0.081 †	1.660 ± 0.139	
Sugar-sweet drinks (c/d)	0.845 ± 0.029	0.958 ± 0.036 †§‡	0.560 ± 0.050 ⊘	0.727 ± 0.101	1.095 ± 0.269	
Fruit Consumption ‡ (c/d)	0.882 ± 0.021	0.88 ± 0.025	0.846 ± 0.045	0.956 ± 0.080	1.153 ± 0.240	
Vegetable Consumption ‡¶ (c/d)	0.609 ± 0.013	0.648 ± 0.015	0.472 ± 0.026	0.651 ± 0.041	0.850 ± 0.139	
Met Recommendation for:						
Fruit Intake	257 (41.35%)	182 (41.08%)	63 (40.65%)	27 (44.26%)	3 (50%)	0.9312
Vegetable Intake	6 (0.90%)	5 (1.13%)	1 (0.65%)	0 (0%)	0 (0%)	0.8064
Parent/Caregiver/Household						
Annual Family Income Level						0.0001
<$20,000	348 (57.91%)	220 (54.18%)	92 (82.88%)	32 (43.24%)	4 (40%)	
$20,000–$34,999	182 (14.81%)	59 (14.53%)	9 (8.11%)	17 (22.97%)	4 (40%)	
$35,000–$59,999	93 (15.47%)	71 (17.49%)	5 (4.51%)	17 (22.97%)	0 (0%)	
>$60,000	71 (11.81%)	56 (13.80%)	5 (7.20%)	8 (10.82%)	2 (20%)	
Receiving any Food Assistance						0.0001
Yes	676 (80.38%)	447 (81.57%)	176 (86.70%)	47 (58.75%)	6 (60%)	
No	165 (19.62%)	101 (18.43%)	27 (13.30%)	33 (41.25%)	4 (40%)	
Type of Food Assistance						
SNAP ∂	585 (67.85%)	401 (71.61%)	146 (69.19%)	33 (40.74%)	5 (50%)	0.0001
Local Food Bank	101 (11.72%)	69 (12.32%)	28 (13.27%)	4 (4.94%)	0 (0%)	0.1319
WIC ∞	274 (31.79%)	162 (28.93%)	86 (40.76%)	22 (27.16%)	4 (40%)	0.0114
Free School Lunch/Breakfast	248 (28.77%)	202 (36.07%)	33 (15.64%)	10 (12.35%)	3 (30%)	0.0001
Food Insecurity δ						0.0001
Always/most times	127 (16.82%)	86 (17.20%)	32 (18.71%)	7 (9.46%)	2 (20%)	
Sometimes	262 (34.70%)	128 (25.6%)	96 (56.16%)	35 (47.29%)	3 (30%)	
Seldom/never	366 (48.48%)	286 (57.20%)	43 (25.15%)	32 (43.24%)	5 (50%)	
Parent/Caregiver Education						0.0001
<12th Grade	281 (32.48%)	184 (32.80%)	79 (37.08%)	17 (20.98%)	1 (10%)	
12th Grade/GED	351 (40.58%)	237 (42.24%)	97 (45.54%)	13 (16.05%)	4 (40%)	
Some college or higher	233 (26.94%)	140 (24.96%)	37 (17.38%)	32 (62.97%)	5 (50%)	
Parent Marital Status						0.0001
Married	340 (39.31%)	190 (33.89%)	90 (42.25%)	55 (67.90%)	5 (50%)	
Not Married	525 (60.69%)	371 (66.13%)	123 (57.75%)	26 (32.10%)	5 (50%)	
Number Children in Household	4.19 ± 0.077	4.29 ± 0.096 §	4.35 ± 0.164 §	3.14 ± 0.151	3.4 ± 0.306	0.0001

Table 1. Cont.

	Total	CHamoru (n = 561)	Other Micronesians (n = 223)	Filipino (n = 81)	Other (n = 10)	p Value
Child Participant						
Household Size						0.008
1–2 children	205 (23.78%)	127 (22.72%)	48 (22.64%)	29 (35.80%)	1 (1%)	
3–4 children	341 (39.56%)	220 (39.36%)	75 (35.38%)	39 (48.15%)	7 (70%)	
5 or more children	316 (36.66%)	212 (37.92%)	89 (41.98%)	13 (16.05%)	2 (20%)	
Acculturation [Y]						0.0565
Integrated	572 (79.89%)	388 (80.15%)	123 (75.00%)	55 (88.71%)	6 (100%)	
Traditional	101 (14.11%)	74 (15.29%)	24 (14.63%)	3 (4.84%)	0	
Assimilated	17 (2.37%)	7 (1.45%)	7 (4.27%)	3 (4.83%)	0	
Marginalized	26 (3.63%)	15 (3.10%)	10 (6.10%)	1 (1.61%)	0	

* Frequency number (%), ¶ Mean ± standard error, ‡ Consumption in cups/day, weighted for weekday/weekend days and adjusted for within person variance, † Significantly ($p < 0.05$) different from Other Micronesians § Significantly ($p < 0.05$) different from Filipino, ∅ Significantly ($p < 0.05$) different from Other, F Sleep Recommendations: at least 11 h/d for 2-year-olds, at least 10 h/d for 3 to 5 year-olds, and at least 9 h/d for 6 to 10 year-olds, Ω Screen-time Recommendation of 2 h/d or less, § BMI percentiles calculated according to CDC reference data and categories assigned as: underweight (<5th percentile), healthy weight (5th–84th percentile), overweight (85th–94th percentile), and obese (95th percentile), ¢ Abdominal obesity defined as waist circumference greater than the International Diabetes Federation cut-point (>90.2 percentile for age and sex), ∂ USDA Supplemental Nutrition Assistance Program (SNAP), ∞ USDA Supplemental Nutrition Assistance Program for Women, Infants, and Children (WIC), δ Question from USDA Core Food Security Module "In the past 12 months how often does money for food run out by the end of the month? Υ What category of acculturation does family consider themselves?

Table 2 shows child participant characteristics by weight status for all ethnic groups combined, and for CHamorus and Other Micronesians separately. Children affected by OWOB reported statistically higher body size parameters as measured by height, weight, WC, BMI, and BMI z-scores, compared to healthy weight children. All children with abdominal obesity, as defined by the International Diabetes Federation [27], were OWOB. Among children in the OWOB weight status, 33.8% had abdominal obesity by this cut-point. It is worth noting that the International Diabetes Federation cut-point is for older children (6–10 years old) and is limited in identifying younger children (2–5 years) with abdominal obesity.

Table 2. Characteristics of child participants from Guam in the Children's Healthy Living (CHL) Program stratified by BMI status.

Participant & Family Characteristics	Total Mean ± SE or n(%)	Healthy Weight * Mean ± SE or n (%)	OWOB * Mean ± SE or n (%)	p Value
Age				0.069
2–5 years old	437 (53.2%)	329 (55.1%)	108 (48%)	
6–8 years old	385 (46.8%)	268 (44.9%)	117 (52%)	
Sex				0.917
Boys	425 (51.7%)	308 (51.6%)	117 (52.0%)	
Girls	397 (48.3%)	289 (48.4%)	108 (48.0%)	
Child Ethnicity				0.455
CHamoru	528 (64.55%)	392 (65.88%)	137 (61.16%)	
Other Micronesians	203 (24.82%)	144 (24.20%)	59 (26.34%)	
Filipino	77 (9.41%)	51 (8.57%)	26 (11.61%)	
Other	10 (1.22%)	8 (1.34%)	2 (0.89%)	
Annual Family Income Level				0.473
<$20,000	331 (57.6%)	234 (56.9%)	97 (59.1%)	
$20,000–$34,999	86 (15%)	63 (15.3%)	23 (14%)	
$35,000–$59,999	89 (15.5%)	60 (14.6%)	29 (17.7%)	
>$60,000	69 (12%)	54 (13.1%)	15 (9.1%)	
Receiving any Food Assistance				0.768
Yes	645 (78.5%)	470 (78.7%)	175 (77.8)	
No	177 (21.5%)	127 (21.3%)	50 (22.2%)	
Type of Food Assistance				
SNAP	556 (67.9%)	408 (68.7%)	148 (65.8%)	0.426
Local Food Bank	99 (12.15%)	72 (72.7%)	27 (27.3%)	0.977
WIC	258 (31.5%)	196 (33.0%)	62 (27.6%)	0.135
Free School Lunch/Breakfast	238 (29.1%)	169 (28.5%)	69 (30.7%)	0.533
Food Insecurity				0.566
Always/most times	120 (16.7%)	88 (16.8%)	32 (16.3%)	
Sometimes	253 (35.2%)	178 (34%)	75 (38.3%)	
Seldom/never	346 (48.1%)	257 (49.1%)	89 (45.4%)	
Parent/Caregiver Education				0.052
<12th Grade	269 (32.7%)	207 (34.7%)	62 (27.6%)	
12th Grade/GED	331 (40.3%)	241 (40.4%)	90 (40%)	
Some college or higher	222 (27%%)	149 (25%)	73 (32.4%)	
Parent Marital Status				0.06
Married	326 (39.7%)	225 (37.7%)	101 (44.9%)	
Not Married	496 (60.3%)	372 (62.3%)	124 (55.1%)	
Number Children in Household	4.19 ± 0.077	4.19 ± 0.094	4.22 ± 0.152	0.838
Household Size				0.491
1–2 children	197 (24.1%)	145 (24.4%)	52 (23.1%)	
3–4 children	319 (38.9%)	224 (37.7%)	95 (42.2%)	
5 or more children	303 (37%)	225 (37.9%)	78 (34.7%)	
Birthplace				0.0070
Guam	685 (84.46%)	505 (85.45%)	180 (81.45%)	
U.S. Mainland	52 (6.41%)	37 (6.26%)	15 (6.79%)	
Saipan, CNMI	31 (3.82%)	20 (3.38%)	13 (5.88%)	
Other Islands in Micronesia	25 (3.08%)	21 (3.55%)	4 (1.81%)	
Philippines	13 (1.60%)	8 (1.35%)	5 (2.26%)	
Other	4 (0.49%)	1 (0.17%)	4 (1.82%)	

Table 2. Cont.

Participant & Family Characteristics	Total Mean ± SE or n(%)	Healthy Weight * Mean ± SE or n (%)	OWOB * Mean ± SE or n (%)	p Value
Acculturation				0.2913
Integrated	542 (80.30%)	394 (79.60%)	148 (82.22%)	
Traditional	94 (13.78%)	72 (14.54%)	21 (12.14%)	
Assimilated	17 (2.52%)	10 (2.02%)	7 (3.89%)	
Marginalized	23 (3.41%)	19 (3.84%)	4 (2.22%)	
Ever Breastfed?				0.2140
Yes	529 (64.59%)	373 (66.13%)	156 (70.59%)	
No	256 (35.41%)	191 (33.87%)	65 (29.41%)	
Exclusively Breastfed?				0.5655
Yes	97 (13.13%)	68 (12.69%)	29 (14.29%)	
No	642 (86.87%)	468 (87.13%)	174 (85.71%)	
Child age (mos) when weaned from breastmilk	9.76 ± 0.438 (n = 495)	10.22 ± 0.542	9.23 ± 0.844	0.3248
Child fed both breastmilk & infant formula				0.5135
Yes	421 (54.39%)	300 (53.67%)	121 (56.28%)	
No	353 (45.61%)	259 (44.33%)	94 (43.72%)	
Average Sleep Duration (h/d)	8.62 ± 0.08	8.54 ± 0.096	8.59 ± 0.142	0.7122
TCSQ Sleep Score	6.34 ± 0.205	6.35 ± 0.257	5.59 ± 0.341	0.0421
Met Sleep Recommendations				0.725
Yes	327 (40.4%)	236 (40%)	91 (41.4%)	
No	483 (59.6%)	354 (60%)	129 (58.6%)	
Average Screen-time (h/d)	5.26 ± 0.132	5.15 ± 0.150	5.55 ± 0.270	0.1743
Met Screen-time Recommendations				0.444
Yes	117 (16.8%)	82 (16.2%)	35 (18.6%)	
No	578 (83.2%)	425 (83.8%)	153 (81.4%)	
Height (cm)	110.52 ± 0.47	108.71 ± 0.528	115.34 ± 0.912	0.0001
Weight (kg)	21.26 ± 0.26	18.77 ± 0.185	27.91 ± 0.635	0.0001
BMI, kg/m²	16.95 ± 0.11	15.64 ± 0.038	20.45 ± 0.280	0.0001
BMI z-score	0.485 ± 0.036	0.007 ± 0.026	1.79 ± 0.045	0.0001
Waist Circumference (cm)	55.07 ± 0.457	51.93 ± 0.188	64.40 ± 0.707	0.0001
Abdominal Obesity				0.0001
Yes	75 (9.2%)	0 (0%)	75 (33.60%)	
No	741 (90.8%)	591 (100%)	148 (66.40%)	
Beverage Consumption ‡				
Water (c/d)	1.31 ± 0.035	1.32 ± 0.043	1.28 ± 0.070	0.5793
Milk (c/d)	1.24 ± 0.24	1.25 ± 0.028	1.21 ± 0.048	0.5394
Sugar-sweetened drinks (c/d)	0.84 ± 0.03	0.31 ± 0.34	0.93 ± 0.061	0.0576
Vegetable Intake ‡ (c/d)	0.61 ± 0.013	0.60 ± 0.015	0.63 ± 0.027	0.2335
Fruit Intake ‡ (c/d)	0.88 ± 0.021	0.87 ± 0.025	0.89 ± 0.040	0.7324
Met Recommendation for				
Fruit Intake	257 (41.35%)	185 (39.96%)	79 (46.20%)	0.1371
Vegetable Intake	6 (0.90%)	4 (0.86%)	2 (1.17%)	0.7242

* Healthy weight defined as BMI between 5th–84th percentile for age and sex; 'OWOB' defined as BMI greater than 85th percentile for age and sex, ‡ Consumption in cups/day, weighted for weekday/weekend days and adjusted for within person variance.

There were no significant differences in the presence of OWOB among children by sex, ethnicity, family income, food insecurity, food assistance, acculturation, screen-time, sleep duration, or intake of fruits, vegetables, water, or milk. OWOB children consumed marginally higher amounts (p value = 0.07) of SSB compared to healthy weight children. There were significant differences in the presence of OWOB among children by certain demographic characteristics, such as parent/caregiver education level, parent/caregiver marital status, and child birthplace (Table 2).

To explore further the relationship between the behavioral factors of interest and OWOB, we calculated ORs separately for CHamorus and Other Micronesians, the two largest ethnic groups in the study (Table 3). Among CHamoru children, those who were older (6–8 years) were 1.63 times more likely to be affected by OWOB than younger children (2–5 years). The highest prevalence of OWOB was seen among Filipino children (33.8%), followed by Other Micronesian children (28.9%), and CHamoru children (25.0%). OWOB was also more likely to occur among children ages 6–8 years

(30.4%) versus children between the ages of 2–5 years (24.7%). No significant associations were found except that association between OWOB and SSB intake, and OWOB and parent education level.

Table 3. Prevalence and Odds of OWOB among child participants from Guam in the Children's Healthy Living (CHL) Program.

Variable	n	% OWOB [†] (95% CI)	Adjusted OR [††] (95% CI)
Overall	822	27.4 (24.3–30.4)	
Child Characteristics			
Sex			
Males	425	27.5 (23.3–31.8)	Referent
Females	397	27.2 (22.8–31.6)	1.001 (0.734–1.366)
Age			
2–5 years	437	24.7 (20.7–28.8)	Referent
6–8 years	385	30.4 (25.8–35.0)	1.337 (0.982–1.821)
Ethnicity			
CHamoru	531	26.0 (22.3–29.7)	Referent
Other Micronesians	204	28.9 (22.7–35.2)	1.186 (0.824–1.706)
Filipino	77	33.8 (23.0–44.6)	1.454 (0.870–2.430)
Other	10	20.0 (−10.2–50.2)	0.693 (0.144–3.329)
Child was breastfed?			
Yes	530	29.4 (25.5–33.3)	1.212 (0.861–1.708)
No	258	25.6 (20.2–30.9)	Referent
Child met sleep standard for his/her age group?			
Yes	327	27.8 (23.0–32.7)	0.994 (0.717–1.378)
No	483	26.7 (22.8–30.7)	Referent
Child met recommendation for screen-time of ≤ 2 h/day?			
Yes	117	29.9 (21.5–38.3)	1.184 (0.757–1.851)
No	578	26.5 (22.9–30.1)	Referent
Child met recommendation for vegetable intake for his/her age group?			
Yes	6	33.3 (−20.9–87.5)	1.342 (0.236–7.649)
No	628	26.9 (23.4–30.4)	Referent
Child met recommendation for fruit intake for his/her age group?			
Yes	264	29.9 (24.4–35.5)	1.274 (0.89–1.823)
No	370	24.9 (20.4–29.3)	Referent
SSB beverage intake [‡] (cups/day)			
(zero intake—referent)	160	21.3 (14.8–27.7)	Referent
Tertile 1 (≤0.42)	54	33.3 (20.4–46.3)	2.064 (1.024–4.160)
Tertile 2 (0.42–1.09)	208	26.4 (20.4–32.5)	1.495 (0.90–2.485)
Tertile 3 (≥1.09)	212	30.2 (24.0–36.4)	1.824 (1.106–3.007)
p-value for trend			0.022
Water beverage intake [‡] (cups/day)			
(zero intake—referent)	26	30.8 (11.8–49.8)	Referent
Tertile 1 (≤0.92)	195	26.2 (19.9–32.4)	0.827 (0.333–2.057)
Tertile 2 (0.92–1.62)	201	28.4 (22.1–34.6)	0.965 (0.388–2.401)
Tertile 3 (≥1.62)	212	25.9 (20.0–31.9)	0.819 (0.330–2.033)
p-value for trend			0.597
Parent/Caregiver/Household Characteristics			
Education Level			
Less than 12th grade (use this as reference)	269	23.1 (18.0–28.1)	Referent
12th grade/GED or higher	553	29.5 (25.7–33.3)	1.415 (1.004–1.994)
Marital Status			
Married	326	31.0 (25.9–36.0)	Referent
Not married	496	25.0 (21.2–28.8)	0.776 (0.564–1.067)
Annual household income			
<$20,000	331	29.3 (24.4–34.2)	Referent
$20,000–$34,999	86	26.7 (17.2–36.3)	0.867 (0.501–1.502)
$35,000–$59,999	89	32.6 (22.7–42.5)	1.121 (0.664–1.892)
$60,000+	69	21.7 (11.8–31.7)	0.600 (0.315–1.143)
Food Insecurity			
Yes	120	26.7 (18.6–34.7)	0.982 (0.627–1.539)
No	599	27.4 (23.8–31.0)	Referent

Table 3. Cont.

Variable	n	% OWOB † (95% CI)	Adjusted OR †† (95% CI)
Receiving any food assistance			
Yes	645	27.1 (23.4–30.6)	1.027 (0.699–1.509)
No	177	28.3 (21.6–35.0)	Referent
Number of children in household			
1–2 children	197	26.4 (20.2–32.6)	Referent
3–4 children	319	29.8 (24.7–34.8)	1.18 (0.789–1.765)
5 or more children	303	25.7 (20.8–30.7)	0.948 (0.622–1.446)
Acculturation—Family considers themselves 'integrated' into culture			
Yes	545	27.3 (23.6–31.1)	1.162 (0.747–1.81)
No	134	24.6 (17.2–32.0)	Referent

† 'Underweight' children excluded from analysis, †† Adjusted for clustering by community, age, sex, and ethnicity, ‡ Consumption in cups/day, weighted for weekday/weekend days and adjusted for within person variance.

3.3. Nutrition Factors

The majority of child participants (80.4%) were receiving some sort of food assistance, including USDA Supplemental Nutrition Assistance Program (SNAP) (67.8%), USDA Supplemental Nutrition Assistance Program for Women, Infants, and Children (WIC) (31.8%), free or reduced school lunch/breakfast (28.8%), and/or assistance from a local food bank (11.7%). Food insecurity was also prevalent as 51.5% of participants reported that food money ran out at the end of the month either always/most times (16.8%) or sometimes (34.7%). Significantly more ($p < 0.001$) Other Micronesian child participants (74.9%) reported that food money ran out at least sometimes compared to CHamoru (42.8%), Filipino (53.7%) and Other (50%) children.

As for OWOB risk factors and CHL related nutrition behaviors, majority of children did not meet recommendations for fruit (58.7%) and vegetable (99.1%) intake and consumed SSB (73.7%). Fruit and vegetable intake did not differ significantly by ethnicity (Table 1) or by the presence of OWOB (Table 2). Mean intake of vegetables was low (0.61 c/d) and only 6 children surveyed (0.09%) consumed the recommended amount of vegetables daily, which equates to ≥1 cup equivalent for children 2 years old and ≥1.5 cup equivalent for children 3–8 years old [34–36]. Mean intake of fruits was somewhat better (0.88 c/d) and more children (41.3%) reported consuming the recommended amount of fruits daily, which equates to ≥1.5 cup equivalent for children 2–8 years old [34].

When asked if the child participant was ever breastfed as a baby, about two-thirds (67%) of all parents/caregivers responded yes. Only 13.1% of children were exclusively breastfed (not shown in table), while 54.2% of children surveyed were fed both breastmilk and infant formula as an infant. CHamoru children (21.32) reported being significantly less likely to be ever breastfed compared to Other Micronesian children (37.2%). Of those children who were ever breastfed, Other Micronesian children were weaned at a significantly older age (12.48 m) compared to children from other ethnic groups. Breastfeeding during infancy, whether exclusive or mixed with infant formula feeding did not differ by the presence of OWOB. Age at weaning also did not differ by presence of OWOB. Among those who were exclusively breastfed, mean age at weaning was significantly higher compared to mixed fed infants (19.27 ± 1.19 m versus 7.56 ± 0.04 m). Risk of OWOB increased significantly with SSB intake. The relationship between presence of OWOB and increasing SSB intake was not monotonic, the ORs (95% CI) for SSB intake for the tertile groups for consumers compared to those with zero intake of SSB were 2.06 (1.02–4.16), 1.50 (0.90–2.48), and 1.82 (1.11–3.01). Only 25% of children surveyed consumed the recommended amount of "zero intake" of SSB [37], and one-third of child participants consumed at least 1.1 cups of SSB per day. Correlation analysis showed that SSB intake was positively and significantly associated with BMI and waist circumference. Among CHamoru children, the relationship between SSB intake and body size was stronger, as SSB intake among CHamoru children was positively and significantly associated with BMI ($r = 0.18$, $p = 0.0002$), waist circumference ($r = 0.16$, $p = 0.0007$), and BMI z-score ($r = 0.11$, $p = 0.023$). In Table 3, although SSB intake was not significantly associated with OWOB for Other Micronesian children, it was significant for CHamoru children. The relationship again was not monotonic, the ORs (95% CI) for SSB intake for the tertile groups of consumers compared to those with zero intake of SSB were 3.15 (1.1–9.08), 2.84 (1.28–6.30) and 3.19 (1.46–6.95).

3.4. Sleep and Screen-Time

Less than half of all children surveyed (40.4%) met the sleep duration recommendations [20]; those recommendations being at least 8–11 h/day for children under the age of 5 years, and 8–10 h per day for children 5 years and older. Sleep duration did not differ by the presence of OWOB, yet we observed TCSQ sleep quality scores (Table 2) were significantly lower ($p = 0.0421$) among children affected by OWOB compared to children with healthy weight (5.59 ± 0.34 versus 6.55 ± 0.26, respectively), meaning that children with OWOB were statistically more likely to suffer from sleep disturbances. Only 30.58% of Other Micronesian children met sleep recommendations (Table 1), which was significantly ($p = 0.014$) less than children from other ethnic groups. Other Micronesian children reported TCSQ sleep quality scores that were lower ($p = 0.056$) compared to children from the other ethnic groups.

The recommended daily screen-time for children is less than 2 h per day [38]. Only one sixth of the children surveyed (16.9%) met this recommendation and meeting screen-time recommendations did not differ between healthy weight children and children affected by OWOB. Average screen-time was slightly more than 5 h per day. When comparisons were made across four ethnic groups, there was a significant difference ($p = 0.007$) in the proportion of children that met the screen-time recommendation: CHamorus (16.7%), Other Micronesian (22.5%), Filipinos (4.6%), and Other (0%). There was also a significant difference in the average daily screen-time among the ethnic groups: CHamorus (5.13 h), Other Micronesians (5.45 h), Filipinos (6.24 h), and Other (3.59 h) (Table 1).

3.5. Acculturation

The majority of study participants (80%) considered their cultural affiliation as integrated, meaning a bicultural orientation where the respondent retains their ethnic cultural identity at the same time moving to join the dominant society (i.e., the US) [22,39]. About 15% of both CHamorus and Other Micronesians considered their cultural affiliation traditional, where the respondent retains their ethnic identity and does not recognize or identify with cultural characteristics of the US [22,39]. The Other Micronesians (6.1%) were most likely of all ethnic groups represented in this study to report having marginalized cultural affiliation, meaning the respondent does not maintain his/her ethnic cultural characteristics and excludes or withdraws him/herself from the dominant society (i.e., the U.S.) [22,39]. Acculturation did not differ by the presence of OWOB (Table 2). However, we observed that among Other Micronesians, children from families who considered their cultural affiliation as integrated into the culture were 2.05 times more likely to be affected by OWOB (CI 0.81–5.20) (Table 3).

4. Discussion

Pacific Islanders were one of the fastest growing racial/ethnic groups in the US in 2000 to 2010 [40], but little is known about OWOB for young children (under 11 year) in the Pacific region [41]. The current prevalence of OWOB in the US is 25% among children between 2–5 years and 32.8% among children between 6–8 years [42]. Findings in this current study on Guam were consistent with previous reports [43] and similar to the US. Unlike previous reports, this study revealed ethnic differences in OWOB presence among children in Guam. Filipino and Other Micronesian had the highest OWOB (33%) and obesity (18%) prevalence compared to other children in Guam.

Some recent studies have shown that obesity among various Pacific Islander groups, such as Samoans, may be linked to specific genes influencing adiposity [40,41,44]; and Pacific Islanders of Polynesian, Micronesian, and Melanesian origin may all carry certain alleles associated with higher body weight, BMI, and risk of obesity [41,45]. Waist circumference-to-height ratio (WHR) and WC have been used as markers of body adiposity in adults and, in children and adolescents (8–18 years), WHR was determined to be better at predicting adiposity [46–48]. One third of this study's participants

(33.8%) were observed to have both, abdominal obesity and OWOB. On the other hand, healthy weight children did not have abdominal obesity (0%). This aligns with other studies that found adiposity indicators, like WC, were associated with being overweight [47]. This is alarming as the location and distribution of body fat are associated with cardiovascular and other disease risks that is likely to continue into adulthood [49–51].

Given the steady rise in obesity over the past few decades on a global scale, environmental (macro and micro) factors promoting obesity are a more likely predominant explanation for racial/ethnic disparities in childhood obesity [52], such as the increase in obesity seen on Guam and other islands in the Pacific. A majority of children in this study exhibited several behaviors that are obesity risk factors such as low intake of fruits and vegetables, high intake of SSB, low sleep duration, and high amounts of sedentary screen-time [52].

From the micro-environment of children, which includes their families and households, in this study, the majority of child participants came from households where their parent/caregivers were unmarried (60.7%) and with at least three or more children (76.2%). Those two factors, compounded by the fact that most of the parents in this study also reported low annual incomes, can lead to an unfavorable home environment. Research shows that family and home environments, whether directly or indirectly, may contribute to the development of child OWOB [53–55], possibly through maternal depression and stress. Further study and more specific questions regarding parent/caregiver psychological health is needed to determine impact of family environment on the presence of OWOB among children in Guam.

Surprisingly, 59.65% of the children surveyed did not meet the recommended sleep duration for their age. Research indicates that short sleep duration puts children at risk for obesity and other metabolic, cardiovascular, and behavior disorders [56–58]. This study did not find sleep duration to differ significantly between children with OWOB and those with healthy weight, possibly due to misinterpretation of the question on sleep duration. Given some of the very low reported levels of sleep hours per day for some of the children and limited English comprehension of the islander parents/caregivers, it is possible that nap times during the day may have been the reported time, rather than sleep over the 24-h period. Future studies should separate questions for nap time sleep from night sleep in determining USAP children's sleep duration and include more qualitative non-subjective measurements for sleep duration. In terms of sleep quality, children affected by OWOB in this study were statistically more likely to suffer from sleep disturbances. This aligns with the research linking poor sleep quality with OWOB and an increased risk for cognitive and behavioral problems [56–58]. Research also links reduced sleep quality with high SSB intake, and in bed screen-time [59].

The proportion of children exceeding screen-time recommendation in this study (83%) was comparable to the 87% reported among a prospective birth cohort of children born in New York led by researchers from the NIH Eunice Kennedy Shriver National Institute of Child Health and Human Development [60]; however, the birth cohort included children below two years of age, which is an age group not represented in the Guam study. Additionally, while screen-time increased with preschool age in the birth cohort, the total hours decreased to below the recommended two hours by 7–8 years old possibly due to school activities [60].

Screen-time has been shown to be associated with other behaviors, especially sleep. Twenge and colleagues [61] found an inverse association, increased screen-time and reduced sleep duration among a population-based sample of 0–17 year-olds in the United States [61]. In the current study, the order of screen-time, from highest to lowest duration, by ethnic group was Filipino (6.24 h), Other Micronesians (5.45 h), CHamorus (5.13 h), and Other (3.59 h). Interestingly, this order was reversed with the TCSQ sleep quality score, where Filipinos reported the highest quality sleep (5.23), and Others reported the lowest quality (8.0), but the pattern was not the same with sleep duration. Researchers are beginning to better understand the impact of screen-time on sleep behaviors. For example, Guerrero and colleagues [62] found a relationship between increased screen-time and increased social problems (e.g., rule-breaking, social problems, aggressive behavior, and thought problems), and the relationship was mediated by sleep duration (every hour increase in sleep = 8.8% to 16.6% decrease in problem behaviors) among 9–10 year-old in the Adolescent Brain Cognitive Development study [63]. Behavioral problems, although complex, are real issues plaguing children and should be considered when building wellness models for healthy families and healthy communities. Further studies on screen-time among children in Guam are warranted.

Childhood behavioral problems have been linked to racial socialization and cultural resilience [64]. Similarly, cultural affiliation, or low acculturation (i.e., traditional), is associated with lower rates of obesity and sedentary behaviors in children from migrant populations [39]. Although CHamorus in this study are not likely migrants, the long history of colonization in Guam lends to multidimensional acculturation for CHamorus and Guamanians alike in the presence of the colonial society (i.e., the US). This considered, CHamoru children had the highest proportion of parents identifying as traditional and the lowest rates of obesity compared to other ethnic groups in this study. Additionally, Filipino children identified most as integrated had the highest average screen-time (hr/d) compared to other ethnic groups. These findings align with previous studies that have found traditional or low acculturation to be protective against obesity and related risk factors [39,65,66]. A greater acculturation (i.e., assimilation) has also shown to be a predictor of lower fruit and vegetable intake among adult populations [67,68]. Therefore, obesity interventions or health programs in Guam should include cultural values and practices to maintain or reinforce healthy cultural behaviors unique to each and shared across ethnic group(s).

Both fruit and vegetable consumption among child participants in this study were low and failed to meet the recommendations set forth by the USDA Dietary Guidelines [34]. Little is known about the food intake, particularly fruits and vegetables, of children on Guam. Pobocik and colleagues [69,70] studied the food intake of over 1000 elementary school-aged children on Guam and reported fruit and vegetable consumption was well below the recommended intake levels [69]. Leon Guerrero and Workman [71] studied health behaviors of adolescents on Guam and reported that only 24.7% of those surveyed reported consumption at least one serving of fruit and/or vegetable, and none reported consuming the recommendations for fruit and vegetable intake set forth by the Dietary Guidelines. Children on Guam are not unlike children from the US mainland. A recent study looking at diet quality by BMI category of US children found that in general, all children's diets in the United States were poor and in need of improvement, regardless of BMI status, age, sex, race/ethnicity, and poverty-to-income ratio classification [72].

CHamorus and Filipinos were less likely to exclusively breastfeed and tended to breastfeed for shorter durations, compared to other Micronesians and Other ethnic groups; mixed feeding was common in all ethnic groups and associated with earlier weaning as would be expected. No relationship of feeding method with overweight and obesity was detected. Breastfeeding is the biologic norm, important for infant nutrition and healthy growth, and protective for child obesity [73–75], although not demonstrated here. Likely other socio-economic (e.g., income) and behavioral factors (e.g., SSB intake) not controlled in this comparison confound the association in this study.

Several studies have shown an association between SSB intake and adverse health outcomes in children, particularly overweight, obesity, unhealthy weight gain, and central adiposity [76–78]. Other longitudinal data indicated that children consuming as little as one SSB serving per day were 55% more likely to be OWOB compared to children with limited SSB consumption [79]. Wojcicki and colleagues looked at the effect of SSB consumption on leukocyte telomere length in preschool children [80]. After adjusting for age sex, and BMI, SSB intake among the preschool children was significantly related to shorter leukocyte length. Shorter telomere length has been associated with a number of adverse health outcomes such as type 2 diabetes, stroke, and myocardial infarction because shortened telomeres start the inflammatory cascade through increased production of cytokines, thus adversely impacting cellular health [80]. SSB consumption during early childhood may not lead immediately to OWOB, as there may be an age effect. It may take a number of years of SSB consumption before the development of OWOB or metabolic changes associated with obesity [77,80–82]. SSB intake may also be a marker of a food and beverage intake pattern and other lifestyle factors that are associated with obesity.

High intake of SSB is common on Guam, and SSBs are readily available in food stores. In a previous study looking at dietary intake of CHamoru and Filipino adults living on Guam, Leon Guerrero and colleagues [11] found that CHamoru adults reported consuming between 7–9% of food energy from SSBs (7% for women and 9% for men). In this same study [11], SSBs were the second largest contributor to energy intake for CHamoru adults; and third largest contributor to energy intake for Filipino adults.

Like most other islands in the Pacific, Guam relies heavily on imported processed foods. A 2013 survey of processed foods available in the Pacific Islands [83] showed that Guam recorded the highest number of available processed food products compared to the other Pacific islands surveyed, with over 2100 products available to Guam consumers. High intake of SSBs is not only a problem for children affected by OWOB. The child participants surveyed on Guam, whether or not they were affected by OWOB, consumed a high amount of SSBs, putting them at risk for developing adverse cardiometabolic outcomes as they grow older.

There were some limitations to this study. The small sample size of Other Micronesian and especially Filipino children made ethnic group comparisons difficult. Some parents/caregivers, Other Micronesians in particular, spoke English as a second language and had limited English comprehension; making it difficult to comprehend and respond to survey tools. This may have affected accuracy of results. Generalizations are limited due to non-randomized cluster sampling. However, recruitment of children at the community-based settings in Guam communities was designed to ensure appropriate representation by age, sex, ethnicity, and geographic location. Since this study reports cross-sectional data, causal association of OWOB with behavioral or demographic factors cannot be conclusively inferred; longitudinal examination is needed to confirm causality. Despite the limitations, we were able to recruit and assess a large sample of children ($n = 865$) from several communities across the island that were representative of the major ethnic groups on Guam. Anthropometric measurements of children surveyed provided a reliable assessment of OWOB status among children on Guam.

In conclusion, the child participants surveyed on Guam, whether or not they are currently affected by OWOB, are at a high risk for developing OWOB in adulthood, as well as other chronic diseases. Specifically, for OWOB risk factors and CHL behaviors, the majority of children surveyed did not meet recommendations for: sleep duration (59.6%), sedentary screen-time (83.11%), or fruit (58.7%) and vegetable (99.1%) intake and consumed SSB (73.7%). The study found children affected by OWOB in this study, were statistically more likely ($p = 0.042$) to suffer from sleep disturbances, and consumed marginally higher amounts (p value = 0.07) of SSB compared to children with healthy weight. The study identified indicators of potentially stressful home situations among participant families that include: high prevalence of the child participants being cared for by a single parent (60.7%), families with three or more children (76.2%), and high prevalence of some level of food insecurity (59.6%) among participant families. These family stressors may also contribute to OWOB among children on Guam. With respect to OWOB prevention guidance, the study found evidence supporting previous studies' findings that traditional or low acculturation to be protective against obesity [39,59,60]. Healthy cultural behaviors, both unique to and shared across ethnic group(s), should be incorporated in future obesity interventions by highlighting healthy cultural values, practices and traditional foods. The obesogenic factors identified in the children in this study provide a basis for health promotion and obesity prevention guidance for children in Guam.

Author Contributions: R.T.L.G. led study concept, acquisition, analysis, and interpretation of data, and writing of manuscript; oversaw and had primary responsibility for final manuscript. L.R.B. assisted in study concept, interpretation of data, and writing of manuscript. M.P.H.-U. assisted in acquisition of data, and providing critical review of manuscript. M.A. assisted in acquisition and entry of data and providing critical review of manuscript. T.F.A. assisted in acquisition, entry and analysis of data, and writing of manuscript. Y.C.P. assisted in acquisition, entry and analysis of data, and writing of manuscript. L.R.W. participated in overall study design, contributed to statistical analysis, interpreted data, and writing of manuscript. R.N. initially assisted in the study concept, participated in design, interpreted data, and writing of manuscript. All authors provided critical review of the manuscript and gave final approval. All authors have read and agreed to the published version of the manuscript.

Funding: This research was funded by the Agriculture and Food Research Initiative grant 2011-68001-30335 from the U.S. Department of Agriculture, National Institute of Food and Agricultural, Science Enhancement Coordinated Agricultural Program and the CHL Center of Excellence is currently funded by the USDA National Institute of Food and Agriculture, Agriculture and Food Research Institute Grant no. 2018-69001-27551.

Acknowledgments: We would like to thank the parents and children who participated in the Children's Healthy Living Program (CHL), as well as our many community partners who assisted.

Conflicts of Interest: The authors declare no conflict of interest.

References

1. Ogden, C.L.; Carroll, M.D.; Kit, B.K.; Flegal, K.M. Prevalence of childhood and adult obesity in the United States, 2011–2012. *JAMA* **2014**, *311*, 806–814. [CrossRef] [PubMed]
2. Ogden, C.L.; Carroll, M.D.; Fryar, C.D.; Flegal, K.M. Prevalence of Obesity among Adults and Youth: United States, 2011–2014. *NCHS Data Brief* **2015**, *219*, 1–8.
3. Yang, L.; Colditz, G.A. Prevalence of Overweight and Obesity in the United States, 2007–2012. *JAMA Intern. Med.* **2015**, *175*, 1412–1413. [CrossRef] [PubMed]
4. Afshin, A.; Forouzanfar, M.H.; Reitsma, M.B.; Sur, P.; Estep, K.; Lee, A.; Marczak, L.; Mokdad, A.H.; Moradi-Lakeh, M.; Naghavi, M.; et al. Health Effects of Overweight and Obesity in 195 Countries over 25 Years. *N. Engl. J. Med.* **2017**, *377*, 13–27. [CrossRef]
5. Ng, M.; Fleming, T.; Robinson, M.; Thomson, B.; Graetz, N.; Margano, C.; Mullany, C.E.; Biryukov, S.; Abbafati, C.; Abera, F.S.; et al. Global, regional, and national prevalence of overweight and obesity in children and adults during 1980–2013: A systematic analysis for the Global Burden of Disease Study 2013. *Lancet* **2014**, *384*, 766–781. [CrossRef]
6. Novotny, R.; Fialkowski, M.K.; Li, F.; Paulino, Y.S.N.; Vargo, D.; Jim, R.; Coleman, P.; Bersamin, A.; Nigg, C.R.; Leon Guerrero, R.T.; et al. Systematic review of prevalence of young child overweight and obesity in the United States Affiliated Pacific region compared to the 48 contiguous states: A the Children's Health Living Program. *Am. J. Pub. Health* **2015**. [CrossRef]
7. Underwood, J. The native origins of the neo-Chamorros of the Mariana Islands. *Micronesia* **1976**, *12*, 203–209.
8. Vilar, M.G.; Chan, C.W.; Santos, D.R.; Lynch, D.; Spathis, R.; Garruto, R.M.; Lum, J.K. The origins and genetic distinctiveness of the Chamorros of the Marianas Islands: An mtDNA perspective. *Am. J. Hum. Biol.* **2013**, *25*, 116–122. [CrossRef]
9. Central Intelligence Agency: The World Factbook. Available online: https://www.cia.gov/library/publications/the-world-factbook/geos/gq.html (accessed on 30 June 2020).
10. *Asian and Pacific Islander American Health Forum Health Briefs: Chamorros in the United States.* Asian and Pacific Islander American Health Forum. 2006. Available online: https://www.apiahf.org/wp-content/uploads/2011/02/APIAHF_Healthbrief08j_2006-1.pdf (accessed on 25 June 2020).
11. Guerrero, R.T.L.; Paulino, Y.C.; Novotny, R.; Murphy, S.P. Diet and obesity among Chamorro and Filipino adults on Guam. *Asia Pac. J. Clin. Nutr.* **2008**, *17*, 216–222.
12. Hankin, J.; Reed, D.; Labarthe, D.; Nichaman, M.; Stallones, R. Dietary and Disease Patterns among Micronesians. *Am. J. Clin. Nutr.* **1970**, *23*, 346–357. [CrossRef]
13. Pollock, N. Food habits in Guam over 500 years. *Pac. Viewp.* **1986**, *27*, 120–143. [CrossRef]
14. Uncangco, A.; Badowski, G.; David, A.; Ehlert, M.; Haddock, R.; Paulino, Y. *First Guam BRFSS Report 2007–2010*; Guam Department of Public Health & Social Services: Mangilao, Guam, USA, 2012.
15. Singh, A.S.; Mulder, C.; Twisk, J.W.; van Mechelen, W.; Chinapaw, M.J. Tracking of childhood overweight into adulthood: A systematic review of the literature. *Obes. Rev.* **2008**, *9*, 474–488. [CrossRef] [PubMed]
16. Barker, D.J.; Osmond, C.; Forsen, T.J.; Kajantie, E.; Eriksson, J.G. Trajectories of growth among children who have coronary events as adults. *N. Engl. J. Med.* **2005**, *353*, 1802–1809. [CrossRef] [PubMed]
17. Wilken, L.R.; Novotny, R.; Fialkowski, M.K.; Boushey, C.J.; Nigg, C.; Paulino, Y.; Leon Guerrero, R.; Bersamin, A.; Vargo, D.; Kim, J.; et al. Children's Healthy Living (CHL) Program for remote underserved minority populations in the Pacific region: Rationale and design of a community randomized trial to prevent early childhood obesity. *BMC Pub. Health* **2013**, *13*, 944. [CrossRef] [PubMed]

18. Novotny, R.; Fialkowski, M.K.; Areta, A.A.; Bersamin, A.; Braun, K.; DeBaryshe, B.; Deenik, J.; Dunn, M.; Hollyer, J.; Kim, J.; et al. The Pacific Way to Child Wellness: The Children's Healthy Living Program for Remote Underserved Minority Populations of the Pacific Region (CHL). *Hawaii J. Med. Pub. Health* **2013**, *72*, 406–408.
19. McGreavey, J.A.; Dornan, P.T.; Pagliari, H.C.; Sullivan, F.M. The tayside children's sleep questionnaire: A simple tool to evaluate sleep problems in young children. *Child Care Health Dev.* **2005**, *31*, 539–544. [CrossRef]
20. Hirshkowitz, M.; Whiton, K.; Albert, S.M.; Alessi, C.; Bruni, O.; DonCarlos, L.; Hazen, N.; Herman, J.; Katz, E.S.; Kheirandish-Gozal, L.; et al. National Sleep Foundation's sleep time duration recommendations: Methodology and results summary. *Sleep Health* **2015**, *1*, 40–43. [CrossRef]
21. Coleman-Jensen, A.; Gregory, C.; Singh, A. *Household Food Security in the United States in 2013*; US Department of Agriculture, Economic Research Service, Ed.; USDA Economic Research Service: Washington, DC, USA, 2014.
22. Kaholokula, J.K.; Iwane, M.K.; Nacapoy, A.H. Effects of perceived racism and acculturation on hypertension in Native Hawaiians. *Hawaii Med. J.* **2010**, *69*, 11–15.
23. Li, F.; Wilkens, L.R.; Novotny, R.; Fialkowski, M.; Paulino, Y.C.; Nelson, R.; Bersamin, A.; Martin, U.; Deenik, J.; Boushey, C. Anthropometric Measurement Standardization in the US-Affiliated Pacific: Report from the Children's Healthy Living Program. *Am. J. Hum. Biol.* **2016**, *28*, 364–371. [CrossRef]
24. Cook, S.; Auinger, P.; Huang, T.T. Growth curves for cardio-metabolic risk factors in children and adolescents. *J. Pediatr.* **2009**, *155*, e15–e26. [CrossRef]
25. Barlow, S. Expert committee recommendations regarding the prevention, assessment, and treatment of child and adolescent overweight and obesity: Summary report. *Pediatrics* **2007**, *120* (Suppl. 4), S164–S192. [CrossRef] [PubMed]
26. *Centers for Disease Control and Prevention A SAS Program for the 2000 CDC Growth Charts (Ages 0 to <20 Years)*; Centers for Disease Control and Prevention; 2014. Available online: https://www.cdc.gov/nccdphp/dnpao/growthcharts/resources/sas.htm (accessed on 6 April 2020).
27. Zimmet, P.; Alberti, K.G.; Kaufman, F.; Tajima, N.; Silink, M.; Arslanian, S.; Wong, G.; Bennett, P.; Shaw, J.; Caprio, S.; et al. The metabolic syndrome in children and adolescents—An IDF consensus report. *Pediatr. Diabetes* **2007**, *8*, 299–306. [CrossRef] [PubMed]
28. Novotny, R.; Nigg, C.; McGlone, K.; Renda, G.; Jung, N.; Matsunaga, M.; Karanja, N. Pacific tracker 2—Expert system (PacTrac2-ES) behavioural assessment and intervention tool for the pacific kids DASH for health (PacDASH) study. *Food Chem.* **2013**, *140*, 471–477. [CrossRef] [PubMed]
29. Martin, C.L.; Murphy, S.P.; Leon Guerrero, R.T.; Davison, N.; Jung, Y.O.; Novotny, R. The Pacific Tracker (PacTrac): Development of a dietary assessment instrument for the Pacific. *J. Food Compost. Anal.* **2008**, *21*, S103–S108. [CrossRef] [PubMed]
30. Murphy, S.; Blitz, C.; Novotny, R. Pacific tracker (PacTrac): An interactive dietary assessment program at the CRCH website. *Hawaii Med. J.* **2006**, *65*, 175–178. [PubMed]
31. Rolland-Cachera, M.F.; Akrout, M.; Peneau, S. Nutrient Intakes in Early Life and Risk of Obesity. *Int. J. Environ. Res. Public Health* **2016**, *13*, 564. [CrossRef]
32. Weihrauch-Blüher, S.; Wiegand, S. Risk Factors and Implications of Childhood Obesity. *Curr. Obes. Rep.* **2018**, *7*, 254–259. [CrossRef]
33. 2015 Poverty Guidelines. Office of the Assistant Secretary for Planning and Evaluation. US Department of Public Health and Social Services. Available online: https://aspe.hhs.gov/2015-poverty-guidelines (accessed on 9 July 2020).
34. U.S. Department of Health and Human Services and U.S. Department of Agriculture. *2015–2020 Dietary Guidelines for Americans*, 8th ed.; December 2015. Available online: http://health.gov/dietaryguidelines/2015/guidelines/ (accessed on 22 April 2020).
35. Bowman, S.; Friday, J.; Moshfegh, A. *MyPyramid Equivalents Database, 2.0 for USDA Survey Foods, 2003–2004 [Online]*; Food Surveys Research Group, Beltsville Human Nutrition Research Center, Agricultural Research Service, U.S. Ed.; Department of Agriculture: Beltsville, MD, USA, 2008.
36. Friday, J.; Bowman, S. *MyPyramid Equivalents Database for USDA Survey Food Codes, 1994–2002 Version 1.0. [Online]*; USDA, Agricultural Research Service, Beltsville Human Nutrition Research Center, Ed.; Community Nutrition Research Group: Beltsville, MD, USA, 2006.
37. Popkin, B.M.; Armstrong, L.E.; Bray, G.M.; Caballero, B.; Frei, B.; Willett, W.C. A new proposed guidance system for beverage consumption in the United States. *Am. J. Clin. Nutr.* **2006**, *83*, 529–542. [CrossRef]

38. American Academy of Pediatrics. Children, adolescents, and television. *Pediatrics* **2001**, *107*, 423–426. [CrossRef]
39. Renzaho, A.M.; Swinburn, B.; Burns, C. Maintenance of traditional cultural orientation is associated with lower rates of obesity and sedentary behaviours among African migrant children to Australia. *Int. J. Obes.* **2008**, *32*, 594–600. [CrossRef]
40. Hixson, L.; Hepler, B.B.; Kim, M.O. *The Native Hawaiian and other Pacific Islander Population: 2010*; US Census Bureau, Ed.; US Census Bureau: Washington, DC, USA, 2012.
41. Wate, J. Chapter 2: The Obesity Pandemic in the Pacific. In *Wealthy but Unhealthy: Overweight and Obesity in Asia and the Pacific: Trends, Costs, and Policies for Better Health*; Helble, M., Sato, A., Eds.; Asian Development Bank Institute: Tokyo, Japan, 2018.
42. Skinner, A.C.; Ravanbakht, S.N.; Skelton, J.A.; Perrin, E.M.; Armstrong, S.C. Prevalence of obesity and severe obesity in US children, 1999–2016. *Pediatrics* **2018**. [CrossRef] [PubMed]
43. Paulino, Y.C.; Guerrero, R.T.; Uncangco, A.A.; Rosadino, M.G.; Quinene, J.C.; Natividad, Z.N. Overweight and obesity prevalence among public school children in Guam. *J. Health Care Poor Underserved* **2015**, *26* (Suppl. 2), 53–62. [CrossRef] [PubMed]
44. Minster, R.L.; Hawley, N.L.; Su, C.T.; Sun, G.; Kershaw, E.E.; Cheng, H.; Buhule, O.D.; Lin, J.; Reupena, M.S.; Viali, S.; et al. A thrifty variant in CREBRF strongly influences body mass index in Samoans. *Nat. Genet.* **2016**, *48*, 1049–1054. [CrossRef] [PubMed]
45. Furusawa, T.; Naka, I.; Yamauchi, T.; Natsuhara, K.; Kimura, R.; Nakazawa, M.; Ishida, T.; Inaoka, T.; Matsumura, Y.; Ataka, Y.; et al. The Q223R polymorphism in LEPR is associated with obesity in Pacific Islanders. *Hum. Genet.* **2010**, *127*, 287–294. [CrossRef]
46. Brambilla, P.; Bedogni, G.; Heo, M.; Pietrobelli, A. Waist circumference-to-height ratio predicts adiposity better than body mass index in children and adolescents. *Int. J. Obes.* **2013**, *37*, 943–946. [CrossRef]
47. Vieira, S.A.; Ribeiro, A.Q.; Hermsdorff, H.H.M.; Pereira, P.F.; Priore, S.E.; Franceschini, S. Waist-to-height ratio index or the prediction of overweight in children. *Rev. Paul. Pediatr.* **2018**, *36*, 7.
48. Rakić, R.; Pavlica, T.; Bjelanović, J.; Vasiljević, P. Predictive ability of waist-to-hip-ratio and waist-to-height-ratio in relation to overweight/obesity in adolescents from Vojvodina (the Republic of Serbia) predictive ability of waist-to-hip-ratio and waist-to-height-ratio: Predictive Ability of Waist-to-Hip-Ratio and Waist-to-Height-Ratio. *Prog. Nutr.* **2019**, *24*, 992–998.
49. Staiano, A.E.; Gupta, A.K.; Katzmarzyk, P.T. Cardiometabolic risk factors and fat distribution in children and adolescents. *J. Pediatr.* **2014**, *164*, 560–565. [CrossRef]
50. Freedman, D.S.; Dietz, W.H.; Srinivasan, S.R.; Berenson, G.S. The relation of overweight to cardiovascular risk factors among children and adolescents: The Bogalusa Heart Study. *Pediatrics* **1999**, *103 Pt 1*, 1175–1182. [CrossRef]
51. Kahn, H.S.; Imperatore, G.; Cheng, Y.J. A population-based comparison of BMI percentiles and waist-to-height ratio for identifying cardiovascular risk in youth. *J. Pediatr.* **2005**, *146*, 482–488. [CrossRef]
52. Dixon, B.; Peña, M.M.; Taveras, E.M. Lifecourse approach to racial/ethnic disparities in childhood obesity. *Adv. Nutr.* **2012**, *3*, 73–82. [CrossRef] [PubMed]
53. Epstein, L.H.; Myers, M.D.; Anderson, K. The association of maternal psychopathology and family socioeconomic status with psychological problems in obese children. *Obes. Res.* **1996**, *4*, 65–74. [CrossRef] [PubMed]
54. Davis, M.; Young, L.; Davis, S.P.; Moll, G. Parental depression, family functioning and obesity among African American children. *J. Cult. Divers.* **2008**, *15*, 61–65. [PubMed]
55. McConley, R.L.; Mrug, S.; Gilliland, M.J.; Lowry, R.; Elliott, M.N.; Schuster, M.A.; Bogart, L.M.; Franzini, L.; Escobar-Chaves, S.L.; Franklin, F.A. Mediators of maternal depression and family structure on child BMI: Parenting quality and risk factors for child overweight. *Obesity* **2011**, *19*, 345–352. [CrossRef]
56. Pacheco, S.R.; Miranda, A.M.; Coelho, R.; Monteiro, A.C.; Braganca, G.; Loureiro, H.C. Overweight in youth and sleep quality: Is there a link? *Arch. Endocrinol. Metab.* **2017**. [CrossRef]
57. Navarro-Solera, M.; Carrasco-Luna, J.; Pin-Arboledas, G.; Gonzalez-Carrascosa, R.; Soriano, J.M.; Codoner-Franch, P. Short Sleep Duration Is Related to Emerging Cardiovascular Risk Factors in Obese Children. *J. Pediatr. Gastroenterol. Nutr.* **2015**, *61*, 571–576. [CrossRef]

58. Sakamoto, N.; Gozal, D.; Smith, D.L.; Yang, L.; Morimoto, N.; Wada, H.; Maruyama, K.; Ikeda, A.; Suzuki, Y.; Nakayama, M.; et al. Sleep duration, snoring prevalence, obesity, and behavioral problems in a large cohort of primary school students in Japan. *Sleep* **2017**, *40*. [CrossRef]
59. Morrissey, B.; Allender, S.; Strugnell, C. Dietary and activity factors influence poor sleep and the sleep-obesity nexus among children. *Int. J. Environ. Res. Public Health* **2019**, *16*, 1778. [CrossRef]
60. Trinh, M.H.; Sundaram, R.; Robinson, S.L.; Lin, T.C.; Bell, E.M.; Ghassabian, A.; Yeung, E.H. Association of trajectory and covariates of children's screen media time. *JAMA Pediatr.* **2019**, *174*, 71–78. [CrossRef]
61. Twenge, J.M.; Hisler, G.C.; Krizan, Z. Associations between screen time and sleep duration are primarily driven by portable electronic devices: Evidence from a population-based study of U.S. children ages 0–17. *Sleep Med.* **2019**, *56*, 211–218. [CrossRef]
62. Guerrero, M.D.; Barnes, J.D.; Chaput, J.P.; Tremblay, M.S. Screen time and problem behaviors in children: Exploring the mediating role of sleep duration. *Int. J. Behav. Nutr. Phys. Act.* **2019**, *16*, 105. [CrossRef] [PubMed]
63. Aflague, T. Boushey, C.; Leon Guerrero, R.; Ahmad, Z.; Kerr, D.; Delp, E. Feasibility and use of the mobile food record for capturing eating occasions among children ages 3–10 years in Guam. *Nutrients* **2015**, *7*, 4403–4415. [CrossRef] [PubMed]
64. Burt, C.H.; Simons, R.L.; Gibbons, F.X. Racial discrimination, ethnic-racial socialization, and crime: A micro-sociological model of risk and resilience. *Am. Sociol. Rev.* **2012**, *77*, 648–677. [CrossRef] [PubMed]
65. Delavari, M.; Sønderlund, A.L.; Swinburn, B.; Mellor, D.; Renzaho, A. Acculturation and obesity among migrant populations in high income countries—A systematic review. *BMC Public Health* **2013**, *13*, 458. [CrossRef] [PubMed]
66. Lind, C.; Mirchandani, G.G.; Castrucci, B.C.; Chávez, N.; Handler, A.; Hoelscher, D.M. The effects of acculturation on healthy lifestyle characteristics among Hispanic fourth-grade children in Texas public schools, 2004–2005. *J. School Health* **2012**, *82*, 166–174. [CrossRef] [PubMed]
67. Bolstad, A.L.; Bungum, T. Diet, acculturation, and BMI in Hispanics living in southern Nevada. *Am. J. Health Behav.* **2013**, *37*, 218–226. [CrossRef]
68. Lee, S.; Sobal, J.; Frongillo, E. Acculturation, food consumption, and diet-related factors among Korean Americans. *J. Nutr. Educ.* **1999**, *31*, 321–330. [CrossRef]
69. Pobocik, R.S.; Richer, J.J. Hentges, D.L. Food sources of macronutrients in the diets of fifth grade children on Guam. *Asian Am. Pac. Isl. J. Health* **1999**, *7*, 25–37.
70. Pobocik, R.S.; Richer, J.J. Estimated intake and food sources of vitamin, A.; folate, vitamin, C.; vitamin, E.; calcium, iron, and zinc for Guamanian children aged 9 to 12. *Pac. Health Dialog* **2002**, *9*, 193–202.
71. LeonGuerrero, R.T.; Workman, R.L. Physical activity and nutritional status of adolescents on Guam. *Pac. Health Dialog* **2002**, *9*, 177–185.
72. Thomson, J.L.; Landry, A.S.; Tussing-Humphreys, L.M.; Goodman, M.H. Diet quality of children in the United States by body mass index and sociodemographic characteristics. *Obes. Sci. Pract.* **2020**, *6*, 84–98. [CrossRef] [PubMed]
73. Koletzko, B.; Godfrey, K.M.; Poston, L.; Szajewska, H.; van Goudoever, J.B.; de Waard, M.; Brands, B.; Grivell, R.M.; Deussen, A.R.; Dodd, J.M.; et al. Nutrition during pregnancy, lactation and early childhood and its implications for maternal and long-term child health: The early nutrition project recommendations. *Ann. Nutr. Metab.* **2019**, *74*, 93–106. [CrossRef] [PubMed]
74. Koletzko, B.; Brands, B.; Grote, V.; Kirchberg, F.F.; Prell, C.; Rzehak, P.; Uhl, O.; Weber, M. Long-term health impact of early nutrition: The power of programming. *Ann. Nutr. Metab.* **2017**, *70*, 161–169. [CrossRef] [PubMed]
75. Horta, B.L.; Loret de Mola, C.; Victora, C.G. Long-term consequences of breastfeeding on cholesterol, obesity, systolic blood pressure and type 2 diabetes: A systematic review and meta-analysis. *Acta. Paediatr.* **2015**, *104*, 30–37. [CrossRef]
76. Keller, A.; Bucher Della Torre, S. Sugar-sweetened beverages and obesity among children and adolescents: A review of systematic literature reviews. *Child. Obes.* **2015**, *11*, 338–346. [CrossRef]
77. Scharf, R.J.; DeBoer, M.D. Sugar-Sweetened Beverages and Children's Health. *Annu. Rev. Public Health* **2016**, *37*, 273–293. [CrossRef]

78. Frantsve-Hawley, J.; Bader, J.D.; Welsh, J.A.; Wright, J.T. A systematic review of the association between consumption of sugar-containing beverages and excess weight gain among children under age 12. *J. Public Health Dent.* **2017**, *77* (Suppl. 1), S43–S66. [CrossRef]
79. Laverty, A.A.; Magee, L.; Monteiro, C.A.; Saxena, S.; Millett, C. Sugar and artificially sweetened beverage consumption and adiposity changes: National longitudinal study. *Int. J. Behav. Nutr. Phys. Act.* **2015**, *12*, 137. [CrossRef]
80. Wojcicki, J.M.; Medrano, R.; Lin, J.; Epel, E. Increased cellular aging by 3 years of age in latino, preschool children who consume more sugar-sweetened beverages: A pilot study. *Child. Obes.* **2018**, *14*, 149–157. [CrossRef]
81. Macintyre, A.K.; Marryat, L.; Chambers, S. Exposure to liquid sweetness in early childhood: Artificially-sweetened and sugar-sweetened beverage consumption at 4–5 years and risk of overweight and obesity at 7–8 years. *Pediatr. Obes.* **2018**, *13*, 755–765. [CrossRef]
82. Dubois, L.; Farmer, A.; Girard, M.; Peterson, K. Regular sugar-sweetened beverage consumption between meals increases risk of overweight among preschool-aged children. *J. Am. Diet. Assoc.* **2007**, *107*, 924–934. [CrossRef] [PubMed]
83. Snowdon, W.; Raj, A.; Reeve, E.; Guerrero, R.; Fesaitu, J.; Cateine, K.; Guignet, C. Processed foods available in the Pacific Islands. *Glob. Health* **2013**, *9*, 53. [CrossRef] [PubMed]

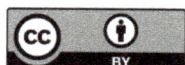

© 2020 by the authors. Licensee MDPI, Basel, Switzerland. This article is an open access article distributed under the terms and conditions of the Creative Commons Attribution (CC BY) license (http://creativecommons.org/licenses/by/4.0/).

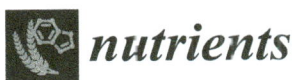

Article

Associations between Subjective and Objective Measures of the Community Food Environment and Executive Function in Early Childhood

Lindsey M. Bryant [1,*], Heather A. Eicher-Miller [2], Irem Korucu [3] and Sara A. Schmitt [1]

1. Human Development & Family Studies, Purdue University, 1202 W. State Street, West Lafayette, IN 47907, USA; saraschmitt@purdue.edu
2. Department of Nutrition Science, Purdue University, 700 W. State Street, West Lafayette, IN 47907, USA; heicherm@purdue.edu
3. Yale Center for Emotional Intelligence, Yale University, 350 George Street, New Haven, CT 065011.3, USA; irem.korucu@yale.edu
* Correspondence: bryant77@purdue.edu

Received: 31 May 2020; Accepted: 24 June 2020; Published: 30 June 2020

Abstract: The present study utilized a cross-sectional design to assess whether two indicators of the community food environment, parent perceptions of the community food environment (i.e., as assessed by parent reports of access to, availability, and affordability of foods) and limited food access (via census data), were related to executive function in preschool children. Children were recruited during the 2014–2015 academic year from Head Start and community-based preschools (N = 102) and children's executive function ability was tested using the Head–Toes–Knees–Shoulders task. Multiple linear regression analysis was used, as well as adjusted standard errors to account for clustering at the classroom level. Parent reports of their food environment were significantly related to children's executive function, such that children living in higher quality community food environments had better executive function. In contrast, limited food access using census data was not significantly related to executive function. The results suggest that parent reports of the community food environment in early childhood may contribute to young children's cognitive outcomes more so than being in a limited food access area, as these data may not represent individual behaviors or capture the variability of the accessibility and affordability of healthy foods. Policy makers should consider correlations between the food environment and early executive functioning when developing new community health, wellness legislation.

Keywords: food access; executive function; preschool children; community food environment

---

1. Introduction

The consumption of foods with a low nutrient density is an important correlate of well-being throughout life and a modifiable risk factor for chronic disease and obesity, which may originate in childhood [1–3]. Previous studies suggest that not eating a healthful diet, adhering to the Dietary Guidelines for Americans (DGA) recommendations, may lead to adverse health outcomes, including iron-deficiency anemia, acute infection, chronic illness, and developmental and mental health problems among children [3–6]. Thus, determining the barriers to health and nutrition among United States (U.S.) children is critical to improving child nutrition and health in both the short and long term [7,8]. The community food environment, conceptualized as the reported availability, affordability, and accessibility (e.g., available transportation) of grocery stores or other entities that sell foods that promote a healthful diet via the DGA [3], has received consideration as a possible determinant of dietary intake and may potentially be associated with health and nutritional outcomes [9,10]. Evidence that U.S. children and adults with access to foods that most children do not consume enough of, such as fruits and vegetables, fare better in terms of their physical health and development compared to those without such access, supports recognition of the community food environment as a potential barrier to health and nutrition [3,11,12].

However, most of the research examining the community food environment in the context of child health and nutrition focuses on the consumption of fruits and vegetables and dietary intake [13–16], but does not consider a potential link between the community food environment and cognitive outcomes. Alternatively, the research related to cognitive outcomes has explicitly evaluated the role of nutrition and obesity (e.g., body mass index (BMI)) in older children and adults on cognition and has not explored the association of the community food environment with cognitive development in young children [16–19]. Thus, very little is known about the potential association between the community food environment and cognition among children. Further, no studies have examined the relation between the community food environment (as assessed both subjectively via parent reports and objectively via census data) and executive function in early childhood, thus warranting further exploration.

Executive function (EF) is defined as the ability to flexibly control automatic thoughts and responses in order to remain goal oriented [20,21] and is considered to have three integrated, cognitive components [22,23]: cognitive flexibility, inhibitory control, and working memory. EF in early childhood is considered an important predictor of short- and long-term health, social–emotional, and academic outcomes [21,24–28]. For instance, children with stronger EF during the preschool years (3–5 years of age) have lower BMIs [25] and demonstrate better social–emotional competence, school readiness, and subsequent academic achievement (e.g., literacy and math [21,26–28]). Furthermore, the preschool years are considered a sensitive period for the development of EF due to structural changes in the prefrontal cortex [20,29]. Thus, EF in this developmental stage may be more susceptible to environmental influences. This may be particularly true for nutritional deficiencies during the preschool period [30,31]. Nutrients provide the necessary components for developmental processes in the brain that impact cognitive development (e.g., neuronal/glial metabolism, myelination, enzyme systems), and deficits to these processes may have a larger impact when the brain is rapidly changing [30,31]. Thus, the community food environment, particularly the availability and affordability of healthful foods, may support EF development in preschool; however, to date, no studies have explored this association.

An Ecological Systems Perspective

The ecological systems perspective illustrates the barriers and opportunities of the community food environment [7,8,32,33]. This perspective posits that, although development is impacted by multiple levels of children's environments, proximal contexts or microsystems (including barriers to healthy food in the home and neighborhood contexts) are the most critical, and often interact to influence developmental outcomes, such as EF [32]. Afshin and colleagues use this perspective to explain an individual's relationship with health and nutrition using a series of microsystems ranging from the most distal, like global impact (e.g., global food availability, international food standards) to sociocultural influences (e.g., social support, social class, social culture norms, social cohesion) to characteristics of an individual (e.g., age, sex, nutritional knowledge, and skills [7]). This framework acknowledges the multiple factors that impact health and nutrition while specifically focusing on associations between individuals and their environments. Barriers to health and healthy diets within the larger ecological system can lead to nutrition risk, which may impact parts of the developing brain that are associated with EF skills [30], thus impacting early EF ability. Though these barriers likely apply more directly to adults, children's food consumption is influenced by parenting behaviors, including parental fruit and vegetable, fat, and soft drink intake [34,35], as well as parental feeding style and eating practices [8]. If parents experience barriers related to the availability and affordability of foods, their children may consequently be impacted when these barriers are linked with developmental trajectories [11,12]. Furthermore, parent experiences and perceptions of the community food environment (via parent reports of access to, availability, and affordability of foods) may be particularly important for evaluating access to healthful foods, relative to more distal assessments of the community food environment (i.e., census tract data of limited access). This may be true given that parents are embedded in their communities, likely understanding the nuances of their access and affordability. In support of this hypothesis, previous literature has identified that adults are able to accurately assess their access to healthful foods, whereas food desert status (as indicated by U.S. Department of Agriculture (USDA) and geographic information systems (GIS) data at the census tract level) does not predict where (e.g., nearest store) and how (e.g., shopping frequency) individuals obtain healthful foods [36]. These discrepancies may be a result of certain assumptions made when evaluating access using census tract data (e.g., assuming individuals buy from the closest stores [37]). Therefore, knowledge of how the community food environment (perceptions or limited access) is related to child development may inform public health programs and policies.

Therefore, the primary aim of this study is to assess whether two indicators of the community food environment, parent reports of the food environment (e.g., access to, availability, and affordability of foods) and limited food access (via census data), are related to EF in children who are three to five years old. We included a subjective (parent reports) and objective measure (census data on limited food access) of the community food environment to test whether differential associations would emerge between these indicators and EF skills. We expected that children with better community food environments across both indicators would have higher scores on an EF task compared with those with worse community food environments.

2. Materials and Methods

2.1. Study Design and Participants

Participants of this cross-sectional study included 102 children (52% female) and one of their parents recruited from 25 Head Start (a federal U.S. preschool program for children from families with low incomes (according to federal U.S. Poverty Guidelines) that provides early child care and education) or center- and community-based preschools located in the central and western regions of a Midwestern state in the U.S. Children ranged from 40 to 66 months (Mean [M] = 53.57, SD = 5.42), and 51% of children were enrolled in Head Start classrooms. Parents' highest level of education ranged from 8th grade to doctoral degree, and approximately 50% of the sample had a high school degree or less. Refer to Table 1 for full descriptive and demographic information.

Table 1. Descriptive means and standard deviations for full sample ($N = 102$).

Variable	Mean or % (SD)	Minimum	Maximum
Age (in months)	53.57 (5.42)	40	66
Sex [a]			
Male ($n = 48$)	48.00%	—	—
Female ($n = 52$)	52.00%	—	—
White ($n = 71$) [b]	69.61%	—	—
Non-white ($n = 26$)	25.49%	—	—
Parent education [c]	4.59 (1.59)	1	9
Home learning environment [d]	2.41 (0.64)	0.80	3.83
HTKS	8.79 (13.53)	0	50
Limited food access [e]			
Yes limited access ($n = 28$)	34.15%		
No limited access ($n = 54$)	65.85%		
Food environment [f]	2.85 (0.91)	0	4

Note. HTKS = Head–Toes–Knees–Shoulders task. Food environment was measured so that affirmative answers to each of the four questions were scored and tallied with scores ranging from 0–4, where 0 = poor food environment. [a] Sex was not reported for two children. [b] Race/ethnicity was not reported for five children. [c] 1 = 8th grade or less, 2 = some high school, 3 = GED, 4 = high school diploma, 5 = some college, 6 = associate's degree, 7 = bachelor's degree, 8 = master's degree, 9 = doctoral/postgraduate degree. [d] Home learning environment was missing for 18 children (84 children). [e] Limited food access was missing for 20 children (82 children). [f] Food environment was missing for 23 children (79 children).

2.2. Procedures

Recruitment occurred during the 2014–2015 academic year after the study was approved by a university Institutional Review Board. Preschools were selected using convenience sampling. Parents of all children within the target age range of 3–5 years old at participating preschools were sent a letter describing the study, inviting them and their child to participate. Written consent was obtained from parents/primary caregivers prior to participation. Children in the study did not have any known pervasive developmental disorders or have severe auditory or visual impairments that were not corrected, and all children were English language speakers who were able to participate in assessments that required an age-appropriate level of English proficiency. All data were collected in the preschool year at one time point. Parents self-reported demographic and family characteristics (e.g., home learning environment) on paper surveys, and children were interviewed in a quiet space in their classrooms for the direct assessment of EF. All participants received a $20 gift card and children received stickers after completing assessments.

2.3. Measures

2.3.1. Food Environment

Parent reports of the food environment were assessed using a four-item survey that included the following items: "My family has access to a grocery store"; "There is public transportation to the grocery store"; "Is healthy food available in your community?"; "Is healthy food affordable in your community?" Responses were scored 0 for "no" and 1 for "yes" and scores were summed (range 0–4) to create the independent variable for use in analysis. Lower scores indicated a poorer food environment based on the U.S. Department of Agriculture's (USDA) definition of food access [38]. Researchers created this parent-report tool because a brief measure, quantifying perceptions of access, transportation, and healthy food availability and affordability was not available [8,11]. The simplicity of the measures (four items), which is similar to other measures that have been used in previous studies [36,39–42], affects the moderate internal reliability for this novel measure ($\alpha = 0.50$).

2.3.2. Limited Food Access

Census tract information for each residential address (parent-reported) in the sample was obtained from the American Community Survey (ACS) data from the U.S. Census Bureau [43], which uses geographical information systems (GIS) software to map addresses to a specific census tract that corresponds with an address. We used tracts from the 2015 data set, the year the data were collected. After identifying what tract families were in, we used a low-access tract variable from the USDA Food Access Research Atlas data set [44]. The Food Access Research Atlas data flagged a tract as low access if at least 500 people within the tract, or 33% of the population, were living more than $\frac{1}{2}$ mile (urban areas) or 10 miles (rural areas) from the nearest supermarket, supercenter, or large grocery store. In the USDA's 2017 report, a directory of supermarkets, supercenters, and large grocery stores within every state was derived by merging the 2015 Store Tracking and Redemption System (STARS) directory of stores authorized to accept Supplemental Nutrition Assistance Program (SNAP) benefits and the 2015 Trade Dimensions TDLinx directory of stores. The block-level population data were derived from the 2010 Census of Population and Housing. A score of 1 indicated a tract was low access and a score of 0 indicated the tract was not considered low access.

2.3.3. Executive Function

Children's executive function was assessed using the Head–Toes–Knees–Shoulders task (HTKS) [45]. The HTKS is a behavioral measure that directly taps into all three components of EF (cognitive flexibility, inhibitory control, working memory), and is typically used with children aged 3–7 [45]. In the practice round, children are first asked to respond by following the directions normally (e.g., "Touch your head"), and then they are asked to respond in the opposite way (e.g., children are asked to touch their heads when the research assistant says, "Touch your toes"). The testing portion consists of 30 items (three sections of ten), and the sections get increasingly complex as the child progresses. In order to progress to the second section, a child has to receive a score of at least 4 on the first section, and similarly, in order to progress to the third section, a child has to receive a score of at least 4 on the second section. Each correct response is worth two points, making the range of possible scores 0–60. Each item is scored as 0 (incorrect), 1 (self-correct), or 2 (correct). The total score of the test is the sum of all the correct items. This task takes approximately 5–10 min to complete. The interrater reliability, scoring agreement, and test–retest reliability is high and shows strong predictive validity [45]. The HTKS has moderate to strong effect sizes, predicting achievement levels and gains across multiple studies in pre-k and kindergarten-aged children [45–47].

2.3.4. Covariates

The characteristics of children and parents, including child sex (1 = female), child age (range: 40–66 months), race/ethnicity (0 = White/Caucasian, 1 = non-White/Caucasian) and parent education (1 = 8th grade or less, 2 = some high school, 3 = GED, 4 = high school diploma, 5 = some college, 6 = associate's degree, 7 = bachelor's degree, 8 = master's degree, 9 = doctoral/postgraduate degree) were also assessed in the participant survey. See Table 1 for details on response categories. The home learning environment was included as a covariate in order to capture other potential confounders that may be related to EF development [48]. Thus, the home learning environment was assessed using 30 parent-reported items that address the frequency of home learning activities that incorporated math, literacy, and general educational practices in which parents engage with their children. Sample items included "playing board games," "using number activity books," "identifying sounds of alphabet letters." Parents reported on the frequency of the activities using the following response options: 0 = never; 1 = a few times per month; 2 = a few times per week; 3 = every day. An average score of all 30 items was used in analyses ($\alpha = 0.89$).

2.4. Analytic Strategy

Data analyses were completed using Stata 16.0 [49]. The classroom intraclass correlation (ICC) was examined to determine between-classroom variance in order to determine whether multilevel modeling would be appropriate. The ICC was 0.002, and thus our models did not require multilevel modeling. However, to be conservative in our statistical approach, in our regression analyses, we adjusted standard errors to account for clustering at the classroom level. In our analysis, we examined the association between the two indicators of the community food environment (parent reports of the food environment and limited food access) and EF among preschool children, while controlling for the home learning environment, child sex, age, race/ethnicity, and parent education. There were very little missing outcome data (< 5% for HTKS); however, full information maximum likelihood (FIML) was employed to handle missing data.

3. Results

Main Results

Means and standard deviations for all study variables can be found in Table 1. On average, participants scored 8.79 points on the HTKS ($SD = 13.53$). A summary of correlations can be found in Table 2. The HTKS was significantly correlated with parent education ($r = 0.28$, $p = 0.007$). Race was significantly correlated with both limited food access ($r = -0.23$, $p = 0.040$) and reports of the community food environment ($r = 0.30$, $p = 0.008$).

Table 2. Correlation matrix for all study variables (N = 102).

Variable	1	2	3	4	5	6	7
1. Age [a]	—						
2. Male	−0.14	—					
3. White	0.08	0.19 [t]	—				
4. Parent education	0.21 *	0.05	0.06	—			
5. Home learning environment	0.06	−0.09	−0.10	0.17	—		
6. HTKS	0.17 [t]	−0.18 [t]	0.06	0.28 **	0.12	—	
7. Limited food access	0.01	−0.15	−0.23 *	0.01	0.08	−0.04	—
8. Food environment	0.22 [t]	−0.00	−0.30 **	0.22 [t]	0.15	0.21	0.13

Note. [a] Child age measured in months. HTKS = Head–Toes–Knees–Shoulders task. [t] $p < 0.10$, * $p < 0.05$, ** $p < 0.01$, *** $p < 0.001$.

It was hypothesized that higher ratings on both indicators of the community food environment would predict stronger EF skills. Partially as expected, parent reports of the food environment were significantly related to children's EF ($\beta = 0.22$, $p = 0.016$) above and beyond limited food access, after controlling for the home learning environment, child sex, child age, race/ethnicity, and parent education. Specifically, a one-unit increase in the community food environment was associated with over three additional points scored on the HTKS. Children normatively gain approximately 1.33 points each month on the HTKS [45]. Thus, what this score indicates is that children experience a fairly substantial increase in EF development (approximately a 3-month gain in EF) with a one-unit increase in parent reports of the food environment. However, contrary to the hypotheses, limited food access was not significantly related to children's EF skills ($\beta = -0.08$, $p = 0.484$). Among the control variables, parent education was significantly and positively associated with EF ($\beta = 0.23$, $p = 0.023$), as well as child sex ($\beta = 0.21$, $p = 0.030$). See Table 3 for all regression estimates.

Table 3. Regression estimates predicting executive functioning.

Variable	β (SE)
Age [a]	0.02 (0.10)
Male	−0.21 (0.10) *
White	0.12 (0.10)
Parent education	0.23 (0.10) *
Home learning environment	0.03 (0.08)
Limited food access	−0.08 (0.11)
Food environment	0.22 (0.09) *

Note. [a] Child age measured in months. * $p < 0.05$, ** $p < 0.01$, *** $p < 0.001$.

4. Discussion

The primary goal of this study was to assess whether two indicators of the community food environment (subjective via parent reports of the food environment and objective via limited food access) were related to EF in preschool-aged children. EF skills in preschool are robust indicators of academic [26,28,50], social–emotional [51], and healthy outcomes [25], and EF deficits during early childhood are related to hyperactivity and attention deficits [52]. Thus, identifying early predictors of EF is critical. Results from our study indicated that, after controlling for the home learning environment, child age, race, sex, and parent education, parent reports of the food environment were significantly positively related to stronger EF skills, whereas limited food access was not related to EF. This suggests that the children of parents who believe they have higher quality community food environments have better EF, regardless of whether families are located in census tracts that are flagged as having limited food access.

4.1. Community Food Environment and Executive Function

As expected, there was an association between the subjective measure of the community food environment (i.e., parent reports of access to, availability, and affordability of foods) and EF in early childhood. This association may be due to the measure encompassing several environmental barriers to healthful foods that put children at greater nutritional risk, thus affecting developmental outcomes like EF. This link between the community food environment and EF development is novel at the distal ecological level, and variables that only examine limited food access at the tract level, rather than the individual level, may not be able to capture these associations. Food insecurity or insufficiency may be a potential mediating factor between the community food environment and EF. Food insufficiency is defined as inadequate food intake due to a lack of environmental resources, and similarly, food insecurity refers to the limited or uncertain availability of or inability to acquire nutritionally adequate, safe, and acceptable foods due to limited resources which may be impacted by environmental constraints (e.g., the community food environment) [53,54]. Food insufficient/insecure families may live in poor food environments where individuals are 22–35% less likely to have a diet conforming to the DGA than those in food environments with a better availability of supermarkets and healthy foods [13]. Additionally, poverty and environmental impacts of poverty (e.g., akin to social class and environmental impacts), as proposed in the sociocultural layer in the larger ecological model [7], may affect nutrition, and in turn, cognitive development [55]. Food insufficiency/insecurity has a limited but growing literature, showing a link with academic achievement in older U.S. children (e.g., poorer math scores, poorer reading scores, grade repetition [53,54,56]), and EF is closely related to these outcomes [26,50]. Further, previous literature that has directly assessed the concurrent and long-term impacts of food insecurity on EF in preschool-aged (3–5) and early elementary-aged children (6–7) has found that global and domain-specific EFs are significantly negatively impacted when children are exposed to any degree of food insecurity [57,58]. Specifically, one of these studies found that any exposure to any level of food insecurity (either marginally insecure or completely food insecure) in either kindergarten or first grade resulted in worse working memory and cognitive flexibility, two components of EF [57].

Alternatively, there was not an association between an objective measure of the food environment (i.e., limited food access; if at least 500 people within the tract, or 33% of the population were, living more than $\frac{1}{2}$ mile (urban areas) or 10 miles (rural areas) from the nearest supermarket, supercenter, or large grocery store) and EF scores. The finding that parent reports were related to EF and an objective measure of food access was not surprising. This may be because our objective measure of limited food access assumes that (1) full-service grocery stores are a proxy for the presence of affordable and nutritionally sufficient food [37], (2) households buy from the closest supermarket [37], (3) alternative store types may not have a similar selection or may not offer as many fruits or vegetables as supermarkets [59], and (4) families are not getting food from alternative food sources like home and community gardens or farmers' markets. Moreover, there is evidence of variability within census tracts related to whether individuals with low incomes shop at a neighborhood store or even the nearest chain store [60]. One study found that while SNAP recipients live 1.8 miles on average from full-service grocery stores, most individuals travel 4.9 miles from home to shop for food [61]. Thus, whether a census tract is flagged as limited food access based on distance from a store may not accurately represent individual behaviors regarding where families are going to buy food or access to foods within a store. Furthermore, this measure may not capture small groceries or small general stores.

Additionally, it may be that parent reports of the food environment are more strongly related to cognitive outcomes, like EF. Indeed, parents' perceptions can be quite powerful influencers on children's development (e.g., reports of praise and school readiness on academic outcomes, perceptions of being overweight on future weight gain) [62,63]. Furthermore, parent reports of the food environment may tap into an emotional or social connectedness of the community they are in, which may then have an effect on EF outcomes. In one study, social cohesion (sense of belonging and unity among members of a community [64]) and reports of food availability (i.e., a large selection of fresh fruits and vegetables is available in my neighborhood grocery/food stores; a large selection of low-fat products is available in my neighborhood grocery/food stores; the fresh fruits and vegetables in my neighborhood are of high quality [39]) were significantly and positively associated [61].

Furthermore, parents may more accurately predict the community food environment because they may be more aware of their experiences and their access to healthful foods. Census data may not be the strongest indicator of the community food environment because they do not take into account factors that contribute to access, like affordability and transportation. In support of this notion, one scholar has proposed that self-reported levels of constructs, like the community food environment (e.g., food insecurity, hunger, access) may be more appropriate when assessing its relations with outcomes because it truly captures the experiences of the phenomena, as opposed to an indirect indicator, like census data [53].

4.2. Limitations and Future Directions

Although this study is the first to document a significant association between parent reports of the community food environment and preschool children's EF skills, limitations must be noted. The study was limited to just one direct assessment of children's EF. Future studies would benefit from the use of multiple measures of early EF, as well as the inclusion of more questions about the social, emotional, and other ecological barriers of the community food environment for exploring the extent to which the community food environment may be differentially related to various components of EF. Additionally, there were missing data for the outcome measure (HTKS), parent reports of the food environment, and the limited food access measure. The missingness of the limited food access measure can be attributed to two things: (1) parents did not provide an address or (2) the address provided could not be matched with a census tract using the GIS software. Furthermore, the missingness of the parent reports of the community food environment can be attributed to a lack of response to the question. Although we cannot force research participants to provide responses to survey questions, future research would benefit from full data on the community food environment. Another limitation was that a definition for healthy food was not provided on the parent report of the community food environment, which may have had an impact on how parents responded to items in the survey. It will be important for future studies to include a definition in parent-report measures of the community food environment to ensure consistency in how parents are conceptualizing a healthy diet. Finally, albeit small, the sample was fairly diverse in terms of socioeconomic status (i.e., parent education), but was rather homogeneous in terms of race/ethnicity. A replication of the findings in future studies with larger samples is necessary to ensure generalizability. Future studies should also consider the intermediary role that food security, food insufficiency, and food intake may play between the community food environment and cognitive outcomes.

5. Conclusions

Results suggest that researchers need to continue efforts to explore the extent to which the community food environment may be linked with EF and other developmental outcomes in early childhood, at both distal and proximal levels. Policy makers may consider the correlation between the parent reports of the food environment and early EF skills when working to improve current legislation around issues related to community health and well-being. Policy measures that not only improve the community food environment broadly, but also consider and take into account parent perceptions of access, affordability, availability and transportation, may have important health and developmental implications, especially in light of the childhood obesity epidemic that exists in the United States [2]. The current findings also have implications for physicians and pediatricians working with families who may be experiencing barriers to a high-quality community food environment. For example, physicians and pediatricians can consider parent perceptions of access, and could provide additional resources for obtaining access to healthful foods that would help to support children's healthy development. This research could help set the stage for the development of effective community- and family-based interventions that target improving access to healthful foods by providing a rationale to intervene in communities by linking families with transportation, economical food access, food delivery, and other policies to promote food access. This study also lays a foundation for future research examining the potential impact of poor community food environments and children's cognitive outcomes.

Author Contributions: Conceptualization, L.M.B. and S.A.S.; methodology, L.M.B. and S.A.S.; formal analysis, L.M.B. and S.A.S.; investigation, S.A.S.; resources, S.A.S.; data curation, S.A.S. and I.K.; writing—original draft preparation, L.M.B. and S.A.S.; writing—review and editing, H.A.E.-M., I.K., and S.A.S.; supervision, S.A.S.; project administration, S.A.S.; funding acquisition, S.A.S. All authors have read and agreed to the published version of the manuscript.

Funding: The research reported in this publication was supported by research funding from the USDA National Institute of Food and Agriculture, Hatch Project (1003434).

Conflicts of Interest: The authors declare no conflict of interest.

References

1. Kawachi, I.; Berkman, L.F. Social ties and mental health. *J. Urban. Health* **2001**, *78*, 458–467. [CrossRef] [PubMed]
2. Morris, A.S.; Robinson, L.R.; Hays-Grudo, J.; Claussen, A.H.; Hartwig, S.A.; Treat, A.E. Targeting parenting in early childhood: A public health approach to improve outcomes for children living in poverty. *Child Dev. Perspect.* **2017**, *88*, 388–397. [CrossRef]
3. U.S. Department of Health and Human Services; U.S. Department of Agriculture. *2015–2020 Dietary Guidelines for Americans*; U.S. Department of Health and Human Services; U.S. Department of Agriculture: Washington, DC, USA, 2015. Available online: http://health.gov/dietaryguidelines/2015/guidelines/ (accessed on 26 June 2019).
4. Kursmark, M.; Weitzman, M. Recent findings concerning childhood food insecurity. *Curr. Opin. Clin. Nutr. Metab. Care* **2009**, *12*, 310–316. [CrossRef] [PubMed]
5. Slack, K.S. Yoo, J. Food hardship and child behavior problems among low-income children. *Soc. Serv. Rev.* **2005**, *79*, 511–536. [CrossRef]
6. Weinreb, L.; Wehler, C.; Perloff, J.; Scott, R.; Hosmer, D.; Sagor, L.; Gundersen, C. Hunger: Its impact on children's health and mental health. *Pediatrics* **2002**, *110*, e41. [CrossRef] [PubMed]
7. Afshin, A.; Micah, R.; Khatibzadeh, S. Dietary policies to reduce noncommunicable diseases. In *The Handbook of Global Health Policy*; Brown, G.W., Yamey, G., Wamala, S., Eds.; John Wiley & Sons, Ltd.: West Sussex, UK, 2014; pp. 175–193.
8. Story, M.; Kaphingst, K.M.; Robinson-O'Brien, R.; Glanz, K. Creating healthy food and eating environments: Policy and environmental approaches. *Annu. Rev. Public Health* **2008**, *29*, 253–272. [CrossRef]
9. Fitzgibbon, M.L.; Stolley, M.R. Environmental changes: May be needed for prevention of overweight in minority children. *Pediatr. Ann.* **2004**, *33*, 45–49. [CrossRef]
10. Sooman, A.; Macintyre, S.; Anderson, A. Scotland's health—A more difficult challenge for some? The price and availability of healthy foods in socially contrasting localities in the west of Scotland. *Health Bull.* **1993**, *51*, 276–284.
11. Morland, K.; Diez Roux, A.V.; Wing, S. Supermarkets, other food stores, and obesity: The atherosclerosis risk in communities study. *Am. J. Prev. Med.* **2006**, *30*, 333–339. [CrossRef]
12. Powell, L.M.; Slater, S.; Mirtcheva, D.; Bao, Y.; Chaloupka, F.J. Food Store Availability and Neighborhood Characteristics in the United States. *Prev. Med.* **2007**, *44*, 189–195. [CrossRef]
13. Moore, L.V; Diez Roux, A.V.; Nettleton, J.A.; Jacobs, D.R. Associations of the local food environment with diet quality—A comparison of assessments based on surveys and geographic information systems. *Am. J. Epidemiol.* **2008**, *167*, 917–924. [CrossRef] [PubMed]
14. Nigg, C.R.; Ul Anwar, M.M.; Braun, K.; Mercado, J.; Kainoa Fialkowski, M.; Ropeti Areta, A.A.; Belyeu-Camacho, T.; Bersamin, A.; Guerrero, R.L.; Castro, R.; et al. A review of promising multicomponent environmental child obesity prevention Intervention strategies by the Children's Healthy Living Program. *J. Environ. Health* **2016**, *79*, 18–26. [CrossRef] [PubMed]

15. Ritchie, L.D.; Woodward-Lopez, G.; Au, L.E.; Loria, C.M.; Collie-Akers, V.L.; Wilson, D.K.; Frongillo, E.A.; Strauss, W.J.; Landgraf, A.J.; Nagaraja, J.; et al. Associations of community programs and policies with children's dietary intakes: The Healthy Communities Study. *Pediatr. Obes.* **2018**. [CrossRef] [PubMed]
16. Woodward-Lopez, G.; Gosliner, W.; Au, L.E.; Kao, J.; Webb, K.L.; Sagatov, R.D.F.; Strauss, W.J.; Landgraf, A.J.; Nagaraja, J.; Wilson, D.K.; et al. Community characteristics modify the relationship between obesity prevention efforts and dietary intake in children: The Healthy Communities Study. *Pediatr. Obes.* **2018**, *13*, 46–55. [CrossRef]
17. Khan, N.A.; Raine, L.B.; Donovan, S.M.; Hillman, C.H. The cognitive implications of obesity and nutrition in childhood. *Monogr. Soc. Res. Child Dev.* **2014**, *79*, 51–71. [CrossRef]
18. Hildreth, K.L.; Van Pelt, R.E.; Schwartz, R.S. Obesity, insulin resistance, and Alzheimer's disease. *Obesity* **2012**, *20*, 1549–1557. [CrossRef]
19. Tascilar, M.E.; Turkkahraman, D.; Oz, O.; Yucel, M.; Taskesen, M.; Eker, I.; Abaci, A.; Dundaroz, R.; Ulas, U.H. P300 auditory event-related potentials in children with obesity: Is childhood obesity related to impairment in cognitive functions? *Pediatr. Diabetes* **2011**, *12*, 589–595. [CrossRef]
20. Garon, N.; Bryson, S.E.; Smith, I.M. Executive function in preschoolers: A review using an integrative framework. *Psychol. Bull.* **2008**, *134*, 31–60. [CrossRef]
21. McClelland, M.M.; Cameron, C.E.; Connor, C.M.D.; Farris, C.L.; Jewkes, A.M.; Morrison, F.J. Links between behavioral regulation and preschoolers' literacy, vocabulary, and math skills. *Dev. Psychol.* **2007**, *43*, 947–959. [CrossRef]
22. Bernier, A.; Beauchamp, M.H.; Carlson, S.M.; Lalonde, G. A secure base from which to regulate: Attachment security in toddlerhood as a predictor of executive functioning at school entry. *Dev. Psychol.* **2015**, *51*, 1177–1189. [CrossRef]
23. Willoughby, M.T.; Blair, C.; Wirth, R.J.; Greenberg, M.T. The measurement of executive function at age 5: Psychometric properties and relationship to academic achievement. *Psychol. Assess.* **2012**, *24*, 226–239. [CrossRef] [PubMed]
24. Hughes, C.H.; Ensor, R.A. How do families help or hinder the emergence of early executive function? *New Dir. Child Adoles.* **2009**, *123*, 35–50. [CrossRef] [PubMed]
25. Schmitt, S.A.; Korucu, I.; Jones, B.L.; Snyder, F.J.; Evich, C.D.; Purpura, D.J. Self-regulation as a correlate of weight status in preschool children. *Early Child Dev. Care* **2017**, *189*, 68–78. [CrossRef]
26. Blair, C.; Razza, R.P. Relating effortful control, executive function, and false belief understanding to emerging math and literacy ability in kindergarten. *Child Dev.* **2007**, *78*, 647–663. [CrossRef]
27. Duckworth, A.L.; Seligman, M.E.P. Self-discipline outdoes IQ in predicting academic performance of adolescents. *Psychol. Sci.* **2005**, *16*, 939–944. [CrossRef] [PubMed]
28. Morrison, F.J.; Ponitz, C.E.C.; McClelland, M.M. Self-regulation and academic achievement in the transition to school. In *Human Brain Development. Child Development at the Intersection of Emotion and Cognition*; Calkings, S.D., Bell, M.A., Eds.; American Psychological Association: Washington, DC, USA, 2010; pp. 203–224. [CrossRef]
29. Carlson, S.M.; Davis, A.C.; Leach, J.G. Less is more—Executive function and symbolic representation in preschool children. *Psychol. Sci.* **2005**, *16*, 609–616. [CrossRef] [PubMed]
30. Nyaradi, A.; Li, J.; Hickling, S.; Foster, J.; Oddy, W.H. The role of nutrition in children's neurocognitive development, from pregnancy through childhood. *Front. Hum. Neurosci.* **2013**, *7*, 97. [CrossRef]
31. Wachs, T.D.; Georgieff, M.; Cusick, S.; Mcewen, B.S. Issues in the timing of integrated early interventions: Contributions from nutrition, neuroscience, and psychological research. In *Prenatal and Childhood Nutrition: Evaluating the Neurocognitive Connections*; Croft, C., Ed.; Apple Academic Press: Oakville, ON, Canada, 2015; pp. 363–397. [CrossRef]
32. Bronfenbrenner, U. Toward an experimental ecology of human development. *Am. Psychol.* **1977**, *32*, 513–531. [CrossRef]
33. Sallis, J.F.; Fisher, E.B.; Owen, N.; Fisher, E.B. Ecological models of health behavior. In *Health Behavior and Health Education*; Glanz, K., Rimer, B.K., Viswanath, K., Eds.; Jossey-Bass: San Francisco, CA, USA, 2015; pp. 465–482.
34. Cook, J.T.; Frank, D.A.; Levenson, S.M.; Neault, N.B.; Heeren, T.C.; Black, M.M.; Berkowitz, C.; Casey, P.H.; Meyers, A.F.; Cutts, D.B.; et al. Child food insecurity increases risks posed by household food insecurity to young children's health. *J. Nutr.* **2006**, *136*, 1073–1076. [CrossRef]

35. Fisher, J.O.; Mitchell, D.C.; Smiciklas-Wright, H.; Birch, L.L. Parental influences on young girls' fruit and vegetable, micronutrient, and fat intakes. *J. Am. Diet. Assoc.* **2002**, *102*, 58–64. [CrossRef]
36. Sohi, I.; Bell, B.A.; Liu, J.; Battersby, S.E.; Liese, A.D. Differences in food environment perceptions and spatial attributes of food shopping between residents of low and high food access areas. *J. Nutr. Educ. Behav.* **2014**, *46*, 241–249. [CrossRef]
37. Breyer, B. Voss-Andreae, A. Food mirages: Geographic and economic barriers to healthful food access in Portland, Oregon. *Heal. Place* **2013**, *24*, 131–139. [CrossRef] [PubMed]
38. U.S. Department of Agriculture. Definitions: Food Access. 2005. Available online: https://www.ers.usda.gov/data-products/food-access-research-atlas/documentation/ (accessed on 26 June 2019).
39. Mujahid, M.S.; Diez Roux, A.V.; Morenoff, J.D.; Raghunathan, T. Assessing the measurement properties of neighborhood scales: From psychometrics to ecometrics. *Am. J. Epidemiol.* **2007**, *165*, 858–867. [CrossRef]
40. Ma, X.; Barnes, T.L.; Freedman, D.A.; Bell, B.A.; Colabianchi, N.; Liese, A.D. Test-retest reliability of a questionnaire measuring perceptions of neighborhood food environment. *Health Place* **2013**, *21*, 65–69. [CrossRef] [PubMed]
41. Co, M.C.; Bakken, S. Influence of the local food environment on Hispanics' perceptions of healthy food access in New York City. *Hisp. Heal. Care Int.* **2018**, *16*, 75–84. [CrossRef] [PubMed]
42. Jayashankar, P.; Raju, S. The effect of social cohesion and social Networks on perceptions of food availability among low-income consumers. *J. Bus. Res.* **2020**, *1*, 316–323. [CrossRef]
43. U.S. Census Bureau. American Community Survey Data. 2005. Available online: https://geocoding.geo.census.gov/geocoder/geographies/addressbatch?form (accessed on 26 June 2019).
44. U.S. Department of Agriculture. Food Access Research Atlas—Download the Data. 2017. Available online: https://www.ers.usda.gov/data-products/food-access-research-atlas/download-the-data/ (accessed on 15 July 2019).
45. McClelland, M.M.; Cameron, C.E.; Duncan, R.J.; Bowles, R.P.; Acock, A.C.; Miao, A.J.; Pratt, M.E. Predictors of early growth in academic achievement: The head-toes-knees-shoulders task. *Front. Psychol.* **2014**, *5*, 599. [CrossRef] [PubMed]
46. Ponitz, C.E.C.; McClelland, M.M.; Jewkes, A.M.; Connor, C.M.D.; Farris, C.L.; Morrison, F.J. Touch your toes! Developing a direct measure of behavioral regulation in early childhood. *Early Child Res. Quart.* **2008** *23*, 141–158. [CrossRef]
47. Wanless, S.B.; McClelland, M.M.; Acock, A.C.; Ponitz, C.E.C.; Son, S.H.; Lan, X.; Morrison, F.J.; Chen, J.L.; Chen, F.M.; Lee, K.; et al. Measuring behavioral regulation in four societies. *Psychol. Assess.* **2011**, *23*, 364–378. [CrossRef]
48. Blair, C.; Cybele Raver, C.; Berry, D.J. Family Life Project Investigators. Two approaches to estimating the effect of parenting on the development of executive function in early childhood. *Dev. Psychol.* **2014**, *50*, 554–565. [CrossRef]
49. StataCorp. *Stata Statistical Software: Release 16*; StataCorp LLC: College Station, TX, USA, 2019.
50. McClelland, M.M.; Acock, A.C.; Piccinin, A.; Rhea, S.A.; Stallings, M.C. Relations between preschool attention span-persistence and age 25 educational outcomes. *Early Child Res. Quart.* **2013**, *28*, 314–324. [CrossRef] [PubMed]
51. Denham, S.A. Social-emotional competence as support for school readiness: What is it and how do we assess it? *Early Educ. Dev.* **2006**, *17*, 57–89. [CrossRef]
52. Pauli-Pott, U.; Becker, K. Neuropsychological basic deficits in preschoolers at risk for ADHD: A meta-analysis. *Clin. Psychol. Rev.* **2011**, *31*, 626–637. [CrossRef]
53. Alaimo, K.; Olson, C.M.; Frongillo, E.A. Food insufficiency and American school-aged children's cognitive, academic, and psychosocial development. *Pediatrics* **2001**, *108*, 44–53. [CrossRef]
54. Jyoti, D.F.; Frongillo, E.A.; Jones, S.J. Community and international nutrition food insecurity affects school children's academic performance, weight gain, and social skills. *J. Nutr.* **2005**, *135*, 2831–2839. [CrossRef]
55. Korenman, S.; Miller, J.E.; Sjaastad, J.E. Long-term poverty and child development in the United States: Results from the NLSY. *Child. Youth Serv. Rev.* **1995**, *17*, 127–155. [CrossRef]
56. Florence, M.D.; Asbridge, M.; Veugelers, P.J. Diet quality and academic performance. *J. Sch. Health* **2008**, *78*, 209–215. [CrossRef]
57. Grineski, S.E.; Morales, D.X.; Collins, T.W.; Rubio, R. Transitional dynamics of household food insecurity impact children's developmental outcomes. *J. Dev. Behav. Pediatr.* **2018**, *39*, 715–725. [CrossRef]

58. Shankar, P.; Chung, R.; Frank, D.A. Association of food insecurity with children's behavioral, emotional, and academic outcomes: A systematic review. *J. Dev. Behav. Pediatr.* **2017**, *38*, 135–150. [CrossRef]
59. Bodor, J.N.; Rice, J.C.; Farley, T.A.; Swalm, C.M.; Rose, D. Disparities in food access: Does aggregate availability of key foods from other stores offset the relative lack of supermarkets in African-American neighborhoods? *Prev. Med.* **2010**, *51*, 63–67. [CrossRef]
60. Hillier, A.; Cannuscio, C.; Karpyn, A.; Mclaughlin, J.; Chilton, M.; Glanz, K. How far do low-income parents travel to shop for food? Empirical evidence from two urban neighborhoods. *Urban Geogr.* **2011**, *32*, 712–729. [CrossRef]
61. U.S. Department of Agriculture. *Access to Affordable and Nutritious Food-Measuring and Understanding Food Deserts and Their Consequences: Report to Congress*; U.S. Department of Agriculture: Washington, DC, USA, 2009. [CrossRef]
62. Lee, H.I.; Kim, Y.H.; Kesebir, P.; Han, D.E. Understanding when parental praise leads to optimal child outcomes: Role of perceived praise accuracy. *Soc. Psychol. Personal. Sci.* **2017**, *8*, 679–688. [CrossRef]
63. Robinson, E.; Sutin, A.R. Parents' perceptions of their children as overweight and children's weight concerns and weight gain. *Psychol. Sci.* **2017**, *28*, 320–329. [CrossRef] [PubMed]
64. Kawachi, I.; Berkman, L. Social cohesion, social capital, and health. In *Social Epidemiology*; Berkman, L.F., Kawachi, I., Eds.; Oxford University Press: New York, NY, USA, 2000; pp. 174–190.

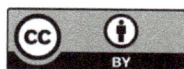

© 2020 by the authors. Licensee MDPI, Basel, Switzerland. This article is an open access article distributed under the terms and conditions of the Creative Commons Attribution (CC BY) license (http://creativecommons.org/licenses/by/4.0/).

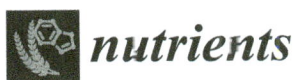

Article

Total Usual Micronutrient Intakes Compared to the Dietary Reference Intakes among U.S. Adults by Food Security Status

Alexandra E. Cowan [1], Shinyoung Jun [1], Janet A. Tooze [2], Heather A. Eicher-Miller [1], Kevin W. Dodd [3], Jaime J. Gahche [4], Patricia M. Guenther [5], Johanna T. Dwyer [4,6], Nancy Potischman [4], Anindya Bhadra [7] and Regan L. Bailey [1,*]

1. Interdepartmental Nutrition Program, Purdue University, 700 W. State Street, West Lafayette, IN 47907, USA; cowan9@purdue.edu (A.E.C.); jun24@purdue.edu (S.J.); heicherm@purdue.edu (H.A.E.-M.)
2. School of Medicine, Wake Forest University, 475 Vine St, Winston-Salem, NC 27101, USA; jtooze@wakehealth.edu
3. NIH National Cancer Institute, 9609 Medical Center Drive, Rockville, MD 20850, USA; doddk@mail.nih.gov
4. NIH Office of Dietary Supplements, 6100 Executive Blvd., Bethesda, MD 20892, USA; jaime.gahche@nih.gov (J.J.G.); dwyerj1@od.nih.gov (J.T.D.); potischn@mail.nih.gov (N.P.)
5. Department of Nutrition and Integrative Physiology, University of Utah, 250 South 850 East, Salt Lake City, UT 84112, USA; PMGuenther@outlook.com
6. Jean Mayer USDA Human Nutrition Research Center on Aging, Tufts University, 711 Washington Street, Boston, MA 02111, USA
7. Department of Statistics, Purdue University, 250 N. University St, West Lafayette, IN 47907, USA; bhadra@purdue.edu
* Correspondence: regan.bailey@purdue.edu; Tel.: +1-765-494-2829

Received: 11 November 2019; Accepted: 16 December 2019; Published: 22 December 2019

Abstract: This study examined total usual micronutrient intakes from foods, beverages, and dietary supplements (DS) compared to the Dietary Reference Intakes among U.S. adults (≥19 years) by sex and food security status using NHANES 2011–2014 data (*n* = 9954). DS data were collected via an in-home interview; the NCI method was used to estimate distributions of total usual intakes from two 24 h recalls for food and beverages, after which DS were added. Food security status was categorized using the USDA Household Food Security Survey Module. Adults living in food insecure households had a higher prevalence of risk of inadequacy among both men and women for magnesium, potassium, vitamins A, B6, B12, C, D, E, and K; similar findings were apparent for phosphorous, selenium, and zinc in men alone. Meanwhile, no differences in the prevalence of risk for inadequacy were observed for calcium, iron (examined in men only), choline, or folate by food security status. Some DS users, especially food secure adults, had total usual intakes that exceeded the Tolerable Upper Intake Level (UL) for folic acid, vitamin D, calcium, and iron. In conclusion, while DS can be helpful in meeting nutrient requirements for adults for some micronutrients, potential excess may also be of concern for certain micronutrients among supplement users. In general, food insecure adults have higher risk for micronutrient inadequacy than food secure adults.

Keywords: NHANES; dietary supplement; micronutrients; DRI; food security

1. Introduction

The 2015–2020 Dietary Guidelines for Americans (DGA) reported a number shortfall nutrients among U.S. adults including calcium, iron, magnesium, potassium, choline, folate and vitamins A, C, D, and E [1,2]. The DGA also recognized food insecurity, defined as limited availability of foods and an individual's inability to access food [3], as a potential barrier to a healthy diet that warrants further research [1]. Indeed, a systematic review concluded that food insecure adults have lower intakes of vitamin A, vitamin B6, calcium, magnesium, and zinc from diet alone when compared to those who were food secure [4]. Dietary supplement (DS) use is also lower in adults living in food insecure U.S. households than in those that are food secure [5], implying that differences in micronutrient intakes between the food secure and food insecure population subgroups might be amplified when total nutrient intakes, inclusive of DS, are considered; however, to our knowledge, no study has compared total usual nutrient intakes by household food security status. Therefore, the purpose of this analysis was to estimate the prevalence of risk of micronutrient inadequacy and excess by comparing total usual micronutrient intake distributions to the Dietary Reference Intakes (DRI); and to parse out the contributions of DS to the total intakes of U.S. adults (1) in the general population and (2) by household food security status, using data from the National Health and Nutrition Examination Survey (NHANES), 2011–2014.

2. Methods

The NHANES is a nationally representative, continuous cross-sectional survey of noninstitutionalized, civilian residents of the U.S. conducted by the National Center for Health Statistics. Complete details of the NHANES survey are publicly available [6]. Briefly, the NHANES protocol includes an in-person household interview that queries health information and demographics as well as a follow-up health examination in a Mobile Examination Center (MEC) for each participant. Written informed consent was obtained for all participants or their proxies, and the NHANES protocol (and publicly released de-identified data) was approved by the Research Ethics Review Board at the CDC/National Center for Health Statistics. For the purposes of this analysis, the most recent data on dietary and DS intakes available from the NHANES (2011–2012 and 2013–2014 cycles) were combined to form an analytic sample of 19,151 participants. These survey years were combined in order to increase the statistical reliability of estimates across population subgroups [6]. Participants who were <19 years of age (n = 7939), did not complete or had incomplete 24 h dietary recall or dietary supplement questionnaire data (n = 1088), or who were pregnant and/or lactating (n = 170) were excluded, yielding a final analytic sample size of 9954 adults.

All demographic data used for this analysis were collected from participants in NHANES using the Computer-Assisted Personal Interview system during the household interview. Household food security status was measured using the USDA's Household Food Security Survey Module; one household reference person responded to 18 items for households with children, or 10 items for households without children. The USDA's Household Food Security Survey Module is on a continuum comprised of four different food security classifications, ranging from full, marginal, low, to very low household food security. "Full food security" describes a household with very little trouble or anxiety regarding household members gaining access to food, while "marginal food security" refers to anxiety regarding household members gaining access to food, without a reduction in the quantity, quality, or the variety of foods consumed [7,8]. "Low food security" defines households that reduce the quality, variety, and desirability of foods, yet the quantity of foods consumed remains adequate [7,8]. "Very low food security" exists when the quantity of foods consumed is inadequate, and eating patterns of the household are subsequently disrupted [7,8]. Households that were considered to have full or marginal food security were classified as food secure (<3 affirmative responses); those with low or very low food security were classified as food insecure (≥3 affirmative responses) [9]. Household food security is reflective of conditions over the previous 12 months, that serve as the inherent reference period in the USDA's Household Food Security Survey Module [10].

DS use in the previous 30 days was collected during the household interview via an in-home inventory and the dietary supplement questionnaire. Participants were asked to show interviewers the containers for all products taken in the past 30 days. For each DS reported, interviewers recorded the name, manufacturer, form of the products (e.g., tablet) and dose per serving for selected single nutrient products from the label. Detailed information on the consumption frequency, amount, and duration of

DS use were also collected for each product reported. Mean daily nutrient intakes from supplemental sources for each individual were calculated using the total number of reported days, amount taken per day, and the dose per serving of each product from the label. More information on the NHANES DS component protocol can be found elsewhere [5,11–13]. All information from DS was obtained from the dietary supplement questionnaire in the in-home inventory.

Dietary intake was self-reported in the MEC using an in-person 24 h dietary recall. A second 24 h dietary recall was completed via telephone approximately 3–10 days after the MEC exam. Both 24 h recalls were collected by trained interviewers using the USDA's automated multiple-pass method [14,15]. The USDA Food and Nutrient Database for Dietary Studies and the NHANES Dietary Supplement Database were used to convert foods, beverages, and DS as consumed to their respective nutrient values [16,17].

The micronutrients chosen for presentation in the main tables of this analysis were selected based on under-consumed micronutrients identified in the 2015–2020 Dietary Guidelines for Americans among some subgroups within the U.S. population: calcium, magnesium, iron, potassium, choline, folate and vitamins A, C, D, and E [1,2]. Micronutrients associated with lower intakes from diet alone among the food insecure (calcium, magnesium, zinc, and vitamins A and B6) in a systematic review were also included [4]. However, vitamins A and E were not available in the NHANES 2011–2014 DS data files; thus, total nutrient intakes could not be estimated, and intakes are reflective of food sources only for these vitamins in the supplementary material provided in Tables S1 and S2. Information on all of the additional micronutrients examined are provided in the supplementary material (Tables S1 and S2). It should be noted that the UL for folate only applies to the synthetic form, folic acid, obtained from DS and fortified foods. Thus, folic acid was the only form of folate used to estimate the proportion of the population exceeding the UL. Sodium was excluded since negligible amounts are found in DS [18].

An adaptation of the National Cancer Institute (NCI) method [19,20] was used to estimate (1) distributions of usual micronutrient intakes (from foods alone and total) by men and women and (2) the proportions of the subpopulations (i.e., sex, food security status) whose usual intakes were above or below age and sex-specific DRIs. The NCI method is used to estimate the distributions of "usual" or "long-term mean daily" intakes by accounting for random measurement error (i.e., within-person variation). It was adapted to estimate the contributions of DS to usual micronutrient intake estimates through the incorporation of reported DS intakes from the dietary supplement questionnaire, using the method described by Bailey et al. [18,21]. Covariates incorporated in the usual intake models included day of the week of the dietary recall (weekend/weekday), interview sequence (first or second dietary recall), and DS use overall. Categorical variables for sex and food security status were used for subgroup analyses. Mean daily nutrient intakes from DS and their relative contribution to total intakes were estimated by adding nutrients from supplemental sources to the adjusted distributions of usual intake from dietary sources to estimate the distributions of total usual micronutrient intake among the adult total population (DS users and nonusers combined) [18,22]. The relative contribution of DS to total micronutrient intakes was calculated by dividing the total usual micronutrient intake from DS by the total usual micronutrient intake from all sources (inclusive of foods and DS) at the population level (Table 1).

Total usual micronutrient intake distributions were compared to age and sex-specific DRIs established by the National Academies of Science, Engineering, and Medicine in order to compare total usual micronutrient intakes to the DRIs, including the %< Estimated Average Requirement (EAR), %> Adequate Intake (AI), and %> Tolerable Upper Intake Level (UL) using the cut-point method [23,24]. The EAR cut-point method assumes that the nutrient requirement distribution is symmetric; therefore, it cannot be applied to iron since the requirement distribution for iron is skewed in reproductive-aged women [25]. Therefore, iron estimates are only presented relative to the EAR for men.

All statistical analyses were performed using SAS software (version 9.4; SAS Institute Inc., Cary, NC, USA) accounting for the NHANES complex survey design and sampling weights to adjust for differential non-response and non-coverage, and oversampling and post-stratification. Standard errors

(SE) for all statistics of interest were approximated using Fay's modified Balanced Repeated Replication technique [26,27]. Differences in the proportion of the population with total usual micronutrient intakes < EAR or > AI within sex groups by food security status were compared using pairwise t-tests; a Bonferroni- adjusted *p*-value of <0.005 was considered statistically significant (Table 2, Table S2). Multiple comparisons were conducted using a pairwise t statistic to assess differences in the proportion of U.S. adult supplement users with total usual micronutrient intakes > UL within sex groups by food security status; a Bonferroni-adjusted *p*-value of <0.0125 was considered statistically significant (Figure 2).

3. Results

In general, the proportion of nutrients from dietary sources was greater than the proportion from DS. However, the relative contributions of DS to total intake varied by nutrient, with the lowest contributions for choline, (0.5%), potassium (0.5%), phosphorus (0.5%), vitamin K (7.0%), and magnesium (8.2%) (Table 1, Table S1). DS contributed over half of total intake for vitamins B6 (61%), B12 (93%), C (52%), and D (71%). However, even with high intakes of vitamins C and D from DS, the proportion of adults at risk of inadequacy remains high (Table 1). Most notably, for vitamin D, 98% of women and 92% of men in the U.S. were at risk of inadequate intake from foods alone, yet, the prevalence of vitamin D inadequacy among adults ranged from 59% to 66%, depending on the sex, even when taking into account nutrient intakes from DS. Smaller differences were found for calcium, magnesium, and vitamin C in both men and women, and for zinc and vitamin B6 in women alone. Calcium DS reduced the prevalence of at-risk intakes from 26% (foods alone) to 21% (total) among men and from 58% (foods alone) to 41% (total) among women, although, unlike vitamin D, calcium from supplemental sources varied, accounting for only 4% to 21% of total intake depending on the sex/food security group considered.

DS contributed a larger proportion to total usual intakes among adults living in food secure households compared with those living in food insecure households for all nutrients examined (Figure 1). A higher prevalence of inadequate intakes was observed among adults living in food insecure than in food secure households, especially for magnesium, vitamin C, and vitamin D (Table 2). Adults living in food insecure households also had a lower prevalence of intakes exceeding the AI for potassium when compared with those in food secure households (Table 2). Similar patterns were observed for intakes of copper, niacin, riboflavin, vitamin B12, and vitamin K in men and women, and phosphorous, selenium, and zinc in men alone (Table S2).

A small proportion of supplement users had total usual intakes that exceeded the UL for folic acid, vitamin D, calcium, or iron (Figure 2); but this was only significantly different for women by food security status with regard to calcium.

Table 1. Relative contribution of dietary supplements to total usual nutrient intakes and the estimated percent (%) of usual intakes (foods alone and total) below the Estimated Average Requirement or above the Adequate Intake for select nutrients among adults (≥19 years) in the U.S, 2011–2014. [1]

	All Adults				Men				Women			
	Total Usual Nutrient Intakes		Total Usual Nutrient Intakes		Total Usual Nutrient Intakes		Total Usual Nutrient Intakes		Total Usual Nutrient Intakes		Total Usual Nutrient Intakes	
	% Contribution from DS	%<EAR/>AI (SE)	% Contribution from DS	%<EAR/>AI (SE)	% Contribution from DS	%<EAR/>AI (SE)	Usual Intake from Foods %<EAR/>AI (SE)		% Contribution from DS	%<EAR/>AI (SE)	Usual Intake from Foods %<EAR/>AI (SE)	
Calcium (mg)	13.2%	31.0 (1.0)	7.5%	21.0 (1.0)	19.5%	26.0 (1.2)	19.5%	41.0 (1.3)	58.0 (1.6)			
Iron (mg) [2]	16.9%	—	8.4%	0.1 (0.1)	25.3%	0.1 (0.1)	25.3%	—	—			
Magnesium (mg)	8.2%	45.2 (1.0)	6.6%	46.0 (1.2)	10.1%	52.0 (1.3)	10.1%	43.6 (1.2)	50.7 (1.3)			
Potassium (mg) [3]	0.5%	37.0 (1.0)	0.5%	36.0 (1.3)	0.5%	35.0 (1.3)	0.5%	33.0 (1.5)	33.0 (1.6)			
Zinc (mg)	26.0%	16.8 (0.7)	21.0%	12.7 (1.1)	32.1%	16.3 (1.4)	32.1%	13.2 (1.1)	17.3 (1.2)			
Choline (mg) [3]	0.5%	12.3 (0.6)	0.3%	12.0 (1.1)	0.5%	11.7 (1.1)	0.5%	3.6 (0.7)	3.4 (0.7)			
Folate (DFE, μg) [4]	27.2%	9.0 (0.8)	21.4%	5.0 (0.6)	33.4%	6.0 (0.8)	33.4%	12.0 (1.2)	15.9 (1.6)			
Vitamin B6 (mg)	61.4%	6.2 (0.6)	52.7%	1.9 (0.5)	71.2%	2.6 (0.6)	71.2%	10.6 (0.8)	14.4 (1.0)			
Vitamin C (mg)	51.7%	35.0 (1.1)	48.1%	39.0 (1.7)	55.0%	50.8 (1.7)	55.0%	32.0 (1.2)	44.0 (1.4)			
Vitamin D (μg)	70.6%	63.1 (0.7)	59.8%	66.4 (1.0)	78.2%	91.5 (0.9)	78.2%	59.1 (1.2)	98.1 (0.3)			

Abbreviations: DS, dietary supplement; EAR, Estimated Average Requirement; AI, Adequate Intake; SE, standard error. [1] The analytic sample includes individuals ≥19 years old that were not pregnant or lactating with complete information for the day 1 and 2, 24 h dietary recalls. [2] Proportion of the population below the EAR for iron was unable to be assessed using the cut-point method in women due to a skewed distribution of nutrient requirements. [3] Indicates % > AI rather than % < EAR. This occurs when sufficient scientific evidence is not available to establish an EAR. [4] As dietary folate equivalents (DFEs). 1 DFE = 1 μg food folate = 0.6 μg of folic acid from fortified food or as a supplement consumed with food = 0.5 μg of a supplement taken on an empty stomach.

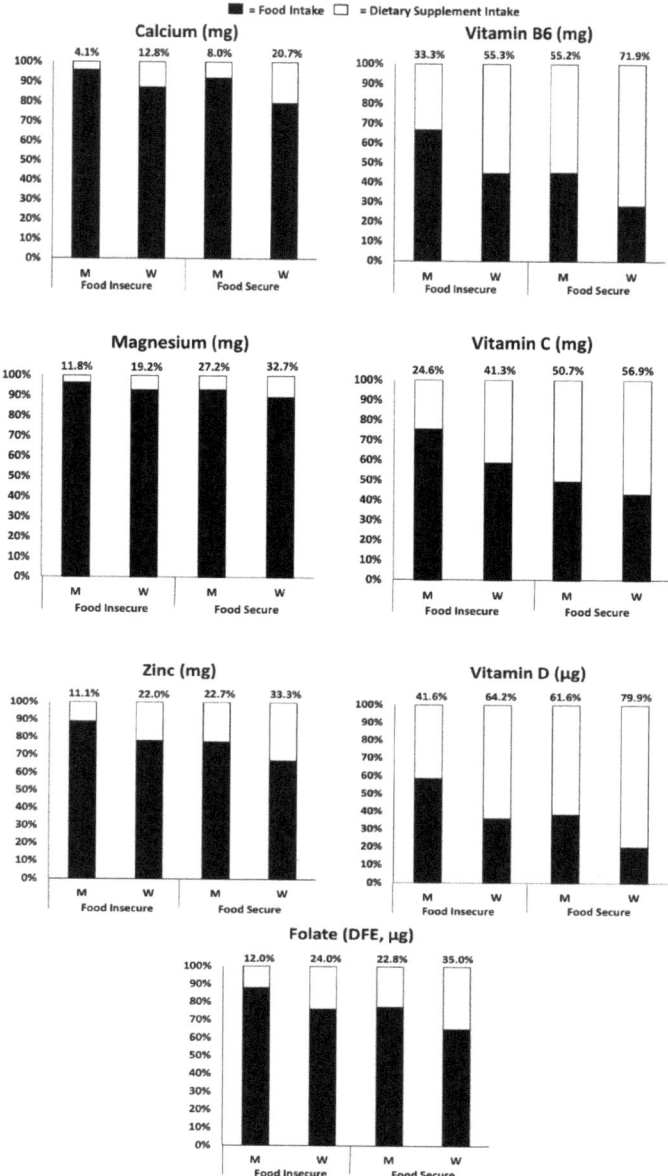

Figure 1. Relative contribution of foods/beverages and dietary supplements to total usual intakes for selected nutrients by age group among men and women by food security status (≥19 years) in the U.S., 2011–2014. [1] ([1] The analytic sample includes individuals ≥19 years old that were not pregnant or lactating with complete information for food security and the day 1 and 2, 24 h dietary recalls. Percentages above each bar represent the relative contribution from dietary supplements). Abbreviations: M, Men; W, Women; DFE, Dietary Folate Equivalents.

Table 2. Proportion of the population falling below the Estimated Average Requirement or above the Adequate Intake from total usual nutrient intakes of select nutrients, by food security status, among adults (≥19 years) in the U.S., 2011–2014. [1,2]

	Food Security Status, % < EAR/> AI (SE)	
	Food Insecure	Food Secure
Men (n, %)	(915, 14.9%)	(3993, 85.1%)
Calcium (mg)	25.0 (2.2)	20.0 (1.3)
Iron (mg) [3]	0.3 (0.2)	0.1 (0.1)
Magnesium (mg)	57.2 (1.7) [a]	43.9 (1.5) [b]
Potassium (mg) [4]	25.0 (2.5) [a]	37.0 (1.6) [b]
Zinc (mg)	20.1 (2.4) [a]	11.3 (1.1) [b]
Choline (mg) [4]	12.6 (2.3)	11.8 (1.1)
Folate (DFE, µg) [5]	7.0 (1.8)	4.0 (0.7)
Vitamin B6 (mg)	6.1 (1.3) [a]	1.4 (0.4) [b]
Vitamin C (mg)	49.0 (3.8) [a]	37.0 (1.7) [b]
Vitamin D (µg)	79.2 (1.5) [a]	64.1 (1.2) [b]
Women (n, %)	(1010, 15.6%)	(4034, 84.4%)
Calcium (mg)	46.0 (3.0)	40.0 (1.3)
Iron (mg) [3]	–	–
Magnesium (mg)	56.9 (2.6) [a]	40.9 (1.4) [b]
Potassium (mg) [4]	24.0 (3.1) [a]	35.0 (1.7) [b]
Zinc (mg)	17.1 (2.8)	12.2 (1.3)
Choline (mg) [4]	4.4 (1.5)	3.5 (0.6)
Folate (DFE, µg) [5]	15.0 (3.5)	11.0 (1.3)
Vitamin B6 (mg)	19.0 (1.6) [a]	8.8 (0.9) [b]
Vitamin C (mg)	42.0 (2.4) [a]	29.0 (1.3) [b]
Vitamin D (µg)	74.7 (1.7) [a]	56.2 (1.2) [b]

Abbreviations: EAR, Estimated Average Requirement; AI, Adequate Intake; SE, standard error. [1] The analytic sample includes individuals ≥19 years old that were not pregnant/lactating with complete information for the day 1 and 2, 24 h dietary recalls. [2] Different superscript letters denote a significant difference between food security categories at a p-value < 0.005. [3] Proportion of the population below the EAR for iron was unable to be assessed using the cut-point method in women due to a skewed distribution of nutrient requirements. [4] Indicates %> AI rather than %< EAR. This occurs when sufficient scientific evidence is not available to establish an EAR. [5] As dietary folate equivalents (DFEs). 1 DFE = 1 µg food folate = 0.6 µg of folic acid from fortified food or as a consumed with food = 0.5 µg of a supplement taken on an empty stomach.

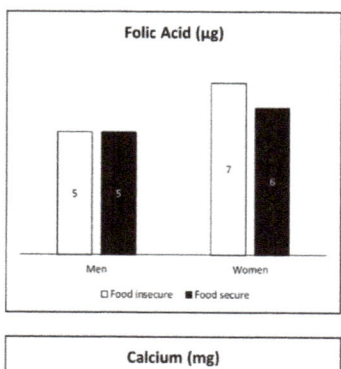
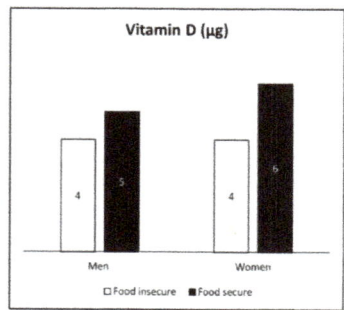
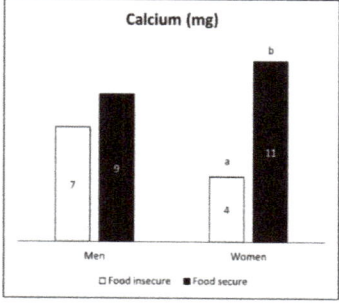
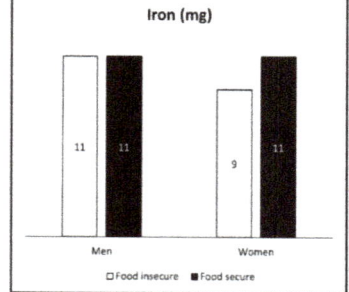

Figure 2. Estimated percent (%) of total micronutrient intakes above the Tolerable Upper Intake Level (UL) by food security status among adult (≥19 years) supplement users in the U.S., 2011–2014. [1,2] ([1] The analytic sample includes individuals ≥19 years old that were not pregnant or lactating with complete information for food security and the day 1 and 2, 24 h dietary recalls. Numerical data labels within each bar represent the estimated proportion (%) of U.S. adult supplement users with intakes greater than the UL. [2] Different superscript letters denote a significant difference between food security categories within sex at a p-value < 0.0125.).

4. Discussion

Our findings suggest that DS aid in reducing the proportion of the population at risk for inadequate intakes, especially for vitamin D, calcium, and vitamin C. However, many Americans still have low intakes of some micronutrients, even with the use of DS, which is especially true among U.S. adults with food insecurity. While this study focuses on individual nutrients, the health effects of a diet, especially those related to chronic diseases, are determined by the sum and interaction of many food constituents in addition to nutrients. Many of these constituents are not yet fully understood and do not have DRIs. Plant products are particularly complex with many bioactive components (flavonoids, various types of fiber, etc.). The recognized health benefits of diets rich in fruits, vegetables, and whole grains, for example, are attributable to more than their nutrient content [1]. Consequently, the Dietary Guidelines for Americans focus on the quality of the overall dietary pattern. To address the problem of food insecurity, the 2015–2020 Dietary Guidelines for Americans call for supporting individuals in making healthy food choices by expanding nutrition-assistance programs and creating networks and partnerships to address the problem. One example is improving the offerings at food pantries [28]. Another is expanding programs, such as the Expanded Food and Nutrition Education Program and SNAP-Ed, which teach food resource management [29].

Two studies have confirmed that total usual nutrient intakes, inclusive of DS, vary by income alone using the family poverty-to-income ratio (PIR) [21,30]. However, as outlined by the Academy of Nutrition and Dietetics, food security results from a constellation of factors that may predispose individuals to nutrition risk beyond income alone, including environmental factors like transportation, food prices, housing costs, unemployment, and social capital, among others [31]. In a previous analysis in Canada, Kirkpatrick et al. revealed a higher prevalence of micronutrient inadequacy for several micronutrients among adolescents and adults living in food insecure as compared with food secure households, specifically for vitamin A, thiamin, riboflavin, vitamin B6, folate, vitamin B12, magnesium, phosphorus, and zinc [32]. The present analysis extends prior foods-based work by examining total micronutrient intakes, inclusive of DS, by food security status. Adults living with food insecurity had a higher risk of micronutrient inadequacy for most micronutrients examined, except for calcium, iron (examined only in men), folate, or choline, when compared with food secure adults. Most notably, in addition to the micronutrients identified by Kirkpatrick et al. [32], the present analysis observed a higher prevalence of micronutrient inadequacy among adults living with food insecurity for copper, potassium, niacin, and vitamins C, D, E, and K in both men and women, and selenium in men alone. While nutrient inadequacy was more of a concern among adults living in food insecure households, all DS users, regardless of food security status, had an increased likelihood of usual intakes above the UL for iron, calcium, vitamin D, and folic acid, increasing risk of adverse health effects [25,33,34].

A strength of this analysis is that the models applied to examine total usual intakes adjust for the effects of random measurement error to the extent possible, in addition to using the recommended method of adding mean daily nutrient intakes from supplemental sources to the adjusted usual nutrient intakes from dietary sources [18,22]. USDA's automated multiple-pass method is a state-of-the-art method for capturing dietary data, as is the Food and Nutrient Database for Dietary Studies that supports it. However, self-reported dietary data are prone to systematic measurement error, like energy underreporting, that may result in an underestimation of micronutrient intakes from the diet. Furthermore, the analysis of nutrients in DS relies on label declarations on products, rather than analytically derived values, that are likely to result in an underestimation of micronutrients from DS [35]. Furthermore, we assume that the DS intake reported for the past 30 days during the in-home interview reflects long-term, habitual DS intake, but little is known about the measurement error structure of DS reporting [18]. NHANES is a nationally representative survey of the U.S. noninstitutionalized population. However, the response rates for the years 2011–2012 and 2013–2014 for adults were 56% and 65%, respectively [36,37], and total usual nutrient intakes could not be estimated for vitamins A and E, as these nutrients are not included in the current NHANES DS data files. An additional limitation is that the bioavailability of nutrients from DS compared to the bioavailability of nutrients from foods remains largely unknown.

5. Conclusions

In summary, our findings are consistent with previous reports that demonstrate that many U.S. adults have inadequate intakes of potassium, magnesium, calcium, vitamin D, and/or vitamin C, even with the use of DS, and that those living with food insecurity have a higher prevalence of micronutrient risk than those not living with food insecurity. These findings suggest that, while DS can be helpful in meeting nutrient requirements for adults for some nutrients, potential excess may also be of concern for certain nutrients among supplement users.

Supplementary Materials: The following are available online at http://www.mdpi.com/2072-6643/12/1/38/s1, Table S1: Relative contribution of dietary supplements to total usual nutrient intakes and the estimated percent (%) of usual intakes (foods alone and total) below the Estimated Average Requirement or above the Adequate Intake for other nutrients among adults (≥19 years) in the U.S., 2011–2014, Table S2: Proportion of the population falling below the Estimated Average Requirement or above the Adequate Intake from total usual nutrient intakes of other nutrients, by food security status among adults (≥ 19 years) in the U.S., 2011–2014.

Author Contributions: A.E.C., S.J., and R.L.B. designed the research and concepts presented, and performed the analysis. A.E.C., S.J., and R.L.B. wrote sections of the paper. J.A.T., H.A.E.-M., K.W.D., J.J.G., P.M.G., J.T.D., N.P., and A.B. provided critical review and insights presented. All authors read and approved the final version of the manuscript. All authors have read and agreed to the published version of the manuscript.

Funding: This research was funded by NIH/NCI, grant number U01CA215834.

Conflicts of Interest: A.E.C., S.J., J.A.T., K.W.D., J.J.G., H.A.E.-M., P.M.G., A.J.M., D.G.R., and A.B. have no conflicts of interest. R.L.B. is a consultant to the NIH Office of Dietary Supplements, reports grants from National Institutes of Health/National Cancer Institute; in the past she has served as a consultant to Nestle/Gerber, the General Mills Bell Institute, RTI International, and Nutrition Impact; Dr. Bailey is a trustee of the International Food Information Council and a board member of International Life Sciences Institute- North America. In the past she has received travel support to present her research on dietary supplements. J.T.D reports personal fees from McCormick Spice, The Mushroom Council, Bay State Milling, ConAgra Foods (until 2018), and Nestlé, on topics outside the submitted work, and stock in several food and drug companies. The funders had no role in the design of the study; in the collection, analyses, or interpretation of data; in the writing of the manuscript; or in the decision to publish the results.

References

1. U.S. Department of Health and Human Services and U.S. Department of Agriculture. In *2015–2020 Dietary Guidelines for Americans*, 8th ed.; Skyhorse Publishing Inc.: New York, NY, USA, 2017.
2. Scientific report of the 2015 Dietary Guidelines Advisory Committee. Available online: https://health.gov/dietaryguidelines/2015-scientific-report/ (accessed on 12 December 2019).
3. Anderson, S.A. Core indicators of nutritional state for difficult-to-sample populations. *J. Nutr.* **1990**, *120*, 1555–1600. [CrossRef] [PubMed]
4. Hanson, K.L.; Connor, L.M. Food insecurity and dietary quality in US adults and children: A systematic review. *Am. J. Clin. Nutr.* **2014**, *100*, 684–692. [CrossRef] [PubMed]
5. Cowan, A.E.; Jun, S.; Gahche, J.J.; Tooze, J.A.; Dwyer, J.T.; Eicher-Miller, H.A.; Bhadra, A.; Guenther, P.M.; Potischman, N.; Dodd, K.W.; et al. Dietary supplement use differs by socioeconomic and health-related characteristics among US adults, NHANES 2011–2014. *Nutrients* **2018**, *10*, 1114. [CrossRef] [PubMed]
6. Johnson, C.L.; Dohrmann, S.M.; Burt, V.L.; Mohadjer, L.K. National Health and Nutrition Examination Survey: Sample design, 2011–2014. *Vital Health Stat. 2* **2014**, *162*, 1–33.
7. National Research Council. *Food Insecurity and Hunger in the United States: An Assessment of the Measure*; National Academies Press: Washington, DC, USA, 2006.
8. Eicher-Miller, H.A.; Mason, A.C.; Weaver, C.M.; McCabe, G.P.; Boushey, C.J. Food insecurity is associated with iron deficiency anemia in US adolescents. *Am. J. Clin. Nutr.* **2009**, *90*, 1358–1371. [CrossRef]
9. Bickel, G.; Nord, M.; Price, C.; Hamilton, W.; Cook, J. *Measuring Food Security in the United States: Guide to Measuring Household Food Insecurity*; United States Department of Agriculture: Washington, DC, USA, 2000.
10. U.S. Adult Food Security Survey Module: Three-Stage Design, With Screeners Economic Research Service. Available online: https://www.ers.usda.gov/media/8279/ad2012.pdf/ (accessed on 12 December 2019).
11. Bailey, R.L.; Fulgoni, V.L., 3rd; Keast, D.R.; Dwyer, J.T. Dietary supplement use is associated with higher intakes of minerals from food sources. *Am. J. Clin. Nutr.* **2011**, *94*, 1376–1381. [CrossRef]
12. Gahche, J.J.; Bailey, R.L.; Potischman, N.; Dwyer, J.T. Dietary supplement use was very high among older adults in the United States in 2011–2014. *J. Nutr.* **2017**, *147*, 1968–1976. [CrossRef]
13. Bailey, R.L.; Gahche, J.J.; Miller, P.E.; Thomas, P.R.; Dwyer, J.T. Why US adults use dietary supplements. *JAMA Intern. Med.* **2013**, *173*, 355–361. [CrossRef]
14. Blanton, C.A.; Moshfegh, A.J.; Baer, D.J.; Kretsch, M.J. The USDA automated multiple-pass method accurately estimates group total energy and nutrient intake. *J. Nutr.* **2006**, *136*, 2594–2599. [CrossRef]
15. Moshfegh, A.J.; Rhodes, D.G.; Baer, D.J.; Murayi, T.; Clemens, J.C.; Rumpler, W.V.; Paul, D.R.; Sebastian, R.S.; Kuczynski, K.J.; Ingwersen, L.A.; et al. The US Department of Agriculture automated multiple-pass method reduces bias in the collection of energy intakes. *Am. J. Clin. Nutr.* **2008**, *88*, 324–332. [CrossRef]
16. Food and Nutrient Database for Dietary Studies 2011–2012. Available online: https://www.ars.usda.gov/ARSUserFiles/80400530/pdf/fndds/fndds_2011_2012.pdf (accessed on 10 October 2019).
17. Centers for Disease Control and Prevention—National Center for Health Statistics. NHANES 2013–2014 Dietary Data. Available online: https://wwwn.cdc.gov/nchs/nhanes/Search/DataPage.aspx?Component=Dietary&CycleBeginYear=2013 (accessed on 10 October 2019).
18. Bailey, R.L.; Dodd, K.W.; Gahche, J.J.; Dwyer, J.T.; Cowan, A.E.; Jun, S.; Eicher-Miller, H.A.; Guenther, P.M.; Bhadra, A.; Thomas, P.R.; et al. Best practices for dietary supplement assessment and estimation of total usual nutrient intakes in population-level research and monitoring. *J. Nutr.* **2019**, *149*, 181–197. [CrossRef] [PubMed]

19. Dodd, K.W.; Guenther, P.M.; Freedman, L.S.; Subar, A.F.; Kipnis, V.; Midthune, D.; Tooze, J.A.; Krebs-Smith, S.M. Statistical methods for estimating usual intake of nutrients and foods: A review of the theory. *J. Am. Diet. Assoc.* **2006**, *106*, 1640–1650. [CrossRef] [PubMed]
20. Tooze, J.A.; Midthune, D.; Dodd, K.W.; Freedman, L.S.; Krebs-Smith, S.M.; Subar, A.F.; Guenther, P.M.; Carroll, R.J.; Kipnis, V. A new statistical method for estimating the usual intake of episodically consumed foods with application to their distribution. *J. Am. Diet. Assoc.* **2006**, *106*, 1575–1587. [CrossRef] [PubMed]
21. Bailey, R.L.; Akabas, S.R.; Paxson, E.E.; Thuppal, S.V.; Saklani, S.; Tucker, K.L. Total usual intake of shortfall nutrients varies with poverty among US adults. *J. Nutr. Educ. Behav.* **2017**, *49*, 639–646.e3. [CrossRef]
22. Garriguet, D. Combining nutrient intake from food/beverages and vitamin/mineral supplements. *Health Rep.* **2010**, *21*, 71–84.
23. Institute of Medicine. *Dietary Reference Intakes: Applications in Dietary Assessment*; The National Academies Press: Washington, DC, USA, 2000; p. 306.
24. Institute of Medicine. *Dietary Reference Intakes: The Essential Guide to Nutrient Requirements (2006)*; National Academies Press: Washington, DC, USA, 2006.
25. Institute of Medicine Panel on Micronutrients. *Dietary Reference Intakes for Vitamin A, Vitamin K, Arsenic, Boron, Chromium, Copper, Iodine, Iron, Manganese, Molybdenum, Nickel, Silicon, Vanadium, and Zinc*; National Academies Press (US): Washington, DC, USA, 2001.
26. Burt, V.L.; Cohen, S.B. A comparison of methods to approximate standard errors for complex survey data. *Rev. Public Data Use* **1984**, *12*, 159–168.
27. Shao, J.; Rao, J. Modified balanced repeated replication for complex survey data. *Biometrika* **1999**, *86*, 403–415.
28. Wright, B.N.; Bailey, R.L.; Craig, B.A.; Mattes, R.D.; McCormack, L.; Stluka, S.; Franzen-Castle, L.; Henne, B.; Mehrle, D.; Remley, D.; et al. Daily dietary intake patterns improve after visiting a food pantry among food-insecure rural midwestern adults. *Nutrients* **2018**, *10*, 583. [CrossRef]
29. Rivera, R.L.; Maulding, M.K.; Eicher-Miller, H.A. Effect of supplemental nutrition assistance program-education (snap-ed) on food security and dietary outcomes. *Nutr. Rev.* **2019**, *77*, 903–921. [CrossRef]
30. Blumberg, J.B.; Frei, B.; Fulgoni, V.L.; Weaver, C.M.; Zeisel, S.H. Contribution of dietary supplements to nutritional adequacy by socioeconomic subgroups in adults of the United States. *Nutrients* **2017**, *10*, 4. [CrossRef]
31. Holben, D.H.; Marshall, M.B. Position of the Academy of Nutrition and Dietetics: Food insecurity in the united states. *J. Acad. Nutr. Diet.* **2017**, *117*, 1991–2002. [CrossRef] [PubMed]
32. Kirkpatrick, S.I.; Tarasuk, V. Food insecurity is associated with nutrient inadequacies among Canadian adults and adolescents. *J. Nutr.* **2008**, *138*, 604–612. [CrossRef] [PubMed]
33. Institute of Medicine Standing Committee on the Scientific Evaluation of Dietary Reference Intakes. *Dietary Reference Intakes for Thiamin, Riboflavin, Niacin, Vitamin B6, Folate, Vitamin B12, Pantothenic Acid, Biotin, and Choline*; National Academies Press (US): Washington, DC, USA, 1998.
34. Institute of Medicine Committee to Review Dietary Reference Intakes for Calcium and Vitamin D. In *Dietary Reference Intakes for Calcium and Vitamin D*; Ross, A.C.; Taylor, C.L.; Yaktine, A.L.; Del Valle, H.B. (Eds.) National Academies Press (US) National Academy of Sciences: Washington, DC, USA, 2011.
35. Andrews, K.W.; Gusev, P.A.; McNeal, M.; Savarala, S.; Dang, P.T.V.; Oh, L.; Atkinson, R.; Pehrsson, P.R.; Dwyer, J.T.; Saldanha, L.G.; et al. Dietary Supplement Ingredient Database (DSID) and the application of analytically based estimates of ingredient amount to intake calculations. *J. Nutr.* **2018**, *148*, 1413S–1421S. [CrossRef] [PubMed]
36. Unweighted Response Rates for NHANES 2011–2012 by Age and Gender. Available online: https://wwwn.cdc.gov/nchs/data/nhanes3/ResponseRates/rrt1112.pdf (accessed on 12 December 2019).
37. Unweighted Response Rates for NHANES 2013–2014 by Age and Gender. Available online: https://wwwn.cdc.gov/nchs/data/nhanes3/ResponseRates/2013_2014_response_rates.pdf (accessed on 12 December 2019).

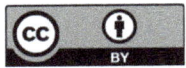

© 2019 by the authors. Licensee MDPI, Basel, Switzerland. This article is an open access article distributed under the terms and conditions of the Creative Commons Attribution (CC BY) license (http://creativecommons.org/licenses/by/4.0/).

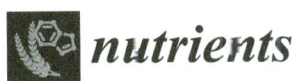

Article

Household Food Insecurity and the Association with Cumulative Biological Risk among Lower-Income Adults: Results from the National Health and Nutrition Examination Surveys 2007–2010

Cindy W. Leung * and Megan S. Zhou

Department of Nutritional Sciences, School of Public Health, University of Michigan, Ann Arbor, MI 48109, USA; zhoumeg@umich.edu
* Correspondence: cindyleung@post.harvard.edu; Tel.: +1-734-647-9087

Received: 10 April 2020; Accepted: 20 May 2020; Published: 23 May 2020

Abstract: Household food insecurity has been associated with adverse health outcomes; however, the mechanisms underlying these associations are not well-defined. Using data from 5005 adults from the 2007–2010 National Health and Nutrition Examination Surveys (NHANES), we examined associations between household food insecurity and cumulative biological risk, a measure of the body's physiological response to chronic stress. Household food security was assessed using the 18-item Household Food Security Survey Module. Marginal food security refers to 1–2 positive responses, and food insecurity refers to ≥3 positive responses. The cumulative biological risk scores were calculated based on the distributions of ten biomarkers from the cardiovascular, metabolic, and immune systems. Elevated biological risk was defined as a risk score of ≥3. Multivariable regression models were used to examine associations between food security and cumulative biological risk scores, adjusting for sociodemographic characteristics. After multivariable adjustment, food insecurity was associated with a 0.14-unit higher cumulative biological risk score (95% CI 0.05–0.22, p-trend = 0.003) and higher odds of elevated biological risk (OR 1.20, 95% CI 1.05–1.37, p-trend = 0.003). These associations differed by gender. Among women, food insecurity was associated with 0.30-unit higher cumulative biological risk score (95% CI 0.14–0.45, p-trend = 0.0004) and higher odds of elevated biological risk (OR 1.61, 95% CI 1.29–2.00, p-trend < 0.0001). These associations were not observed in men. Women experiencing food insecurity demonstrated elevated levels of biological risk. These findings support the hypothesis that food insecurity may be associated with women's chronic health outcomes through the pathway of chronic stress. Further research is needed to understand why these associations were not observed in men.

Keywords: food insecurity; allostatic load; biological risk; chronic stress; National Health and Nutrition Examination Surveys

1. Introduction

Food insecurity, defined as inadequate access and availability of food due to a lack of monetary resources, has persisted in the United States since its routine measurement in national population surveys in the 1990s [1]. In 2018, it was estimated that 14.3 million households or 11.1% of U.S. households experienced food insecurity during the year [1]. Household food insecurity has been associated with numerous physical and mental health outcomes among low-income adults, including higher levels of obesity [2–4], hypertension [5], diabetes [6,7] and poorer diabetes management [8,9], metabolic syndrome [10], lower cognitive function [11,12], depression [13,14], and poorer overall health [15,16]. The mechanisms underlying these associations have not been fully elucidated; however, a number of studies have demonstrated associations between household food insecurity and modifiable health behaviors, such as poorer diet quality [17–19], lower levels of physical activity [20], higher rates of smoking [21–23], and poorer sleep outcomes [24,25]. Several researchers have also alluded to the role of chronic stress in explaining the observed associations [14,26–30], though none of these studies have been able to test the association between food insecurity and chronic stress directly.

Chronic stress refers to the repeated activation of major body systems in response to external stimuli perceived to be threatening [31]. In response to a stressor, the hypothalamic–pituitary–adrenal (HPA) axis and the sympathetic–adrenal–medullary (SAM) systems are activated, triggering a release of hormones and cytokines that act on multiple organ systems [31,32]. The concept of allostatic load has been used to describe how repeated exposure and prolonged response to stress can dysregulate these organ systems, resulting in "wear and tear" on the body over time [32]. Operationally, there is no single, gold-standard approach for measuring allostatic load, though allostatic load scores often include a combination of biomarkers from neuroendocrine, immune, metabolic, and cardiovascular systems—all known to be affected by the secretion of stress hormones and inflammatory markers [33]. Thus, allostatic load is theorized to represent the body's cumulative physiological response to chronic stress and to account for individual variability in the appraisal of different stress exposures, which may be more relevant to predicting subsequent health outcomes than the perception of stress [34].

Prior research has explored the role of the allostatic load as a framework through which to understand health disparities. Greater socioeconomic adversity [35–38] and minority race/ethnicity [39–41] have both been associated with elevated allostatic load in numerous studies. Household food insecurity is both a form of socioeconomic adversity and an issue with relatively high prevalence in low-income and minority racial/ethnic households [1]. However, its relation to allostatic load has only been explored in one study [42]. In an analysis of 733 Puerto Rican adults residing in Boston, food insecurity was associated with greater dysregulation of the neuroendocrine and inflammatory systems, but not total allostatic load [42]. In order to understand the pathways connecting food insecurity and adverse health outcomes, more research is needed to examine this association in a larger and more representative sample of adults.

In the present study, neuroendocrine markers are important components of allostatic load measurement but were unavailable in the National Health and Nutrition Examination Surveys (NHANES). Thus, we created a score to represent a cumulative biological risk, guided by the allostatic load framework. The objective of the present study was to examine the association between household food insecurity and cumulative biological risk in a national sample of adults. We hypothesized that adults who experienced more severe household food insecurity would demonstrate greater cumulative biological risk.

2. Materials and Methods

2.1. Study Population

Administered by the National Center for Health Statistics, NHANES is an ongoing, multistage survey designed to be representative of the civilian, noninstitutionalized U.S. population. NHANES collects information on demographic indicators and health outcomes through interviews, in-person examinations, and laboratory testing. Data from 2007 to 2008 and from 2009 to 2010 were combined in the present study, representing the most recent years in which all markers of cumulative biological risk were routinely collected (e.g., C-reactive protein was not assessed in NHANES 2011–2012 or 2013–2014). The analytic population was further restricted to adults between the ages of 20–65 and with household incomes ≤300% of the federal poverty level (FPL). An income threshold of 300% FPL was chosen because household food insecurity is relatively uncommon among households with incomes >300% FPL, and inclusion of a lower-income sample reduces the potential for confounding by socioeconomic status, as has been done in prior studies [6,17,43]. Pregnant women were also excluded, as body mass index (BMI) was one of the markers of biological risk. The analytic sample included 5005 adults.

2.2. Food Security Status

The primary exposure of interest was household food security, measured using the 18-item U.S. Household Food Security Survey Module [44]. Questions were asked in three stages and attribute related experiences or behaviors to insufficient resources to buy food over the past 12 months. A score was created by summing the affirmative responses of the 18 questions, with higher scores indicating more severe food insecurity. Food security was defined as 0 affirmative responses, meaning the household had no indicators of insufficient food access. Marginal food security was defined as 1–2 affirmative responses and refers to mild indicators of insufficient food access such as anxiety over the food supply. Food insecurity was defined as three or more affirmative responses and refers to multiple indicators of insufficient food access, including reducing the quality and the variety of the amount of food consumed by at least one member of the household. Food insecurity refers to the combined categories of low food security (i.e., 3–5 affirmative responses in households without children or 3–7 affirmative responses in households with children) and very low food security (i.e., 6–10 affirmative responses in households without children or 8–18 affirmative responses in households with children). Food insecurity categorizations and definitions are in accordance with the U.S. Department of Agriculture [44].

2.3. Cumulative Biological Risk

To assess cumulative biological risk, we included the following ten biomarkers: (1) systolic blood pressure, (2) diastolic blood pressure, (3) body mass index (BMI), (4) glycohemoglobin, (5) total cholesterol, (6) high-density lipoprotein (HDL) cholesterol, (7) total/HDL cholesterol ratio, (8) C-reactive protein, (9) albumin, and (10) estimated glomerular filtration rate (eGFR). The selection of biomarkers for the present study was guided by the availability of data within NHANES and on the basis of previous research [45–48]. Systolic blood pressure, diastolic blood pressure, total cholesterol, HDL cholesterol, and pulse represented the cardiovascular system. BMI, glycohemoglobin, albumin, and eGFR represented the metabolic system. C-reactive protein represented the immune system.

Each biomarker was categorized using clinically-relevant guidelines for low-risk, moderate-risk, and high-risk categories [47]. The cut-points used were: (1) systolic blood pressure: <120 mmHg, 120–<150 mmHg, and ≥150 mmHg; (2) diastolic blood pressure: <80 mmHg, 80–<90 mmHg, and ≥90 mmHg; (3) BMI: <25 kg/m^2, 25–<30 kg/m^2, ≥30 kg/m^2; (4) glycohemoglobin: <5.7%, 5.7–<6.5%, and ≥6.5%; (5) total cholesterol: <200 mg/dL, 200–<240 mg/dL, ≥240 mg/dL; (6) HDL cholesterol: ≥60 mg/dL, 40–<60 mg/dL, and <40 mg/dL; (7) total/HDL ratio: <5; 5–<6, ≥6; (8) C-reactive protein: <1 mg/L, 1–<3 mg/L, and ≥3 mg/L; (9) albumin: ≥3.8, 3.0–<3.8, and <3.0; and (10) eGFR: ≥60 mL/min/1.73 m^2, 30–<60 mL/min/1.73 m^2, and <30 mL/min/1.73 m^2. Each biomarker was scored as zero points for low risk, 0.5 points for moderate risk, and one point for high risk. Adults who reported taking medication for high blood pressure, high cholesterol, or diabetes were also assigned to the high-risk groups for systolic and diastolic blood pressure, total cholesterol, and glycohemoglobin, respectively. A cumulative biological risk score was then created as the sum of the risk scores across the ten components, ranging from 0 (lowest) to 10 (highest). Similar to prior studies [45,46], elevated biological risk was defined as a score ≥3. Both continuous and dichotomous cumulative biological risk scores were examined as primary outcomes.

2.4. Study Covariates

Sociodemographic covariates were selected as variables hypothesized to be joint predictors of the association between food insecurity and cumulative biological risk, guided by the prior literature. These included age (continuous), gender, race/ethnicity (Non-Hispanic White, Non-Hispanic Black, Hispanic, Other), educational attainment (<12 years, high school graduate or equivalent, some college, or college graduate), household income relative to the federal poverty line (continuous), and marital status (married or living with a partner, never married, or separated, widowed, or divorced).

2.5. Statistical Analysis

Complex sampling weights for the mobile examination center were recalculated and used to account for different sampling probabilities and participation rates across the four-year period. Sampling weights were used in all subsequent analyses. Differences in sociodemographic characteristics by household food security were compared using univariate regression for continuous variables and χ^2 tests for categorical variables. Next, the distributions in individual biomarkers by household food security were compared using univariate regression and χ^2 tests. Multivariable linear and logistic regression models were used to examine associations between food security and cumulative biological risk. Differences in these associations by gender were evaluated by testing the significance of the interaction terms between household food security and gender on the outcomes. Models were first adjusted for age and gender, and second for all other sociodemographic covariates (race/ethnicity, educational attainment, household income, and marital status). In all models, age and household income were modeled as linear and quadratic terms to allow for a curvilinear relationship with cumulative biological risk. In a sensitivity analysis, we further examined the associations between the household food security and cumulative biological risk using a four-category household food security variable. Statistical tests were two-sided, and significance was considered at $p < 0.05$. Statistical analyses were performed with SAS 9.3 (SAS Institute Inc., Cary, NC, USA).

3. Results

In the analytic population of 5005 adults, 59.3% were food-secure, 14.4% were marginally food secure, and 26.2% were food-insecure. Table 1 shows the differences in the sociodemographic characteristics by household food security. Compared to food-secure adults, marginally food-secure and food-insecure adults were more likely to be of younger age, of minority race/ethnicity background, have lower educational attainment, have lower household income, and were more likely to be never married, or separated, divorced, or widowed.

Bivariate comparisons of biomarkers comprising cumulative biological risk and household food security are shown in Table 2. Compared to food-secure adults, marginally food-secure and food-insecure adults were more likely to have higher mean glycohemoglobin ($p = 0.01$), C-reactive protein ($p = 0.005$), and albumin ($p = 0.0002$). Significant differences were also evident for some risk categories. Marginally food-secure adults were more likely to be at moderate- or high-risk for systolic blood pressure ($p = 0.04$), and both marginally food-secure and food-insecure adults were more likely to be at moderate- or high-risk for HDL cholesterol ($p = 0.05$). There were no other significant bivariate associations between individual biomarkers and food security status.

Table 3 shows the associations between household food security and cumulative biological risk. Food insecurity was associated with a 0.22-point greater cumulative biological risk score (95% CI 0.11–0.32, p-trend = 0.0002), which remained significant after multivariate adjustment ($\beta = 0.14$, 95% CI 0.05–0.22, p-trend = 0.003). Although the associations between marginal food security and cumulative biological risk and between food insecurity and cumulative biological risk both appeared stronger in women than in men, the interaction was not statistically significant (p-interaction = 0.09).

When examining elevated biological risk (score ≥3), food insecurity was associated with higher odds of elevated biological risk (OR 1.20, 95% CI 1.05–1.37, p-trend = 0.003), after adjusting for sociodemographic characteristics. This association was significantly modified by gender (p-interaction = 0.03). Among women, food insecurity was associated with elevated biological risk (OR 1.61, 95% CI 1.29–2.00, p-trend < 0.0001). Among men, no association was observed between food insecurity and elevated biological risk (OR 0.93, 95% CI 0.72–1.20, p-trend = 0.70). A sensitivity analysis using a four-category household food security variable showed similar results with cumulative biological risk scores and elevated biological risk (Supplemental Table S1).

Table 1. Household food security and sociodemographic characteristics of 5005 adults (20–65 year) with household incomes ≤300% of the federal poverty level: National Health and Nutrition Examination Surveys 2007–2010.

	Food Secure (n = 2599)	Marginal Food Secure (n = 819)	Food Insecure (n = 1587)	p-Value
Age, mean (SE)	39.8 (0.5)	38.2 (0.5)	37.9 (0.5)	0.05
Women, n (%)	1336 (51.6)	445 (55.1)	844 (52.8)	0.24
Race/ethnicity, n (%)				<0.0001
Non-Hispanic White	1101 (62.9)	235 (41.3)	531 (44.0)	
Non-Hispanic Black	511 (12.4)	189 (20.4)	357 (21.2)	
Hispanic	832 (16.9)	365 (31.9)	625 (29.3)	
Other race/ethnicity	155 (7.8)	30 (6.4)	74 (5.5)	
Educational attainment, n (%)				<0.0001
<12 years	793 (23.1)	313 (32.8)	728 (40.6)	
High school diploma or equivalent	667 (26.4)	220 (30.3)	402 (27.0)	
Any college	756 (31.6)	202 (26.5)	390 (27.6)	
College graduate or higher	383 (19.0)	84 (10.4)	67 (4.8)	
Household income (as ratio to federal poverty level), mean (SE)	1.68 (0.02)	1.38 (0.03)	1.15 (0.03)	<0.0001
Marital status, n (%)				0.0009
Married or living with partner	1475 (57.4)	457 (53.2)	819 (51.5)	
Never married	637 (26.8)	192 (25.2)	388 (26.4)	
Separated, divorced, or widowed	407 (15.8)	170 (21.7)	80 (22.0)	

Table 2. Household food security and biomarkers of cumulative biological risk: National Health and Nutrition Examination Surveys 2007–2010.

	Food-Secure	Marginal Food Secure	Food-Insecure	p
Systolic blood pressure				
Mean (SE)	118.7 (0.4)	118.9 (0.6)	118.1 (0.6)	0.52
Low-risk (<120 mmHg), n (%)	1212 (52.2)	352 (51.0)	753 (56.6)	0.04
Moderate-risk (120–<150 mmHg), n (%)	692 (28.6)	238 (31.7)	383 (24.3)	
High-risk (≥120 mmHg), n (%)	535 (19.2)	160 (17.3)	317 (19.1)	
Diastolic blood pressure				
Mean (SE)	70.8 (0.6)	70.7 (0.5)	70.7 (0.6)	0.99
Low-risk (<80 mmHg), n (%)	1597 (67.4)	502 (69.6)	954 (68.9)	0.69

Table 2. Cont.

	Food-Secure	Marginal Food Secure	Food-Insecure	p
Moderate-risk (80–<90 mmHg), n (%)	288 (12.0)	87 (12.3)	178 (11.6)	
High-risk (≥90 mmHg), n (%)	554 (20.6)	161 (18.0)	321 (19.5)	
Body mass index (kg/m^2)				
Mean (SE)	28.8 (0.2)	29.6 (0.3)	29.4 (0.3)	0.06
Low-risk (<25 kg/m^2), n (%)	770 (32.8)	216 (29.0)	420 (29.5)	0.19
Moderate-risk (25–<30 kg/m^2), n (%)	829 (31.4)	267 (30.7)	505 (31.7)	
High-risk (≥30 kg/m^2), n (%)	972 (35.7)	328 (40.3)	648 (38.8)	
Glycohemoglobin				
Mean (SE)	5.53% (0.03%)	5.57% (0.04%)	5.66% (0.03%)	0.01
Low-risk (<5.7%), n (%)	1664 (72.6)	497 (67.7)	975 (68.8)	0.18
Moderate-risk (5.7–<6.5%), n (%)	522 (19.2)	198 (23.0)	360 (21.8)	
High-risk (≥6.5%), n (%)	278 (8.2)	90 (9.3)	181 (9.4)	
Total cholesterol (mg/dL)				
Mean (SE)	196.3 (1.0)	193.1 (1.6)	196.5 (1.8)	0.23
Low-risk (<200 mg/dL), n (%)	1277 (53.4)	418 (56.9)	792 (54.2)	0.38
Moderate-risk (200–<240 mg/dL), n (%)	680 (26.9)	222 (27.7)	424 (27.3)	
High-risk (≥240 mg/dL), n (%)	495 (19.7)	139 (15.4)	293 (18.5)	
HDL cholesterol (mg/dL)				
Mean (SE)	51.0 (0.5)	50.0 (0.8)	49.8 (0.6)	0.07
Low-risk (≥60 mg/dL), n (%)	628 (26.2)	177 (23.0)	334 (21.6)	0.05
Moderate-risk (40–<60 mg/dL), n (%)	1207 (48.8)	377 (48.0)	775 (52.1)	
High-risk (<40 mg/dL), n (%)	608 (25.0)	221 (29.0)	398 (26.3)	
Total/HDL cholesterol ratio				

Table 2. Cont.

	Food-Secure	Marginal Food Secure	Food-Insecure	p
Mean (SE)	4.21 (0.04)	4.26 (0.08)	4.34 (0.06)	0.1
Low-risk (<5), n (%)	1838 (76.0)	567 (73.0)	1103 (73.1)	0.24
Moderate-risk (5–<6), n (%)	313 (11.9)	98 (12.7)	187 (11.9)	
High-risk (≥6), n (%)	292 (12.1)	110 (14.3)	217 (15.0)	
C-reactive protein				
Mean (SE)	0.37 (0.01)	0.46 (0.03)	0.46 (0.03)	0.005
Low-risk (<1 mg/L), n (%)	2197 (90.5)	691 (89.5)	1319 (87.8)	0.12
Moderate-risk (1–<3 mg/L), n (%)	232 (8.5)	81 (9.7)	164 (10.5)	
High-risk (≥3 mg/L), n (%)	25 (1.0)	8 (0.8)	29 (1.6)	
Albumin				
Mean (SE)	4.29 (0.01)	4.28 (0.02)	4.22 (0.02)	0.0002
Low-risk (≥3.8 mg/mL), n (%)	2302 (95.8)	731 (94.1)	1380 (92.3)	n/A
Moderate-risk (3.0–<3.8 ug/mL), n (%)	129 (4.2)	41 (5.9)	115 (7.0)	
High-risk <3.0 mg/mL), n (%)	2 (0.1)	0	8 (0.7)	
Estimated Glomerular Filtration Rate (mL/min)				
Mean (SE)	101.1 (0.6)	102.6 (0.9)	102.2 (0.8)	0.3
Low-risk (≥60 mL/min/1.73 m^2), n (%)	2378 (98.5)	751 (97.5)	1455 (97.4)	0.08
Moderate-risk (30–<60 mL/min/1.73 m^2), n (%)	45 (1.3)	16 (2.0)	39 (2.3)	
High-risk (<30 mL/min/1.73 m^2), n (%)	10 (0.2)	5 (0.5)	8 (0.4)	

Table 3. Associations between household food security and cumulative biological risk: National Health and Nutrition Examination Surveys 2007–2010.

	Cumulative Biological Risk Score				Elevated Biological Risk (Score ≥ 3)			
	Age- and Gender-Adjusted		Multivariable-Adjusted		Age- and Gender-Adjusted		Multivariable-Adjusted	
	β	95% CI	β	95% CI	OR	95% CI	OR	95% CI
All adults								
Food secure	Ref.	-	Ref.	-	Ref.	-	Ref.	-
Marginal food secure	0.18	−0.02, 0.38	0.13	−0.05, 0.30	1.26	0.97, 1.64	1.22	0.97, 1.55
Food insecure	0.22	0.11, 0.32	0.14	0.05, 0.22	1.27	1.10, 1.47	1.20	1.05, 1.37
p-trend		0.0002		0.003		0.0003		0.003
Men								
Food secure	Ref.	-	Ref.	-	Ref.	-	Ref.	-
Marginal food secure	0.13	−0.21, 0.47	0.07	−0.25, 0.39	1.25	0.77, 2.02	1.16	0.72, 1.88
Food insecure	0.02	−0.17, 0.22	−0.02	−0.20, 0.15	0.98	0.75, 1.28	0.93	0.72, 1.20
p-trend		0.72		0.86		0.95		0.70
Women								
Food secure	Ref.	-	Ref.	-	Ref.	-	Ref.	-
Marginal food secure	0.23	0.04, 0.42	0.18	0.01, 0.35	1.30	0.94, 1.80	1.31	0.95, 1.79
Food insecure	0.41	0.24, 0.58	0.30	0.14, 0.45	1.71	1.39, 2.10	1.61	1.29, 2.00
p-trend		<0.0001		0.0004		<0.0001		<0.0001

Multivariable model further adjusted for race/ethnicity, educational attainment, household income, and marital status. p-interaction for multivariable-adjusted model of cumulative biological risk by gender was 0.09, and for multivariable-adjusted model of elevated biological risk by gender was 0.03.

4. Discussion

In this national sample of lower-income adults, food insecurity was significantly associated with elevated biological risk in women. Significant associations were also observed between marginal food security and food insecurity and higher cumulative biological risk scores, supporting the notion that marginal food security is similar to food insecurity with respect to adverse health risks [30,49]. These findings suggest that food insecurity, and potentially even experiences of marginal food security are associated with the dysregulation of the major body systems in women [31,50].

To date, only one other study has examined the association between food insecurity and allostatic load. Among 733 Puerto Rican adults in the Boston Puerto Rican Health Study (BPHC), McClain and colleagues found that food insecurity was associated with greater dysregulation of the neuroendocrine and immune systems over a five-year follow-up period, but not with the total allostatic load [42]. The differences in these findings may be due to BPHC study participants being older and already having higher burden of chronic disease at baseline than the general NHANES population, and the lack of neuroendocrine markers within NHANES to investigate this specific association.

The results of the present study also highlight differences in the associations between food insecurity and cumulative biological risk between men and women. Although it is unclear why the associations were significant among women and not significant among men, prior research on the connections between food insecurity and stress may provide insight into these differences. The development of the early Radimer/Cornell hunger scale drew primarily from women's experiences of household food insecurity and demonstrated that one of the earliest indicators was worrying about the household food resources being depleted [51]. This item, now in the U.S. Household Food Security Survey Module, is consistently endorsed by the vast majority of food-insecure households [1]. Qualitative research studies exploring the lived experiences of women have also expanded our understanding of the stressful experience of food insecurity. In a study of predominantly mothers from Quebec City, participants described the "psychological suffering" of food insecurity, as feelings of powerlessness, guilt, shame, feelings of inequity, and fears of being judged or labeled [29]. Mothers from another study in Philadelphia and Minneapolis discussed the continual trade-off between food and other basic necessities due to limited financial resources, characterizing their psychological response as sadness, frustration, resignation, worry and fear, and shame [52]. In quantitative studies of pregnant women, food insecurity has been related to higher reported levels of perceived stress, disordered eating behaviors, trait anxiety, and depressive symptoms, and lower self-esteem and mastery [53,54]. Furthermore, a systematic review on social position, stress, and obesity-related risk factors concluded that women not only perceive stress more strongly but also exhibit a greater physiological response to social stressors when compared to men [55]. At the present time, more qualitative and quantitative research is needed to better understand how men's psychological and physiological responses to food insecurity may differ from the responses of women and how those differences may translate into subsequent implications for health.

Although the present study did not include dietary intake as a mediator or outcome, the inverse association between food insecurity and diet quality has been well-established in prior studies. In a study of food pantry clients in Connecticut, food insecurity was associated with a lower likelihood of consuming fruits, vegetables, and fiber [56]. Another study in Texas found that urban and rural adults experiencing food-related hardship were more likely to consume sugar-sweetened beverages [57]. Within NHANES, a previous analysis showed inverse associations between household food insecurity and adult's dietary quality, as indicated by the lower scores on the Healthy Eating Index and the Alternate Healthy Eating Index [17]. The results from the present study on household food insecurity and some biomarkers of cumulative biological risk, e.g., glycohemoglobin, HDL cholesterol, and systolic blood pressure, may be driven, in part, by differences in dietary quality rather than chronic stress. However, the chronic stress and dietary pathways stemming from food insecurity are not mutually exclusive, and several studies have demonstrated how chronic stress could also alter eating behaviors to negatively impact dietary quality. Chronic stress activates the hypothalamus–pituitary–adrenal

(HPA) axis, which triggers a cascade of hormones, leading to the release of cortisol [32,58]. Cortisol stimulates food intake, particularly foods high in fat and sugar, and can lead to excessive caloric intake and cardiometabolic disease over time [59,60]. When food is available, food-insecure individuals may overeat not simply in response to the physical sensation of hunger, but as physiological and behavioral coping strategies to chronic stress. In a qualitative study by Tester and colleagues, food-insecure parents discussed disordered eating habits observed in their children, including binge eating, hiding food, and night-time eating behaviors not discussed by food-secure parents [61]. To date, there have been few studies on the associations between household food insecurity and disordered eating among adults, with most research limited to children [62,63] and pregnant women [54,63]. Further research, particularly using longitudinal study designs and robust measurement of food insecurity, chronic stress, diet quality and eating behaviors, and multiple systems comprising allostatic load, are needed to better understand the relationship between food insecurity and allostatic load and elucidate the pathways of chronic stress and dietary intake in the general population.

The results of this study have potential clinical and policy implications. The finding that even marginal food security was associated with higher cumulative biological risk scores among women is consistent with research showing that children in households with marginal food security exhibit poorer health and developmental outcomes than children in food-secure households [49]. Screening of food insecurity in health care settings using the validated Hunger Vital Sign measure can help identify adults with marginal food security for the referral to community food programs and social services [64]. Economic and nutrition programs and policies aimed at improving food security should also ensure that they are reaching populations with marginal food security to ameliorate any adverse health outcomes related to anxiety over household food resources and milder indicators of food insecurity that precede behavioral adaptations.

The primary limitation of this study is the cross-sectional design, which limits the ability to make causal inferences about the findings. Although we restricted the analytic sample to adults with household incomes ≤300% of the federal poverty level and further adjusted for household income in statistical analyses, we cannot rule out the potential for residual confounding by income or other proxies of socioeconomic status, which are known to have salient relationships with health behaviors, physical health, and mental health [65]. Relatedly, we cannot exclude the potential for reverse causation, where elevated biological risk might lead to increased health care costs, subsequently influencing household food security. Another limitation is the assessment of household food security in NHANES, which occurs over a 12-month period. By aggregating over the past year, our understanding is limited as to whether experiences of food insecurity were episodic or chronic. Prior research suggests food-insecure individuals may exhibit disordered eating behaviors corresponding to a monthly cycle of when food is plentiful or scarce [61,66]. How food insecurity-induced disordered eating is associated with cumulative biological risk is unknown given the long period over which food insecurity indicators are measured. Further, no information is available on the history of food insecurity in the family, as cumulative experiences of food insecurity experienced before the study window may have also contributed to biological risk.

Another important limitation of the NHANES dataset is that it lacks neuroendocrine markers to better measure allostatic load. Further research is needed to understand how food insecurity is associated with neuroendocrine dysregulation and the primary system of allostatic load to better understand its relationship with chronic stress.

5. Conclusions

Understanding the mechanisms underlying food insecurity and adverse health outcomes is critical to designing effective interventions to reduce socioeconomic and health disparities. The findings of the present study show higher cumulative biological risk scores among marginally food-secure and food-insecure women, providing additional evidence to suggest even mild experiences of food insecurity may affect physical and mental health outcomes through chronic stress. Further research is needed to understand why these associations were not observed in men and to better elucidate the role of food insecurity in promoting chronic stress independent of other forms of socioeconomic adversity in women.

Supplementary Materials: The following are available online at http://www.mdpi.com/2072-6643/12/5/1517/s1, Table S1: Associations between household food security (using the four-category variable) and cumulative biological risk: National Health and Nutrition Examination Surveys 2007–2010.

Author Contributions: Conceptualization, C.W.L. and M.S.Z.; Formal analysis, C.W.L.; Writing—original draft, C.W.L. and M.S.Z.; Writing—reviewing & editing, C.W.L. and M.S.Z. All authors have read and agreed to the published version of the manuscript.

Funding: C.W.L. was supported by grant 4R00 HD084758 from NIH.

Conflicts of Interest: The authors have no conflict of interest to disclose.

References

1. Coleman-Jensen, A.; Rabbitt, M.P.; Gregory, C.A.; Singh, A. *Household Food Security in the United States in 2018, ERR-270*; U.S. Department of Agriculture, Economic Research Service: Washington, DC, USA 2019.
2. Pan, L.; Sherry, B.; Njai, R.; Blanck, H.M. Food insecurity is associated with obesity among US adults in 12 states. *J. Acad. Nutr. Diet.* **2012**, *112*, 1403–1409. [CrossRef] [PubMed]
3. Franklin, E.; Jones, A.; Love, D.; Puckett, S.; Macklin, J.; White-Means, S. Exploring Mediators of Food Insecurity and Obesity: A Review of Recent Literature. *J. Community Health* **2012**, *37*, 253–264. [CrossRef] [PubMed]
4. Adams, E.J.; Grummer-Strawn, L.; Chavez, G. Food Insecurity Is Associated with Increased Risk of Obesity in California Women. *J. Nutr.* **2003**, *133*, 1070–1074. [CrossRef] [PubMed]
5. Seligman, H.K.; Laraia, B.A.; Kushel, M. Food insecurity is associated with chronic disease among low-income NHANES participants. *J. Nutr.* **2009**, *140*, 304–310. [CrossRef] [PubMed]
6. Seligman, H.K.; Bindman, A.B.; Vittinghoff, E.; Kanaya, A.M.; Kushel, M. Food Insecurity is Associated with Diabetes Mellitus: Results from the National Health Examination and Nutrition Examination Survey (NHANES) 1999–2002. *J. Gen. Intern. Med.* **2007**, *22*, 1018–1023. [CrossRef]
7. Fitzgerald, N.; Hromi-Fiedler, A.; Segura-Pérez, S.; Pérez-Escamilla, R. Food insecurity is related to increased risk of type 2 diabetes among Latinas. *Ethn. Dis.* **2011**, *21*, 328–334.
8. Seligman, H.K.; Davis, T.C.; Schillinger, D.; Wolf, M.S. Food insecurity is associated with hypoglycemia and poor diabetes self-management in a low-income sample with diabetes. *J. Health Care Poor Underserved* **2010**, *21*, 1227–1233.
9. Berkowitz, S.A.; Baggett, T.P.; Wexler, D.J.; Huskey, K.W.; Wee, C.C. Food Insecurity and Metabolic Control Among U.S. Adults with Diabetes. *Diabetes Care* **2013**, *36*, 3093–3099. [CrossRef]
10. Stuff, J.E.; Casey, P.H.; Connell, C.; Champagne, C.M.; Gossett, J.M.; Harsha, D.; McCabe-Sellers, B.; Robbins, J.; Simpson, P.M.; Szeto, K.L.; et al. Household Food Insecurity and Obesity, Chronic Disease, and Chronic Disease Risk Factors. *J. Hunger. Environ. Nutr.* **2007**, *1*, 43–62. [CrossRef]
11. Gao, X.; Scott, T.; Falcon, L.M.; Wilde, P.E.; Tucker, K.L. Food insecurity and cognitive function in Puerto Rican adults. *Am. J. Clin. Nutr.* **2009**, *89*, 1197–1203. [CrossRef]
12. Portela-Parra, E.T.; Leung, C.W. Food Insecurity Is Associated with Lower Cognitive Functioning in a National Sample of Older Adults. *J. Nutr.* **2019**, *149*, 1812–1817. [CrossRef] [PubMed]
13. Leung, C.W.; Epel, E.S.; Willett, W.C.; Rimm, E.B.; Laraia, B.A. Household Food Insecurity Is Positively Associated with Depression among Low-Income Supplemental Nutrition Assistance Program Participants and Income-Eligible Nonparticipants. *J. Nutr.* **2014**, *145*, 622–627. [CrossRef] [PubMed]
14. Whitaker, R.C.; Phillips, S.M.; Orzol, S.M. Food Insecurity and the Risks of Depression and Anxiety in Mothers and Behavior Problems in their Preschool-Aged Children. *Pediatrics* **2006**, *118*, e859–e868. [CrossRef] [PubMed]
15. Stuff, J.E.; Casey, P.H.; Szeto, K.L.; Gossett, J.M.; Robbins, J.; Simpson, P.M.; Connell, C.; Bogle, M.L. Household Food Insecurity Is Associated with Adult Health Status. *J. Nutr.* **2004**, *134*, 2330–2335. [CrossRef] [PubMed]
16. Gucciardi, E.; Vogt, J.A.; DeMelo, M.; Stewart, D.E. Exploration of the Relationship Between Household Food Insecurity and Diabetes in Canada. *Diabetes Care* **2009**, *32*, 2218–2224. [CrossRef]

17. Leung, C.W.; Epel, E.S.; Ritchie, L.D.; Crawford, P.B.; Laraia, B.A. Food Insecurity Is Inversely Associated with Diet Quality of Lower-Income Adults. *J. Acad. Nutr. Diet.* **2014**, *114*, 1943–1953.e2. [CrossRef]
18. Mello, J.A.; Gans, K.; Risica, P.M.; Kirtania, U.; Strolla, L.O.; Fournier, L. How Is Food Insecurity Associated with Dietary Behaviors? An Analysis with Low-Income, Ethnically Diverse Participants in a Nutrition Intervention Study. *J. Am. Diet. Assoc.* **2010**, *110*, 1906–1911. [CrossRef]
19. Hanson, K.L.; Connor, L.M. Food insecurity and dietary quality in US adults and children: A systematic review. *Am. J. Clin. Nutr.* **2014**, *100*, 684–692. [CrossRef]
20. To, Q.G.; Frongillo, E.A.; Gallegos, D.; Moore, J.B. Household food insecurity is associated with less physical activity among children and adults in the U.S. population. *J. Nutr.* **2014**, *144*, 1797–1802. [CrossRef]
21. Kim-Mozeleski, J.E.; Tsoh, J.Y. Cigarette Smoking Among Socioeconomically Disadvantaged Young Adults in Association with Food Insecurity and Other Factors. *Prev. Chronic Dis.* **2016**, *13*, E08.
22. Kim-Mozeleski, J.E.; Seligman, H.K.; Yen, I.H.; Shaw, S.J.; Buchanan, D.R.; Tsoh, J.Y. Changes in Food Insecurity and Smoking Status over Time: Analysis of the 2003 and 2015 Panel Study of Income Dynamics. *Am. J. Health Promot.* **2018**, *33*, 698–707. [CrossRef] [PubMed]
23. Armour, B.S.; Pitts, M.M.; Lee, C.-W. Cigarette Smoking and Food Insecurity among Low-Income Families in the United States, 2001. *Am. J. Health Promot.* **2008**, *22*, 386–392. [CrossRef] [PubMed]
24. Ding, M.; Keiley, M.K.; Garza, K.B.; Duffy, P.A.; Zizza, C.A. Food Insecurity Is Associated with Poor Sleep Outcomes among US Adults. *J. Nutr.* **2014**, *145*, 615–621. [CrossRef] [PubMed]
25. Liu, Y.; Njai, R.S.; Greenlund, K.J.; Chapman, D.P.; Croft, J.B. Relationships Between Housing and Food Insecurity, Frequent Mental Distress, and Insufficient Sleep Among Adults in 12 US States, 2009. *Prev. Chronic Dis.* **2014**, *11*, E37. [CrossRef]
26. Hromi-Fiedler, A.; Bermúdez-Millán, A.; Segura-Pérez, S.; Pérez-Escamilla, R. Household food insecurity is associated with depressive symptoms among low-income pregnant Latinas. *Matern. Child Nutr.* **2010**, *7*, 421–430. [CrossRef]
27. Lent, M.D.; Petrovic, L.E.; Swanson, J.A.; Olson, C.M. Maternal Mental Health and the Persistence of Food Insecurity in Poor Rural Families. *J. Health Care Poor Underserved* **2009**, *20*, 645–661. [CrossRef]
28. Siefert, K.A.; Heflin, C.M.; Corcoran, M.E.; Williams, D.R. Food insufficiency and physical and mental health in a longitudinal survey of welfare recipients. *J. Health Soc. Behav.* **2004**, *45*, 171–186. [CrossRef]
29. Hamelin, A.-M.; Beaudry, M.; Habicht, J.-P. Characterization of household food insecurity in Québec: Food and feelings. *Soc. Sci. Med.* **2002**, *54*, 119–132. [CrossRef]
30. Lee, J.S.; Gundersen, C.; Cook, J.; Laraia, B.; Johnson, M.A. Food Insecurity and Health across the Lifespan12. *Adv. Nutr.* **2012**, *3*, 744–745. [CrossRef]
31. McEwen, B.; Seeman, T.E. Available online: https://macses.ucsf.edu/research/allostatic/allostatic.php#stress (accessed on 23 May 2019).
32. McEwen, B.S. Stress, adaptation, and disease. Allostasis and allostatic load. *Ann. N. Y. Acad. Sci.* **1998**, *840*, 33–44. [CrossRef]
33. Duong, M.; Bingham, B.A.; Aldana, P.C.; Chung, S.T.; E Sumner, A. Variation in the Calculation of Allostatic Load Score: 21 Examples from NHANES. *J. Racial Ethn. Health Disparities* **2016**, *4*, 455–461. [CrossRef] [PubMed]
34. Seeman, T.E.; McEwen, B.S.; Rowe, J.W.; Singer, B.H. Allostatic load as a marker of cumulative biological risk: MacArthur studies of successful aging. *Proc. Natl. Acad. Sci. USA* **2001**, *98*, 4770–4775. [CrossRef] [PubMed]
35. Merkin, S.S.; Karlamangla, A.; Roux, A.V.D.; Shrager, S.; Seeman, T.E. Life course socioeconomic status and longitudinal accumulation of allostatic load in adulthood: Multi-ethnic study of atherosclerosis. *Am. J. Public Health* **2014**, *104*, e48–e55. [CrossRef] [PubMed]
36. McCrory, C.; Fiorito, G.; Cheallaigh, C.N.; Polidoro, S.; Karisola, P.; Alenius, H.; Layte, R.; Seeman, T.; Vineis, P.; Kenny, R.A. How does socio-economic position (SEP) get biologically embedded? A comparison of allostatic load and the epigenetic clock(s). *Psychoneuroendocrinology* **2019**, *104*, 64–73. [CrossRef]
37. Gruenewald, T.L.; Karlamangla, A.S.; Hu, P.; Stein-Merkin, S.; Crandall, C.; Koretz, B.; Seeman, T.E. History of socioeconomic disadvantage and allostatic load in later life. *Soc. Sci. Med.* **2011**, *74*, 75–83. [CrossRef]
38. Seeman, T.; Epel, E.; Gruenewald, T.; Karlamangla, A.; McEwen, B.S. Socio-economic differentials in peripheral biology: Cumulative allostatic load. *Ann. N. Y. Acad. Sci.* **2010**, *1186*, 223–239. [CrossRef]

39. Upchurch, D.M.; Stein, J.; Greendale, G.A.; Chyu, L.; Tseng, C.-H.; Huang, M.-H.; Lewis, T.T.; Kravitz, H.M.; Seeman, T. A Longitudinal Investigation of Race, Socioeconomic Status, and Psychosocial Mediators of Allostatic Load in Midlife Women. *Psychosom. Med.* **2015**, *77*, 402–412. [CrossRef]
40. Geronimus, A.T.; Hicken, M.; Keene, D.; Bound, J. "Weathering" and Age Patterns of Allostatic Load Scores Among Blacks and Whites in the United States. *Am. J. Public Health* **2006**, *96*, 826–833. [CrossRef]
41. Duru, O.K.; Harawa, N.T.; Kermah, D.; Norris, K.C. Allostatic load burden and racial disparities in mortality. *J. Natl. Med Assoc.* **2012**, *104*, 89–95. [CrossRef]
42. McClain, A.C.; Xiao, R.S.; Gao, X.; Tucker, K.L.; Falcon, L.M.; Mattei, J. Food Insecurity and Odds of High Allostatic Load in Puerto Rican Adults. *Psychosom. Med.* **2018**, *80*, 733–741. [CrossRef]
43. Gamba, R.J.; Leung, C.W.; Guendelman, S.; Lahiff, M.; Laraia, B.A. Household Food Insecurity Is Not Associated with Overall Diet Quality Among Pregnant Women in NHANES 1999–2008. *Matern. Child Health J.* **2016**, *20*, 2348–2356. [CrossRef] [PubMed]
44. U.S. Household Food Security Survey Module: Three-Stage Design, With Screeners. Available online: ers.usda.gov/media/8271/hh2012.pdf (accessed on 22 May 2020).
45. Chen, X.; Redline, S.; Shields, A.E.; Williams, D.R.; Williams, M.A. Associations of allostatic load with sleep apnea, insomnia, short sleep duration, and other sleep disturbances: Findings from the National Health and Nutrition Examination Survey 2005 to 2008. *Ann. Epidemiol.* **2014**, *24*, 612–619. [CrossRef] [PubMed]
46. Parente, V.; Hale, L.; Palermo, T. Association between breast cancer and allostatic load by race: National Health and Nutrition Examination Survey 1999–2008. *Psycho-Oncology* **2012**, *22*, 621–628. [CrossRef] [PubMed]
47. Rodriquez, E.J.; Livaudais-Toman, J.; Gregorich, S.E.; Jackson, J.S.; Nápoles, A.M.; Perez-Stable, E.J. Relationships between allostatic load, unhealthy behaviors, and depressive disorder in U.S. adults, 2005–2012 NHANES *Prev. Med.* **2018**, *110*, 9–15. [CrossRef] [PubMed]
48. Morrison, S.; Shenassa, E.D.; Mendola, P.; Wu, T.; Schoendorf, K. Allostatic load may not be associated with chronic stress in pregnant women, NHANES 1999–2006. *Ann. Epidemiol.* **2013**, *23*, 294–297. [CrossRef]
49. Cook, J.T.; Black, M.; Chilton, M.; Cutts, D.; De Cuba, S.E.; Heeren, T.; Rose-Jacobs, R.; Sandel, M.; Casey, P.H.; Coleman, S.; et al. Are Food Insecurity's Health Impacts Underestimated in the U.S. Population? Marginal Food Security Also Predicts Adverse Health Outcomes in Young U.S. Children and Mothers123. *Adv. Nutr.* **2013**, *4*, 51–61. [CrossRef]
50. Meijer, J. Stress in the Relation between Trait and State Anxiety. *Psychol. Rep.* **2001**, *88*, 947–964. [CrossRef]
51. Radimer, K.L.; Olson, C.M.; Greene, J.C.; Campbell, C.C.; Habicht, J.-P. Understanding hunger and developing indicators to assess it in women and children. *J. Nutr. Educ.* **1992**, *24*, 36S–44S. [CrossRef]
52. Knowles, M.; Rabinowich, J.; Ettinger de Cuba, S.; Cutts, D.B.; Chilton, M. "Do You Wanna Breathe or Eat?": Parent Perspectives on Child Health Consequences of Food Insecurity, Trade-Offs, and Toxic Stress. *Matern. Child Health J.* **2016**, *20*, 25–32. [CrossRef]
53. Laraia, B.A.; Siega-Riz, A.M.; Gundersen, C.; Dole, N. Psychosocial factors and socioeconomic indicators are associated with household food insecurity among pregnant women. *J. Nutr.* **2006**, *136*, 177–182. [CrossRef]
54. Laraia, B.; Vinikoor-Imler, L.C.; Siega-Riz, A.M. Food insecurity during pregnancy leads to stress, disordered eating, and greater postpartum weight among overweight women. *Obesity* **2015**, *23*, 1303–1311. [CrossRef] [PubMed]
55. Moore, C.J.; Cunningham, S. Social Position, Psychological Stress, and Obesity: A Systematic Review. *J. Acad. Nutr. Diet.* **2012**, *112*, 518–526. [CrossRef] [PubMed]
56. Robaina, K.A.; Martin, K.S. Food Insecurity, Poor Diet Quality, and Obesity among Food Pantry Participants in Hartford, CT. *J. Nutr. Educ. Behav.* **2013**, *45*, 159–164. [CrossRef] [PubMed]
57. Sharkey, J.R.; Johnson, C.M.; Dean, W.R. Less-healthy eating behaviors have a greater association with a high level of sugar-sweetened beverage consumption among rural adults than among urban adults. *Food Nutr. Res.* **2011**, *55*, 5819. [CrossRef] [PubMed]
58. Cohen, S.; Janicki-Deverts, D.; Miller, G.E. Psychological Stress and Disease. *JAMA* **2007**, *298*, 1685–1687. [CrossRef]
59. Adam, T.C.; Epel, E. Stress, eating and the reward system. *Physiol. Behav.* **2007**, *91*, 449–458. [CrossRef]
60. Dallman, M.F. Stress-induced obesity and the emotional nervous system. *Trends Endocrinol. Metab.* **2009**, *21*, 159–165. [CrossRef]

61. Tester, J.; Lang, T.C.; Laraia, B.A. Disordered eating behaviours and food insecurity: A qualitative study about children with obesity in low-income households. *Obes. Res. Clin. Pract.* **2015**, *10*, 544–552. [CrossRef]
62. Oberle, M.M.; Willson, S.R.; Gross, A.C.; Kelly, A.S.; Fox, C.K. Relationships among Child Eating Behaviors and Household Food Insecurity in Youth with Obesity. *Child. Obes.* **2019**, *15*, 298–305. [CrossRef]
63. Laraia, B.; Epel, E.; Siega-Riz, A.M. Food insecurity with past experience of restrained eating is a recipe for increased gestational weight gain. *Appetite* **2013**, *65*, 178–184. [CrossRef]
64. Gundersen, C.; Engelhard, E.E.; Crumbaugh, A.S.; Seligman, H.K. Brief assessment of food insecurity accurately identifies high-risk US adults. *Public Health Nutr.* **2017**, *20*, 1367–1371. [CrossRef] [PubMed]
65. Adler, N.E.; Boyce, T.; Chesney, M.A.; Cohen, S.; Folkman, S.; Kahn, R.L.; Syme, S.L. Socioeconomic status and health. The challenge of the gradient. *Am. Psychol.* **1994**, *49*, 15–24. [CrossRef] [PubMed]
66. Bruening, M.; MacLehose, R.; Loth, K.A.; Story, M.; Neumark-Sztainer, D. Feeding a Family in a Recession: Food Insecurity Among Minnesota Parents. *Am. J. Public Health* **2012**, *102*, 520–526. [CrossRef] [PubMed]

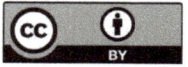

© 2020 by the authors. Licensee MDPI, Basel, Switzerland. This article is an open access article distributed under the terms and conditions of the Creative Commons Attribution (CC BY) license (http://creativecommons.org/licenses/by/4.0/).

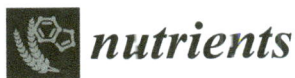

Article

Food Insecurity and COVID-19: Disparities in Early Effects for US Adults

Julia A. Wolfson [1,2,*] and Cindy W. Leung [2]

[1] Department of Health Management and Policy, University of Michigan School of Public Health, Ann Arbor, MI 48109, USA
[2] Department of Nutritional Sciences, University of Michigan School of Public Health, Ann Arbor, MI 48109, USA; cinleung@umich.edu
* Correspondence: jwolfson@umich.edu; Tel.: +1-734-764-6036

Received: 15 May 2020; Accepted: 29 May 2020; Published: 2 June 2020

Abstract: The COVID-19 pandemic has dramatically increased food insecurity in the United States (US). The objective of this study was to understand the early effects of the COVID-19 pandemic among low-income adults in the US as social distancing measures began to be implemented. On 19–24 March 2020 we fielded a national, web-based survey (53% response rate) among adults with <250% of the federal poverty line in the US ($N = 1478$). Measures included household food security status and COVID-19-related basic needs challenges. Overall, 36% of low-income adults in the US were food secure, 20% had marginal food security, and 44% were food insecure. Less than one in five (18.3%) of adults with very low food security reported being able to comply with public health recommendations to purchase two weeks of food at a time. For every basic needs challenge, food-insecure adults were significantly more likely to report facing that challenge, with a clear gradient effect based on severity of food security. The short-term effects of the COVID-19 pandemic are magnifying existing disparities and disproportionately affecting low-income, food-insecure households that already struggle to meet basic needs. A robust, comprehensive policy response is needed to mitigate food insecurity as the pandemic progresses.

Keywords: covid-19; food insecurity; low-income adults; disparities; survey

1. Introduction

Food insecurity, a condition defined by limited or uncertain access to sufficient, nutritious food for an active, healthy life, disproportionately affects low-income communities and communities of color [1]. Food is a core social determinant of health [2] and food insecurity is associated with numerous poor health outcomes in both the short and long term [3–9]. The unprecedented COVID-19 pandemic, and the associated social and economic response [10] (e.g., school closures, stay at home orders, business closures, and job losses) have the potential to dramatically increase food insecurity and its related health disparities among already at-risk populations. Early evidence suggests that food insecurity is indeed rapidly rising above pre-epidemic levels [11–13]. Household food insecurity has risen from 11% in 2013 to 38% in March 2020; in April 2020, 35% of households with a child aged 18 and under were food insecure [12,13]. Households already struggling with food insecurity may find their current situations exacerbated by COVID-19 with fewer resources to comply with social distancing recommendations. Food insecure individuals also may have less flexibility in their jobs to allow them to earn income while staying home, or may be at higher risk of losing their jobs completely, thereby decreasing (or eliminating) their incomes. These factors may put food insecure households both at higher risk of contracting COVID-19 and of greater food insecurity due to the economic effects of COVID-19 mitigation efforts.

In addition to the long-term health and economic effects of the COVID-19 pandemic, it is important to understand the immediate impact of social distancing measures to fight COVID-19 on vulnerable populations who already struggle to meet their basic needs. To do so, we fielded a national survey of low-income adults in the US on 19–24 March 2020 to understand the immediate effects of how COVID-19 was impacting low-income Americans and any disparities in its effects based on food security status.

2. Materials and Methods

We designed a web-based (Qualtrics) survey to measure the initial effects of COVID-19 on low-income adults in the United States (US) in mid-March 2020, just as some states were beginning to implement school closures and "stay at home" orders. The web-based survey was formatted to be accessible when access both via smart phones and on a personal computer or laptop. The survey was fielded using TurkPrime, an online crowdsourcing platform that is designed to be used for academic research [14]. TurkPrime allows researchers to use quotas to recruit a sample that matches their specific needs and has been used in numerous academic studies from a variety of disciplines published in the peer-reviewed literature [15–19]. In the present study, we used a census matched panel of US adults (matched on age, gender, and race/ethnicity to the overall population) and limited the sample to low-income adults with household incomes <250% of the federal poverty line (FPL). The FPL is calculated based on both household size and annual household income. For example, 100% of the FPL for a four-person household is $26,200, and 250% of the FPL for a four-person household is $655,000 per year. The annual income for a two-person household at 250% FPL is $43,100.

The survey was open to participants on 19–24 March 2020. We invited 2840 eligible panel members to participate and 1497 participants completed the survey (53% completion rate). Additional exclusions included participants who completed the survey in <4 min ($n = 7$), indicated they did not live in the US ($n = 3$), and were missing food insecurity data ($n = 9$) resulting in a final analytic sample size of 1478. Forty-four percent of participants took the survey on a personal computer or laptop and 56% took the survey on a smart phone or mobile device. This study was determined to be exempt by the Institutional Review Board at the University of Michigan.

2.1. Measures

Food security: Food security status over the past 30 days was measured using the 18-item US Household Food Security Module [20]. Questions are ordered by severity and include three levels of screening for adults, and an additional level of questions only for households with children. Affirmative responses to questions were summed to create a total food security score (out of 10 for adults and out of 18 for households with children). Food security categories (high, marginal, low, very low) were assigned according to US Department of Agriculture scoring guidelines [21]. The term food insecurity refers to the combined categories of low and very low food security.

COVID-19-related basic needs challenges: We inquired about challenges related to meeting basic needs people may have faced in the early weeks of the US COVID-19 epidemic and response. First, we asked about participants' ability to comply with recommendations to purchase two weeks of food (which was recommended by public health efforts to limit grocery shopping trip and facilitate social distancing). We also asked participants whether they had encountered any of the following challenges due to the coronavirus: the ability to feed their family, availability of household items such as toilet paper, access to healthcare, access to medications, the ability to pay bills, ability to rent or pay mortgages, whether they had been unable to work due to lack of childcare, and whether they had been unable to work due to illness.

COVID-19-related workplace reactions: At the time of data collection, some, but not all, states had begun issuing stay at home orders and mandatory business closures. Even in states without stay at home mandates, some businesses were making adjustments to operations due to COVID-19. We asked working adults (i.e., those with full- or part-time work outside the home) what their employer was doing to adjust to the pandemic. Specifically, we asked "Workplaces in the US are adjusting to the coronavirus situation in different ways. What is your workplace doing to adjust?" Participants were given the following response options: nothing, my workplace is proceeding as normal; all employees are encouraged to work at home; all employees must work at home; essential employees must come in to work but others can work from home; hours are being reduced for hourly employees; my place of employment has temporarily closed due to the coronavirus; my place of employment has closed and I have been laid off; work is busier and employees need to work longer hours; other.

Expected impact of COVID-19 on employment and income: We asked working adults what they expected would happen at their job if they or someone in their family became ill with COVID-19. Response options focused on whether they would be able to stay home, whether they had vacation or sick days they could use, and what they expected would happen if they missed work due to illness.

2.2. Analysis

All analyses were conducted in 2020 with Stata, Version 15 (StataCorp LP, College Station TX, USA). First, we describe the socio-demographic characteristics of the study sample overall and by food security status using cross tabulations and chi-squared tests of significant differences. Next, we examine differences in COVID-19-related basic needs and workplace challenges (among participants working full or part time), by food security status using cross tabulations. Missing data was treated using listwise deletion. Significant differences by food security status were assessed using chi-squared tests. All tests were two tailed and significance was considered at $p < 0.05$.

3. Results

The characteristics of the sample of low-income adults are presented in Table 1. Overall, 36% of this sample was food secure, 20% had marginal food security, and 44% were food insecure (17% low food security; 27% very low food security). Individuals with low or very low food security were more likely to be non-Hispanic Black or Hispanic, to have children in the home, and have less than a college education. Individuals with very low food insecurity were also more likely to rent their homes, not have health insurance or have Medicaid, and were more likely to be receiving SNAP benefits. The distribution of the sample by state of residence is shown in Appendix A.

Table 1. Demographic characteristics of the study sample overall and by food security status ($n = 1478$).

	Overall	Food Security Status				p-Value
		High	Marginal	Low	Very Low	
	n (%) [a]	n (%) [b]	n (%) [b]	n (%) [b]	n (%) [b]	
Total	1478 (100)	532 (36)	290 (20)	256 (17)	400 (27)	
Age						
18–39	635 (43)	168 (26)	116 (18)	140 (22)	211 (33)	<0.001
40–59	429 (29)	152 (35)	88 (21)	62 (14)	127 (30)	
≥60	414 (28)	212 (51)	86 (21)	54 (13)	62 (15)	
Sex						
Male	733 (50)	285 (39)	135 (18)	128 (17)	185 (25)	0.100
Female	745 (50)	247 (33)	155 (21)	128 (17)	215 (29)	
Race/ethnicity						
NH White	990 (67)	384 (39)	185 (19)	160 (16)	261 (26)	0.026
NH Black	161 (11)	47 (29)	36 (22)	36 (22)	42 (26)	
Hispanic	186 (13)	55 (30)	35 (19)	39 (21)	57 (31)	
Asian	73 (5)	24 (33)	23 (32)	11 (15)	15 (21)	
Other	68 (5)	22 (32)	11 (16)	10 (15)	25 (37)	
Household Size						
1–3 people	1113 (75)	416 (37)	219 (20)	177 (16)	301 (27)	0.054
≥4 people	365 (25)	116 (32)	71 (19)	79 (22)	99 (27)	

Table 1. Cont.

	Overall	Food Security Status				p-Value
		High	Marginal	Low	Very Low	
	n (%) [a]	n (%) [b]	n (%) [b]	n (%) [b]	n (%) [b]	
Marital Status						
Single, never married	564 (38)	199 (35)	108 (19)	118 (21)	139 (35)	<0.001
Married	448 (30)	180 (40)	91 (20)	68 (15)	109 (24)	
Separated, divorced, widowed	311 (21)	124 (40)	58 (19)	43 (14)	86 (28)	
Living with a partner	150 (10)	27 (18)	32 (21)	26 (17)	65 (43)	
Children < 18 years in home						
Yes	445 (30)	120 (27)	85 (19)	92 (21)	148 (33)	<0.001
No	1033 (70)	412 (40)	205 (20)	164 (16)	252 (24)	
Income						
<$35,000/year	894 (60)	297 (33)	175 (20)	165 (18)	257 (29)	0.015
$35,000 ≤ $59,000/year	418 (28)	162 (39)	75 (18)	69 (17)	112 (27)	
≥$59,000/year	166 (11)	73 (44)	40 (24)	22 (13)	31 (19)	
Education						
High school/GED	439 (30)	122 (28)	83 (19)	91 (21)	143 (33)	<0.001
Some college	524 (35)	197 (38)	104 (29)	75 (14)	148 (28)	
College/grad degree	515 (35)	213 (41)	103 (20)	90 (17)	109 (21)	
Employment status						
Full time job (hourly or salary)	408 (29)	139 (34)	68 (17)	81 (20)	120 (29)	0.002
Part time job (hourly or salary)	239 (17)	83 (35)	51 (21)	41 (17)	64 (27)	
Not working, looking for work	197 (14)	58 (29)	38 (19)	38 (19)	63 (32)	
Not working, not looking for work	415 (30)	186 (45)	86 (21)	55 (13)	88 (21)	
Home-maker	141 (10)	46 (33)	27 (19)	21 (15)	47 (33)	
Student						
Yes	95 (6)	29 (31)	26 (27)	20 (21)	20 (21)	0.106
No	1383 (94)	503 (36)	264 (19)	236 (17)	380 (27)	
Home ownership						
Rent	744 (50)	201 (27)	144 (19)	154 (21)	245 (33)	<0.001
Own	538 (43)	287 (45)	128 (20)	89 (14)	134 (21)	
Other	96 (7)	44 (46)	18 (19)	13 (14)	21 (22)	
Health insurance						
None	231 (16)	68 (29)	40 (17)	35 (15)	88 (38)	<0.001
Yes, through work	260 (18)	97 (37)	45 (17)	57 (22)	61 (23)	
Yes, Medicare	437 (30)	189 (43)	83 (19)	73 (17)	92 (21)	
Yes, Medicaid	338 (23)	91 (27)	73 (22)	55 (16)	119 (35)	
Yes, other	212 (14)	87 (41)	49 (23)	35 (17)	40 (19)	
Political party affiliation						
Republican	396 (27)	174 (44)	76 (19)	50 (13)	96 (24)	0.004
Democrat	594 (40)	190 (32)	124 (21)	115 (19)	165 (28)	
Independent	488 (33)	168 (34)	90 (18)	91 (19)	139 (28)	
SNAP benefits						
No	1065 (72)	452 (42)	207 (19)	182 (17)	224 (21)	<0.001
Yes	413 (28)	80 (19)	83 (20)	74 (18)	176 (43)	
Region of residence						
Northeast	273 (18)	90 (33)	57 (21)	59 (22)	67 (25)	0.406
Midwest	332 (22)	127 (38)	69 (21)	47 (14)	89 (27)	
South	542 (37)	196 (36)	95 (18)	97 (18)	154 (28)	
West	331 (22)	119 (36)	69 (21)	53 (16)	90 (27)	

[a] Column percentage; [b] Row percentage.

Figure 1 shows the ability of low-income US adults to comply with public health recommendations to stock up on two weeks of food to avoid excess grocery store trips and facilitate social distancing. Nearly 2/3 (60%) of food-secure, low-income adults reported being able to comply with that recommendation, compared to less than one in five (18.8%) of low-income adults with very low food security. Adults with very low food security were more likely to report their local stores were sold out of products, and not being able to afford to purchase an extra two weeks of food at one time.

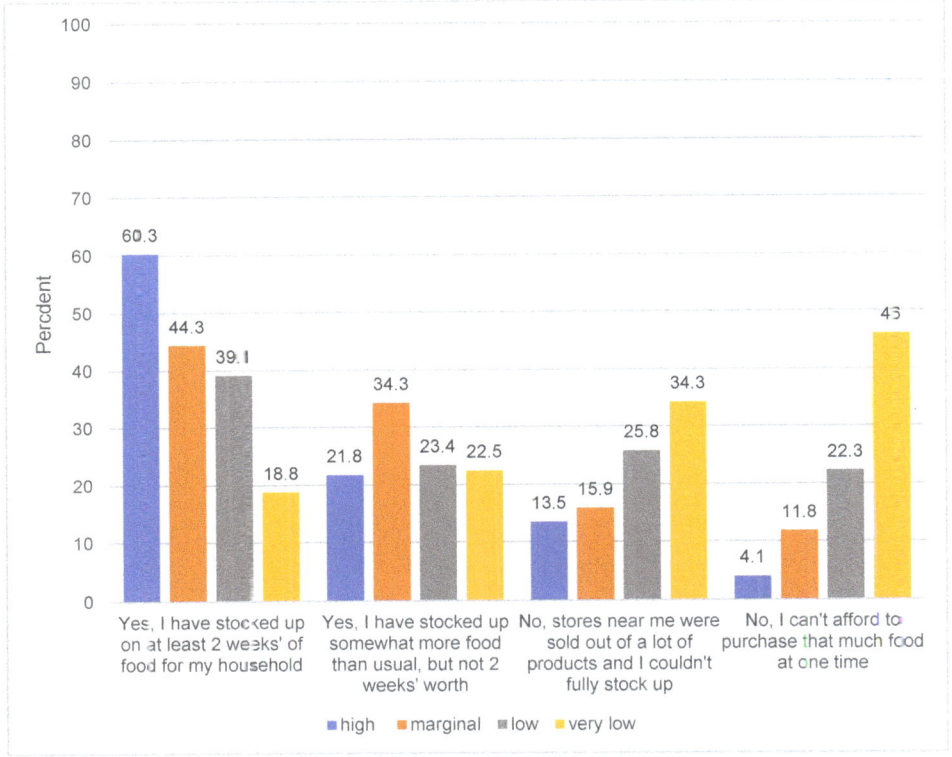

Figure 1. Ability to comply with recommendation to stock up on two weeks of food among low-income US adults, by food security status ($n = 1478$). Question text: "Experts have recommended stocking up on two weeks of food for your household to prepare for the coronavirus. Have you been able to do this" [Please check all that apply. One respondent was missing data for this question and was excluded from analysis. Differences within each response option by food security status are significant at $p < 0.001$ based on chi-squared tests.

Potential basic needs challenges related to COVID-19 are displayed in Figure 2. For every challenge asked about, food-insecure adults were significantly more likely to report dealing with that challenge, with a clear gradient effect based on severity of food security status. Strikingly, 41.3% of adults with very low food security reported not having enough food to feed themselves or their family compared to 10.7% of adults with low food security, 3.1% of adults with marginal food security and 1.6% of adults with high food security. Half (49.9%) of adults with very low food security did not have enough money to pay their bills compared to 36.9% of those with low food security, 23.1% of those with marginal food security and 8.8% of food secure adults.

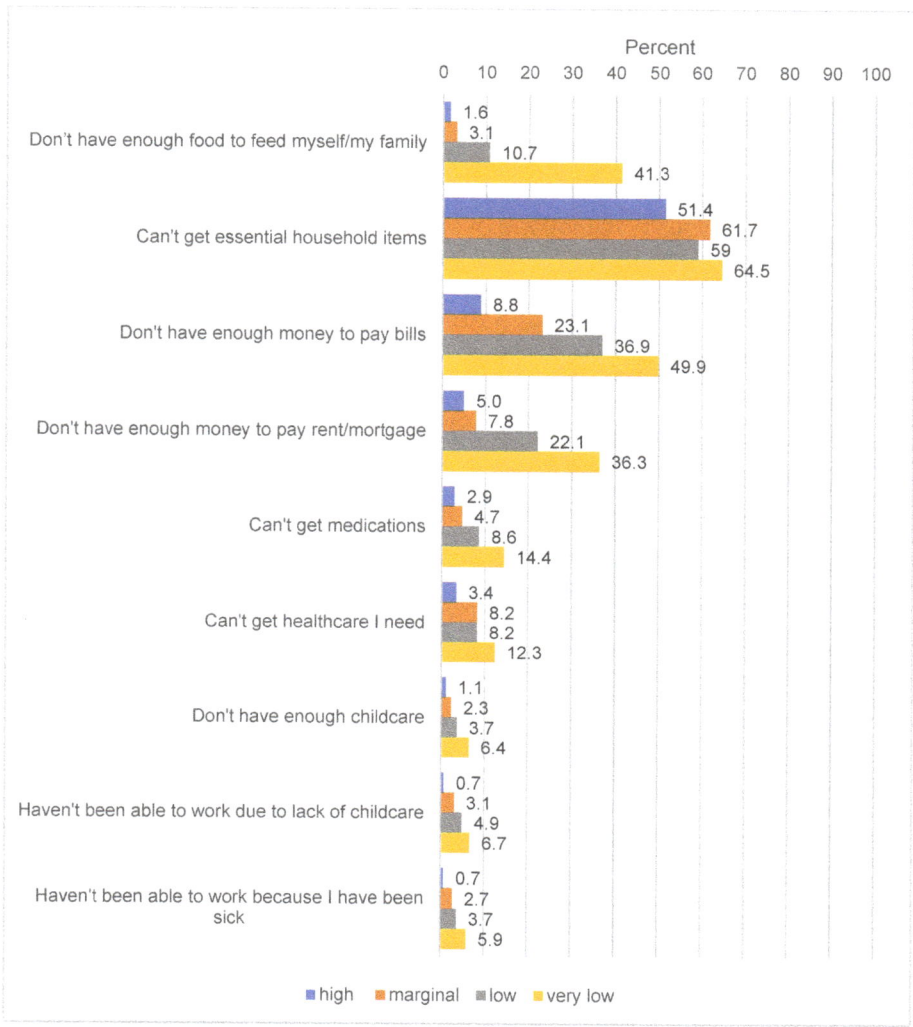

Figure 2. Challenges encountered by low-income US adults as a result of COVID-19, as of 19–24 March, by food security status (*n* = 1478). Question text: "Have you experienced any of the following challenges due to the coronavirus (COVID-19) so far?" [Please check all that apply] Percentages reflect the percent of respondents in each food security category that said they encountered that problem. Ten percent of respondents (*n* = 161) did not indicate any of the response options were challenges for them and are counted as 'missing'.

Food-secure, low-income adults working full or part time (44.3% of the overall sample) were more likely than their food-insecure counterparts to work in jobs that were either proceeding as normal, were busier than usual, or had closed and laid off employees. In contrast, working adults with food insecurity were more likely to have their hours reduced (Table 2). When asked what they thought would happen if they or someone in their family got sick with COVID-19, working adults with very low food security were less likely than their food-secure counterparts to have sick days or vacation days they could use, and were more likely to say they would lose their job if they missed too many days of work (52% very low food security vs. 18% high food security, $p < 0.001$).

Table 2. COVID-19 effects on workplaces among low-income adults working full or part time in the US overall and by food security status as of 19–24 March 2020 ($n = 655$).

	Overall ($n = 655$)	Food Security Status				p-Value
		High $n = 225$ (34%)	Marginal $n = 120$ (18%)	Low $n = 124$ (19%)	Very Low $n = 186$ (28%)	
	n (%) [a]	n (%) [b]	n (%) [b]	n (%) [b]	n (%) [b]	
What is your workplace doing to adjust to COVID-19? [c]						
Nothing, proceeding as normal	152 (23)	64 (42)	27 (18)	25 (16)	36 (24)	0.004
Employees encouraged to work at home	69 (11)	15 (22)	17 (25)	17 (25)	20 (29)	
Employees must work at home	69 (11)	17 (25)	14 (20)	16 (23)	22 (32)	
Essential employees must come in, others work from home	58 (9)	29 (50)	5 (9)	14 (24)	10 (32)	
Hours are reduced	79 (12)	20 (25)	11 (14)	17 (22)	31 (39)	
Temporarily closed	131 (20)	44 (34)	27 (21)	21 (16)	39 (30)	
Closed and I have been laid off	25 (4)	11 (44)	6 (24)	3 (12)	5 (20)	
Busier, employees working extra hours	47 (7)	21 (45)	9 (19)	8 (17)	9 (19)	
If you or someone in your family becomes ill with COVID-19, what do you expect will happen regarding your job? [c] (check all that apply)						
I will be able to stay home without using sick or vacation days	162 (26)	71 (44)	31 (19)	31 (19)	29 (18)	0.003
I will be able to use sick days to stay home without losing income	123 (19)	55 (45)	22 (18)	23 (19)	23 (19)	0.022
I will be able to use vacation days to stay home without losing income	74 (12)	27 (36)	11 (15)	17 (23)	19 (26)	0.573
I do not have sick days so if I am not able to work I will lose income	260 (41)	72 (28)	49 (19)	45 (17)	94 (36)	0.002
I will have to go into work even if I am sick	33 (5)	6 (18)	6 (18)	8 (24)	13 (39)	0.180
If I miss too many days of work I could lose my job	61 (10)	11 (18)	9 (15)	9 (15)	32 (52)	<0.001

[a] Column percentage; [b] Row percentage; [c] Asked among respondents who are working full or part time.

4. Discussion

This study presents results from a national survey of low-income adults in the US in the days immediately following the first major policy steps to enforce COVID-19-related social distancing measures on a wide scale in the US. Though large-scale school and business closures were only beginning to be implemented [22], we find that the effects of the COVID-19 pandemic were already impacting low-income adults, with disproportionately negative effects for low-income adults experiencing food insecurity. This initial evidence from a time period before even greater economic effects and job losses took place demonstrate that the COVID-19 pandemic threatens to greatly exacerbate existing health disparities related to food security status. Indeed, evidence from later surveys show that food insecurity in the US has dramatically increased well beyond levels seen during the Great Recession [12,13].

Results from this study illuminate the extent to which, very early in the COVID-19 trajectory in the US, individuals with food insecurity were disproportionately vulnerable to the severe economic and health consequences of the crisis. Our findings show that as early as mid-March 2020, food-insecure adults currently working outside the home were at greater risk of losing their income or their jobs if they got sick from COVID-19. Regardless of whether they get sick or their employment status, food-insecure individuals were also more likely to report expecting that they will lose income during the pandemic. For already low-income households, loss of income puts them at high risk of severe food insecurity and an inability to meet other basic needs, both of which can lead to future physical and mental health problems [23–26]. Compared to low-income, food-secure adults, food-insecure adults were more likely to report that they had already been laid off, and that their income would go down substantially. Fifty-four percent of food secure adults reported they expected their income would remain the same compared to 23% of adults with very low food security (results not shown, but available upon request). Subsequent massive job losses [27] and more extensive social distancing measures [10] after data collection ended have likely exacerbated the trends we document in our results.

Across the lifespan, food insecurity is associated with a range of negative health outcomes over the short and long term, including poor mental health outcomes such as depression, stress, and anxiety [4,9,28], poor diet quality [7,29], high rates of chronic diseases such as diabetes and obesity [6,30,31], and lower overall health status [3,5,32]. Food insecurity is also associated with higher healthcare expenditures, in part due to the higher burden of chronic health conditions among food-insecure patients and the known tradeoffs between food and medicine [24,26]. As the COVID-19 pandemic and the associated economic fallout progress, it will be critical for policymakers, health systems, and the public health community to proactively and comprehensively address access to food and other basic needs, particularly for populations at risk of, and already experiencing, food insecurity. Failure to do so will have long-term implications for population health, health disparities, and the health care system as a whole.

Food-insecure adults are more likely to be people of color, with lower social standing, who have less flexible and secure jobs, and are more vulnerable to chronic stress and other basic needs insecurities [1]. In 2018, 11.1% of adults in the US were food insecure; among low-income adults (<185% FPL), 29.1% were food insecure [1]. We find that, as of mid-March, 2020, 44% of adults with an income <250% of the FPL were food insecure in the past 30 days, and these individuals were more likely to be non-Hispanic Black or Hispanic. This disparity in food security status based on race/ethnicity is an additional way in which COVID-19 is disproportionately impacting communities of color in the US. Since mid-March, adult and child food insecurity rates in the US have dramatically risen [12,13]. In our study, adults currently experiencing food insecurity were not able to buy food in bulk quantities and therefore are at greater risk of exposure to the virus (due to the need for more frequent food shopping trips) as well as being at greater risk of an acute hunger crisis (due to lack of financial resources to purchase sufficient food). In addition, as individuals already at risk for food insecurity are more vulnerable to losing their jobs, rates of food insecurity will climb higher as the pandemic progresses.

Direct income support, expanded unemployment benefits, and additional support for federal food assistance programs included in the CARES act (passed on 27 March 2020) and the Families First Coronavirus Response Act (passed on 18 March 2020) are important first steps to supporting low-income families in the US [33,34]. However, longer-term support for individuals, as well as institutions and organizations that provide food, is needed. Some communities are already experiencing unprecedented demand in the emergency food system [35], and the federal government, states, and cities are scrambling to ensure that families with children who depend on free or reduced price meals at school do not go hungry [36]. Given the scale of the pandemic and the likely duration of social distancing measures and the associated economic impacts, more support is urgently needed to mitigate the toll of COVID-19 on the most vulnerable members of society. In particular, in addition to direct economic support to individuals, financial support for the emergency food system, greater flexibility for school systems to provide food to families, and long-term, expanded food assistance support via the Supplemental Nutrition Assistance Program (SNAP) are all urgently needed. Expanded SNAP benefits were critical for providing needed support for low-income families during the Great Recession, and were effective at reducing food insecurity [37]. Congress and the Trump administration should urgently increase SNAP benefits and expand eligibility for the program to help low-income families afford food during this extraordinary time.

Limitations

Results from this study should be considered in light of some limitations. First, the web-based survey panel does not use probability-based sampling and is not nationally representative. However, the TurkPrime panel is national in scope, and uses census-matched quotas to achieve a sample that closely aligns with the demographics of the population in the US which mitigates some of this concern. However, because we limited our sample to households <250% of the FPL (based on income and household size), and because the survey was only available in English, the demographics of our sample may be more similar to the US population overall and undercount some key demographic groups, particularly non-Hispanic Blacks and Hispanics, non-English speakers, and immigrants. Relatedly, this data was collected via a web-based survey which by definition required participants to have internet access via a computer or a smart phone. This method of data collection could also have undercounted some groups (e.g., those with very low income, without high school degrees, and those living in rural areas without broadband internet access) [38], likely those especially vulnerable to food insecurity. It is important to note, however, that any bias introduced from these factors would have biased results into the direction of undercounting, rather than overcounting, food insecurity and the other outcomes we document here. Second, respondents could choose whether or not to participate in the survey which may introduce some selection bias. Third, all measures in the study are self-reported and may be subject to a social-desirability bias. However, the fact that the survey was fielded online and was completely anonymous may mitigate this concern. Fourth, this survey is cross-sectional and we cannot make any statements about causal relationship between the coronavirus and our measure of food insecurity in the past 30 days. Finally, data were collected very quickly after social distancing measures and business and school closures began to be implemented in some (but not all) states. This is a strength as we were able to capture the immediate, real-time impacts on low-income adults. However, some measures also focused on anticipated effects. It is possible that the respondents did not accurately assess the likely effect of the coronavirus pandemic on their employment and income. However, initial evidence in the weeks after our data were collected show clearly that unemployment and rates of food insecurity have skyrocketed. The longer-term effects on low-income adults in the US, and associated disparities based on food insecurity, may be better or worse than those expected by participants in this survey. It will be imperative for future research to examine the long-term effects of the coronavirus pandemic and associated social distancing measures on food insecurity and associated health outcomes, particularly among vulnerable communities that were already struggling at the start of the pandemic.

The strengths of our study include the fact that we were able to collect these data so quickly after a national emergency was declared and states began implementing policies to slow the spread of COVID-19. Our large national sample of low-income adults is another key strength as is our use of the gold standard 18-question USDA food security screener module.

5. Conclusions

The social and economic upheaval caused by the COVID-19 pandemic is magnifying existing disparities and disproportionately affecting low-income, food-insecure households that already struggle to meet basic needs. The early effects documented in the present study are likely to continue to worsen as the pandemic continues unless extensive policy and economic supports are swiftly implemented.

Author Contributions: Conceptualization, J.A.W. and C.W.L.; Methodology, J.A.W.; Formal analysis, J.A.W.; Data curation, J.A.W.; Writing—Original draft preparation, J.A.W.; Writing—Review and editing, J.A.W. and C.W.L.; project administration, J.A.W.; funding acquisition, J.A.W. All authors have read and agreed to the published version of the manuscript.

Funding: Funding for this study was provided by a Faculty Research Grant from the University of Michigan Poverty Solutions. J.A.W. was also supported by the National Institutes of Diabetes and Digestive and Kidney Diseases of the National Institutes of Health (Award #K01DK119166) and C.W.L. was supported by the Eunice Kennedy Shriver National Institute for Child Health and Human Development (Award #4R00HD084758).

Conflicts of Interest: The authors declare no conflict of interest. The funders had no role in the design of the study; in the collection, analyses, or interpretation of data; in the writing of the manuscript, or in the decision to publish the results.

Appendix A

Table A1. Distribution of the Sample by State.

State	N	Percent
Alabama	22	1.49
Alaska	3	0.2
Arizona	35	2.37
Arkansas	16	1.08
California	150	10.15
Colorado	19	1.29
Connecticut	10	0.68
Delaware	7	0.47
District of Columbia	2	0.14
Florida	102	6.9
Georgia	50	3.38
Hawaii	7	0.47
Idaho	8	0.54
Illinois	62	4.19
Indiana	28	1.89
Iowa	11	0.74
Kansas	19	1.29
Kentucky	27	1.83
Louisiana	17	1.15
Maine	10	0.68
Maryland	20	1.35
Massachusetts	26	1.76
Michigan	58	3.92
Minnesota	21	1.42
Mississippi	14	0.95
Missouri	30	2.03
Montana	4	0.27

Table A1. Cont.

State	N	Percent
Nebraska	5	0.34
Nevada	26	1.76
New Hampshire	6	0.41
New Jersey	37	2.5
New Mexico	13	0.88
New York	100	6.77
North Carolina	52	3.52
North Dakota	0	0
Ohio	68	4.6
Oklahoma	25	1.69
Oregon	17	1.15
Pennsylvania	72	4.87
Puerto Rico	0	0
Rhode Island	3	0.2
South Carolina	30	2.03
South Dakota	3	0.2
Tennessee	31	2.1
Texas	90	6.09
Utah	21	1.42
Vermont	3	0.2
Virginia	29	1.96
Washington	28	1.89
West Virginia	13	0.88
Wisconsin	28	1.89
Wyoming	0	0
Total	1478	100

References

1. Coleman-Jensen, A.; Rabbitt, M.; Gregory, C.; Singh, A. Household Food Security in the United States in 2018; ERR-270; USDA, Economic Research Service: Washington, DC, USA, 2019.
2. Marmot, M. Social determinants of health inequalities. Lancet 2005, 365, 1099–1104. [CrossRef]
3. Gundersen, C.; Ziliak, J.P. Food Insecurity And Health Outcomes. Health Aff. (Millwood) 2015, 34, 1830–1839. [CrossRef]
4. Martinez, S.M.; Frongillo, E.A.; Leung, C.; Ritchie, L. No food for thought: Food insecurity is related to poor mental health and lower academic performance among students in California's public university system. J. Health Psychol. 2018. [CrossRef]
5. Pooler, J.A.; Hartline-Grafton, H.; DeBor, M.; Sudore, R.L.; Seligman, H.K. Food Insecurity: A Key Social Determinant of Health for Older Adults. J. Am. Geriatr. Soc. 2019, 67, 421–424. [CrossRef]
6. Cheung, H.C.; Shen, A.; Oo, S.; Tilahun, H.; Cohen, M.J.; Berkowitz, S.A. Food Insecurity and Body Mass Index: A Longitudinal Mixed Methods Study, Chelsea, Massachusetts, 2009–2013. Prev. Chronic Dis. 2015, 12, E125. [CrossRef]
7. Leung, C.W.; Epel, E.S.; Ritchie, L.D.; Crawford, P.B.; Laraia, B.A. Food insecurity is inversely associated with diet quality of lower-income adults. J. Acad. Nutr. Diet. 2014, 114, 1943–1953.e2. [CrossRef]
8. Berkowitz, S.A.; Berkowitz, T.S.Z.; Meigs, J.B.; Wexler, D.J. Trends in food insecurity for adults with cardiometabolic disease in the United States: 2005–2012. PLoS ONE 2017, 12, e0179172. [CrossRef]
9. Bruening, M.; Dinour, L.M.; Chavez, J.B.R. Food insecurity and emotional health in the USA: A systematic narrative review of longitudinal research. Public Health Nutr. 2017, 20, 3200–3208. [CrossRef]
10. Kaiser Family Foundation. State Data and Policy Actions to Address Coronavirus. 2020. Available online: https://www.kff.org/health-costs/issue-brief/state-data-and-policy-actions-to-address-coronavirus/ (accessed on 12 April 2020).

11. Niles, M.T.; Bertmann, F.; Morgan, E.H.; Wentworth, T.; Biehl, E.; Neff, R. Food Access and Security during Coronavirus: A Vermont Study. In *College of Agriculture and Life Sciences Faculty Publications*; University of Vermont: Burlington, VT, USA, 2020.
12. Fitzpatrick, K.; Harris, C.; Drawve, G. Assessing U.S. Food Insecurity in the United States during COVID-19 Pandemic. 2020. Available online: https://fulbright.uark.edu/departments/sociology/research-centers/community-family-institute/_resources/community-and-family-institute/revised-assessing-food-insecurity-brief.pdf (accessed on 28 April 2020).
13. Bauer, L. The COVID-19 Crisis Has Already Left Too Many Children Hungry in America. 6 May 2020. Available online: https://www.brookings.edu/blog/up-front/2020/05/06/the-covid-19-crisis-has-already-left-too-many-children-hungry-in-america/ (accessed on 7 May 2020).
14. Litman, L.; Robinson, J.; Abberbock, T. TurkPrime.com: A versatile crowdsourcing data acquisition platform for the behavioral sciences. *Behav. Res. Methods* **2017**, *49*, 433–442. [CrossRef]
15. Zimmerman, M.; Kerr, S. How should the severity of depression be rated on self-report depression scales? *Psychiatry Res.* **2019**, *280*, 112512. [CrossRef]
16. Yap, K.; Grisham, J.R. Unpacking the construct of emotional attachment to objects and its association with hoarding symptoms. *J. Behav. Addict.* **2019**, *8*, 249–258. [CrossRef]
17. Wolfson, J.A.; Lahne, J.; Raj, M.; Insolera, N.; Lavelle, F.; Dean, M. Food Agency in the United States: Associations with Cooking Behavior and Dietary Intake. *Nutrients* **2020**, *12*, 877. [CrossRef]
18. Skrzynski, C.; Creswell, K.G.; Bachrach, R.L.; Chung, T. Social discomfort moderates the relationship between drinking in response to negative affect and solitary drinking in underage drinkers. *Addict. Behav.* **2018**, *78*, 124–130. [CrossRef]
19. Minen, M.T.; Jalloh, A.; Begasse de Dhaem, O.; Seng, E.K. Behavioral Therapy Preferences in People with Migraine. *Headache* **2020**, *32*, 196–200. [CrossRef]
20. Bickel, G.; Nord, M.; Price, C.; Hamilton, W.; Cook, J. *Guide to Measuring Household Food Security*; Revised 2000; U.S. Department of Agriculture: Washington, DC, USA, 2000. Available online: https://www.fns.usda.gov/guide-measuring-household-food-security-revised-2000 (accessed on 27 May 2020).
21. United States Department of Agriculture Economic Research Service. Definition of Food Insecurity. 2019. Available online: https://www.ers.usda.gov/topics/food-nutrition-assistance/food-security-in-the-us/definitions-of-food-security/ (accessed on 13 April 2020).
22. Aljazeera. Lockdowns, Closures: How Is Each US State Handling Coronavirus? 2020. Available online: https://www.aljazeera.com/news/2020/03/emergencies-closures-states-handling-coronavirus-200317213356419.html (accessed on 14 April 2020).
23. Sachs-Ericsson, N.; Schatschneider, C.; Blazer, D.G. Perception of Unmet Basic Needs as a Predictor of Physical Functioning Among Community-Dwelling Older Adults. *J. Aging Health* **2006**, *18*, 852–868. [CrossRef]
24. Berkowitz, S.A.; Seligman, H.K.; Choudhry, N.K. Treat or eat: Food insecurity, cost-related medication underuse, and unmet needs. *Am. J. Med.* **2014**, *127*, 303–310.e3. [CrossRef]
25. Berkowitz, S.A.; Meigs, J.B.; DeWalt, D.; Seligman, H.K.; Barnard, L.S.; Bright, O.J.; Schow, M.; Atlas, S.J.; Wexler, D.J. Material need insecurities, control of diabetes mellitus, and use of health care resources: Results of the Measuring Economic Insecurity in Diabetes study. *JAMA Intern. Med.* **2015**, *175*, 257–265. [CrossRef]
26. Berkowitz, S.A.; Basu, S.; Meigs, J.B.; Seligman, H.K. Food Insecurity and Health Care Expenditures in the United States, 2011–2013. *Health Serv. Res.* **2018**, *53*, 1600–1620. [CrossRef]
27. Long, H.; Dam, A.V. America is in a depression, the challenge now is to make it short-lived. *The Washington Post*, 9 April 2020.
28. Martin, M.S.; Maddocks, E.; Chen, Y.; Gilman, S.E.; Colman, I. Food insecurity and mental illness: Disproportionate impacts in the context of perceived stress and social isolation. *Public Health* **2016**, *132*, 86–91. [CrossRef]
29. Leung, C.W.; Wolfson, J.A.; Lahne, J.; Barry, M.R.; Kasper, N.; Cohen, A.J. Associations between Food Security Status and Diet-Related Outcomes among Students at a Large, Public Midwestern University. *J. Acad. Nutr. Diet.* **2019**, *119*, 1623–1631. [CrossRef]
30. Smith, T.M.; Colon-Ramos, U.; Pinard, C.A.; Yaroch, A.L. Household food insecurity as a determinant of overweight and obesity among low-income Hispanic subgroups: Data from the 2011–2012 California Health Interview Survey. *Appetite* **2016**, *97*, 37–42. [CrossRef] [PubMed]

31. Seligman, H.K.; Laraia, B.A.; Kushel, M.B. Food insecurity is associated with chronic disease among low-income NHANES participants. *J. Nutr.* **2009**, *140*, 304–310. [CrossRef] [PubMed]
32. Lee, J.S.; Gundersen, C.; Cook, J.; Laraia, B.; Johnson, M.A. Food insecurity and health across the lifespan. *Adv. Nutr.* **2012**, *3*, 744–745. [CrossRef] [PubMed]
33. Coronavirus Aid, Relief, and Economic Security (CARES) Act. Public Law 116-136. 2020.
34. Families First Coronavirus Response Act. Public Law 116-127. 2020.
35. Kulish, N. 'Never Seen Anything Like It': Cars Line up for Miles at Food Banks. 2020. Available online: https://www.nytimes.com/2020/04/08/business/economy/coronavirus-food-banks.html?referringSource=articleShare (accessed on 14 April 2020).
36. United States Department of Agriculture Food and Nutrition Service. Find Meals for Kids When Schools are Closed. 2020. Available online: https://www.fns.usda.gov/meals4kids (accessed on 14 April 2020).
37. Nord, M.; Prell, M. *Food Security Improved Following the 2009 ARRA Increase in SNAP Benefits*; ERR-116 Report No. 1477-2017-4088; US Department of Agriculture, Economic Research Service: Washington, DC, USA, 2011.
38. Anderson M.; Perrin A.; Jiang, J.L.; Kumar, M. 10% of Americans Don't Use the Internet. Who Are They? *Pew Research Center*. 2019. Available online: https://www.pewresearch.org/fact-tank/2019/04/22/some-americans-dont-use-the-internet-who-are-they/ (accessed on 27 May 2020).

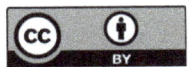

© 2020 by the authors. Licensee MDPI, Basel, Switzerland. This article is an open access article distributed under the terms and conditions of the Creative Commons Attribution (CC BY) license (http://creativecommons.org/licenses/by/4.0/).

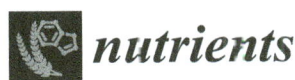

Article

Caregiver's Self-Confidence in Food Resource Management Is Associated with Lower Risk of Household Food Insecurity among SNAP-Ed-Eligible Head Start Families

Lamis Jomaa [1,2], **Muzi Na** [2], **Sally G. Eagleton** [2,3], **Marwa Diab-El-Harake** [1] and **Jennifer S. Savage** [2,3,*]

1. Department of Nutrition and Food Sciences, Faculty of Agricultural and Food Sciences, American University of Beirut, Riad El-Solh, P.O. Box 11-0236, Beirut 1107-2020, Lebanon; lj18@aub.edu.lb (L.J.); md106@aub.edu.lb (M.D.-E.-H.)
2. Department of Nutritional Sciences, Penn State College of Health and Human Development, 108C Chandlee Laboratory, University Park, PA 16802, USA; muzi.na@psu.edu (M.N.); sge5@psu.edu (S.G.E.)
3. Center for Childhood Obesity Research, Penn State College of Health and Human Development, University Park, PA 16802, USA
* Correspondence: jfs195@psu.edu

Received: 26 June 2020; Accepted: 29 July 2020; Published: 31 July 2020

Abstract: Food resource management (FRM) behaviors are key components within nutrition education programs designed to help food insecure households maximize their food dollars. However, little is known about the association between FRM self-confidence and financial practices with household food insecurity (HFI) among families with young children. Using a sample of SNAP-Ed-eligible Head Start families, this study examined associations between FRM self-confidence, FRM behaviors and financial practices by HFI. A needs assessment survey was conducted with caregivers of Head Start children ($n = 365$). HFI was measured using the US Household Food Security Survey Module. Chi-square and logistic regression analyses were conducted to examine if FRM self-confidence, FRM behaviors, and financial practices differed by HFI. Participants with high FRM self-confidence had lower odds of HFI (OR = 0.54, 95%CI: 0.33, 0.87), yet FRM behaviors, financial practices, and HFI were not related after adjusting for covariates. All FRM self-confidence questions significantly differed by HFI, whereas only one of six FRM behaviors and two of three financial practices differed by HFI (all p-values < 0.05). Promoting caregivers' self-confidence in FRM skills within nutrition education programs may be explored as a potential strategy to assist low-income households to stretch their food dollars in an attempt to address HFI.

Keywords: food resource management; food insecurity; self-confidence; nutrition education; financial practices; SNAP-Ed; Head Start; young children

1. Introduction

Household food insecurity (HFI), defined as "the inability to provide enough food for a healthy and active lifestyle for all household members [1]", remains a serious social and public health problem in the US [2]. Food insecurity is especially prevalent among low-income families with children. In 2018, 13.9% of American households with children were food insecure, and the prevalence of HFI reached 14.3% among households with children 6 years of age or younger [3]. Food insecurity is associated with a range of negative health outcomes among infants and young children, including poor physical health, increased risk of infections, micronutrient deficiencies [4,5], suboptimal sleep quality [6], adverse behavioral, mental, and academic behaviors [5,7,8], as well as obesity and other chronic conditions during childhood and later in life [7,9].

Federal assistance programs that provide monetary benefits along with nutrition education to low-income households have been shown to alleviate HFI [10]. These nutrition education programs, such as the Supplemental Nutrition Assistance Program Education (SNAP-Ed) and the Expanded Food and Nutrition Education Program (EFNEP), provide participants with trainings on how to maximize the use of their food dollars while providing healthy foods to their families and children [11]. An integral component of these nutrition education programs is to teach individuals how to acquire food resource management (FRM) skills and behaviors defined as "the handling of all foods and the resources that may be used to acquire foods by an individual or family [12]." In addition, FRM trainings cover topics such as meal planning, shopping strategies, food selection, budgeting, food preparation, and cooking strategies to maximize nutrition under resource constraints [12]. Previous studies indicate that integrating FRM within nutrition education (e.g., food preparation tips, healthful food selection, and budgeting) improves the food security status of low-income households [10,13], including those with children [14,15].

Although food assistance programs, such as SNAP and SNAP-Ed, focus on behavioral change in FRM, less emphasis has been placed on assessing participants' self-efficacy and confidence in their FRM skills. Few studies, to date, have reported how nutrition education interventions targeting self-efficacy and confidence in FRM can improve food security [15,16]. Perceived self-efficacy represents a key construct in behavioral change theories, as it refers to an "individual's confidence in their ability to plan and follow through with a series of actions that will result in desired outcomes or achievements" [17]. Research studies examining the effect of self-efficacy on behavioral change related to nutrition, exercise, and weight loss [18], as well as the prevention of chronic diseases [19], have demonstrated the pivotal role that self-efficacy plays in improving health. Knowing that families experiencing food insecurity may face various challenges affecting their confidence in managing their budgets to maintain food sufficiency [20,21], it is integral to further examine the association between FRM self-confidence and HFI [16].

Food insecurity is linked to income [1]; however, food insecurity is not the outcome of income alone. Instead, it is influenced by a myriad of other demographic, environmental, and financial factors [22,23]. To further examine the determinants of HFI, a growing body of literature has been exploring the association between financial management skills and food insecurity [22,24]. It was previously suggested that good financial management practices may safeguard certain households from food insecurity, whereas those with less effective financial skills may be at increased risk of food insecurity [22,25]. To our knowledge, the associations between FRM, financial practices, and HFI have not been adequately explored in the literature, particularly among households with young children. To address this research gap, the present study aimed to first examine the associations between FRM self-confidence and FRM behaviors by HFI status using a sample of SNAP-Ed-eligible Head Start families. A secondary objective of the study was to explore the association between financial practices of caregivers and HFI status in the study sample. Head Start is a federally-funded program that serves just over 900,000 low-income preschool children in the US to optimize their health and nutrition. The Head Start program also provides balanced snacks and meals to children through the Child and Adult Care Food Program [26]. Although previous studies have shown that Head Start programs can help alleviate HFI and improve nutrition outcomes of children [27,28], none, to our knowledge, have examined the potential associations between caregiver's FRM self-confidence and behaviors by HFI. We hypothesized that (1) caregivers with higher self-confidence and better FRM skills would have lower risk of being food insecure; and (2) caregivers with good financial practices would report lower levels of food insecurity.

2. Materials and Methods

2.1. Sampling and Recruitment

Caregiver-child dyads in the present study were recruited from Head Start preschool classrooms in four rural counties in central Pennsylvania. Data used in the present study were drawn from a needs assessment survey that was designed to characterize the home environments of low-income families with young children and to better inform future nutrition education programming for the Head Start participants. The survey was distributed through classrooms to 1297 Head Start families. If parents had more than one child enrolled in Head Start, they were instructed to complete the survey for their oldest child enrolled in the program. Of the 1297 distributed surveys, 379 (30%) were returned in the mail. Caregivers received a $25 gift card for their participation. Data collection spanned May 2017 to May 2018. Among nine families, a survey was completed for two children in the home, thus we excluded the survey for the younger of the two children. Four children were excluded because they were outside the age range of Head Start eligibility, resulting in a final study sample of 365. For the purpose of the present study, a minimum sample size of 134 participants was required to test for the associations between our main variables of interest (FRM behavior, FRM self-confidence, and HFI) at 80% power and with 95% confidence interval. The sample size calculations were done using data from previous studies that examined similar associations [10,16]. Informed consent was obtained from subjects prior to their participation in the study. The study was conducted in accordance with the Declaration of Helsinki, and the protocol was approved by the Institutional Review Board at the Pennsylvania State University (00007467).

2.2. Caregiver and Household Characteristics

The survey included questions related to the caregiver characteristics, such as age and sex, ethnicity, education, employment, and marital status. As for household characteristics, questions included child's age, number of children in the household, number of people supported by household income, participation in assistance programs in the past 12 months (e.g., Special Supplemental Nutrition Program for Women, Infants, and Children (WIC) and Supplemental Nutrition Assistance Program (SNAP)), and household income. Household income was missing in seventy-four of 365 households (20.2%). Missing income was imputed based on WIC and SNAP status, parent education, marital status, and employment using PROC MI in SAS software (SAS Institute Inc., Cary, NC, USA).

2.3. Household Food Insecurity Status

Household food insecurity (HFI) experienced during the previous 12 months was measured using the 18-item US Household Food Security Survey Module [1]. The food security status of households was determined by the number of food-insecure conditions and behaviors the household reports. Households were classified as 'food secure' if participants responded affirmatively to two or fewer items on the 18-item scale and as 'food insecure' if the affirmative responses were on three or more items, such as "cutting the size of meals or skipping meals because there wasn't enough money for food during the past 12 months" or "losing weight because there wasn't enough money for food".

2.4. Food Resource Management (FRM) Self-Confidence and Behaviors

FRM self-confidence and FRM behaviors of caregivers were assessed in the present study using two sets of questions derived from the SNAP-Ed evaluation framework guide and toolkit [11]. These questions were previously used and validated in other studies assessing the impact of nutrition education programs targeting low-income adults, including SNAP-Ed, Cooking Matters, and Expanded Food and Nutrition Education Program (EFNEP), on participants' FRM skills [10,14,29] and confidence [16,29].

The caregivers' self-confidence in FRM abilities (in the past 12 months) was assessed in the present study using five questions. Three questions assessed caregiver confidence to "choose the best-priced form of fruits and vegetables", "buy healthy foods on a budget", and "cook healthy foods on a budget"; and two questions were related to caregiver's confidence in their ability to "make a shopping list and stick to it" and "compare prices of similar foods to find the best value". Responses for these questions were measured using a 4-point Likert scale that ranged from 1 (*not very confident*) to 4 (*very confident*). An average FRM self-confidence score was calculated for each participant based on their responses to the five questions, and a binary score was later created for FRM self-confidence to classify participants into two groups (low/high): participants with scores less than the median were categorized as "low" FRM self-confidence, whereas participants with scores greater than or equal to the median score were categorized as "high" FRM self-confidence. A high FRM self-confidence indicated a greater self-confidence in shopping, preparing foods, and managing food resources on a budget.

The FRM behaviors of participants in the present study were assessed using six questions from the SNAP-Ed evaluation framework and toolkit, asking how often do caregivers "plan meals before shopping", "prepare shopping list", "compare prices before buying", "use grocery store flyers", and "identify foods on sales or use coupons" [11]. A 5-point response scale (1 = *never*, 2 = *rarely*, 3 = *sometimes*, 4 = *usually*, 5 = *always*) was used for each of the FRM behavior items. An average FRM behavior score was first calculated, then a binary score was created to classify participants into two groups: participants with scores less than the median were categorized as "low" FRM behaviors, whereas participants with scores greater than or equal to the median score were categorized as "high" FRM behaviors. A high FRM behavior indicated better practices in meal planning, shopping with a grocery list, and comparing prices.

2.5. Financial Situation, Financial Practices, and Difficulties

To assess the financial situation, respondents were asked to describe their own financial situation with responses including: 1 = "Very comfortable and secure", 2 = "Very comfortable and secure", 3 = "Occasionally have some difficulty making ends meet", 4 = "Tough to make ends meet but keeping head above water", and 5 = "In over your head". As for financial difficulties, these were evaluated based on 5 questions from the USDA national food study [30] to assess difficulties that individuals had in meeting their essential household expenses, such as mortgage or rent payments, utility bills, or important medical care during the past six months.

Financial practices of the caregivers were also assessed using 3 questions that were derived from the USDA national food study [30]. Caregivers were asked to report how frequently they adopted the following practices during the past 6 months: "review your bills for accuracy", "pay your bills on time", and "pay more than the "minimum payment due" on your credit card bills". Response options ranged from 1 = never to 5 = always. An average financial practices score was calculated for each participant based on their responses to the five questions, and a binary score was later created (low/high): participants with scores less than the median were categorized as "low", whereas participants with scores greater than or equal to the median score were categorized as "high", referring to those with better financial practices.

2.6. Statistical Analyses

Descriptive statistics were reported in the present study as frequencies and proportions for categorical variables and as medians and interquartile ranges (IQR) for non-normal continuous variables. Chi-square tests and Mann-Whitney U tests were conducted to explore differences between categorical variables and non-normal continuous variables by HFI status (food secure vs. food insecure households), respectively. Simple and multiple logistic regression analyses were also conducted to examine the association between FRM self-confidence, FRM behaviors, and financial practices by HFI status. Variables included in the multiple logistic regression models were those found to have a significant bivariate relationship with HFI and were statistically significant in the simple logistic models ($p < 0.05$). Sensitivity analyses were also conducted to assess the validity of findings by: (1) adjusting for significant and non-significant sociodemographic variables as potential confounders in the logistic regression models, (2) running linear regression models with HFI and other variables of interest (FRM behavior, FRM self-confidence and financial practices) as continuous variables, and (3) running models using imputed and non-imputed income data. For the models with non-imputed income, we excluded subjects with missing income in the sensitivity analysis. Results from the logistic regression models were expressed as odds ratios with 95% confidence intervals. Statistical analyses were conducted using Stata/MP version 15.1 (StataCorp. College Station, TX, USA). A p-value of 0.05 was used to detect significance in all analyses used in the present study.

3. Results

3.1. Descriptive Characteristics of the Study Sample

The majority of caregivers in our study sample were females (96%), White non-Hispanic (98%), and completed high school education level or less (61%). The median age of caregivers was 30 (IQR = 9) years old. More than half of study participants were married or partnered (57%) and unemployed (54%). In addition, almost three quarters of participants were receiving SNAP benefits (75%) and WIC (70%). The median number of children in the household was 2, and the prevalence of HFI was 37% (see Table 1).

Caregiver and household characteristics of the study sample were also presented by HFI in Table 1. Participation in the SNAP/Food Stamps program was significantly greater among food insecure households compared to food secure ones (84% vs. 69%, $p = 0.001$), whereas participation in WIC was less common among food insecure households (64% vs. 74%, respectively, $p = 0.041$). No other significant associations were noted between HFI and demographic characteristics in the present study.

Table 1. Descriptive characteristics of a sample of low-income Head Start families with preschool-aged children from four rural counties in central Pennsylvania, USA, by household food insecurity status, ($n = 365$) [1,2,3].

	Total Sample ($n = 365$)	Food Secure ($n = 229$)	Food Insecure [4] ($n = 136$)	p-Value
Caregiver characteristics				
Parent's age	30 [9]	30 [9]	30 [8]	0.915
Parent ethnicity				
Hispanic	7 (2)	4 (2)	3 (2)	0.711
Non-Hispanic	330 (98)	209 (98)	121 (98)	
Parent gender				
Female	346 (96)	217 (96)	129 (96)	0.831
Male	15 (4)	9 (4)	6 (4)	
Highest parent education completed				
≤High school	212 (61)	134 (63)	78 (59)	0.461
>High school	135 (39)	80 (37)	55 (41)	
Marital status				
Not married	155 (43)	95 (42)	60 (44)	0.623
Married or partnered	210 (57)	134 (58)	76 (56)	
Employment status				
Unemployed	194 (54)	120 (53)	74 (55)	0.751
Employed	167 (46)	106 (47)	61 (45)	
Household characteristics				
Child's age	4 [1]	4 [1]	5 [1]	0.383
Number of children	2 [1]	2 [1]	2 [1]	0.860

Table 1. Cont.

	Total Sample (n = 365)	Food Secure (n = 229)	Food Insecure [4] (n = 136)	p-Value
Number of people (supported by income)	4 [2]	4 [2]	4 [2]	0.242
Yearly household income				0.635
<$20,000	176 (49)	108 (48)	68 (50)	
≥$20,000	185 (51)	118 (52)	67 (50)	
Participation in assistance program (in the past 12 months) [5]				
SNAP/Food Stamps	270 (75)	156 (69)	114 (84)	0.001
WIC	253 (70)	167 (74)	86 (64)	0.041

[1] Categorical variables were presented as n (%) and non-normal continuous variables were presented as medians and interquartile ranges (IQR). IQR represents the difference between the upper and lower quartiles (Q3–Q1). [2] Chi-square tests were conducted to determine differences between categorical variables and binary food security status. [3] Mann-Whitney U tests were used to determine differences between non-normal continuous variables and binary food security status. [4] Households with low and very low food security status were categorized as food insecure and those with marginal or high food security were classified as food secure [1]. [5] SNAP, Supplemental Nutrition Assistance Program; TANF, Temporary Assistance for Needy Families; WIC, The Special Supplemental Nutrition Program for Women, Infants, and Children.

3.2. Food Resource Management and Household Food Insecurity

Table 2 presents FRM self-confidence and FRM behaviors of caregivers in the study sample and by HFI. Results showed that almost three-quarters of caregivers were *moderately* to *very confident* in choosing best priced food items, comparing food prices for best values, and cooking healthy food items on a budget. In addition, slightly greater than two-thirds of participants were *moderately* or *highly confident* in "buying health foods for their families on a budget" and "making a shopping list and sticking to it". The proportion of participants reporting *usually* or *always* adopting FRM behaviors ranged between 31% and 79%. The less adopted FRM behaviors included "using grocery store flyers to plan meals" (31%), "planning of meals prior to grocery shopping" (57%), and "identifying foods on sale or using coupons to save money" (57%).

Table 2. Food resource management (FRM) self-confidence and FRM behaviors of Head Start caregivers in the study sample by household food insecurity, (n = 365) [1].

	Responses	Total Sample (n = 365)	Food Secure (n = 229)	Food Insecure (n = 136)	p-Value
FRM self-confidence n (%)					
How confident are you that you can choose the best-priced form of fruits and vegetables (fresh, frozen or canned)?	Not very confident	17 (5)	9 (4)	8 (6)	0.046
	Somewhat confident	80 (22)	44 (19)	36 (27)	
	Moderately confident	135 (37)	80 (35)	55 (40)	
	Very confident	131 (36)	94 (42)	37 (27)	
How confident are you that you can buy healthy foods for your family on a budget?	Not very confident	28 (8)	12 (5)	16 (12)	<0.001
	Somewhat confident	85 (23)	44 (20)	41 (30)	
	Moderately confident	127 (35)	78 (34)	49 (37)	
	Very confident	122 (34)	94 (41)	28 (21)	
How confident are you that you can cook healthy foods for your family on a budget?	Not very confident	18 (5)	10 (4)	8 (6)	<0.001
	Somewhat confident	83 (23)	36 (16)	14 (34)	
	Moderately confident	126 (34)	79 (35)	47 (35)	
	Very confident	137 (38)	103 (45)	34 (25)	
How confident are you that you can make a shopping list and stick to it?	Not very confident	31 (8)	16 (7)	15 (11)	0.008
	Somewhat confident	86 (24)	50 (22)	36 (26)	
	Moderately confident	113 (31)	63 (28)	50 (37)	
	Very confident	134 (37)	99 (43)	35 (26)	

Table 2. Cont.

	Responses	Total Sample ($n = 365$)	Food Secure ($n = 229$)	Food Insecure ($n = 136$)	p-Value
How confident are you that you can compare prices of similar foods to find the best value?	Not very confident	21 (6)	9 (4)	12 (9)	0.015
	Somewhat confident	70 (19)	40 (18)	30 (22)	
	Moderately confident	122 (33)	71 (31)	51 (37)	
	Very confident	151 (42)	108 (47)	43 (32)	
FRM behaviors n (%)					
How often do you compare prices before buying food?	Never	17 (5)	13 (6)	4 (3)	0.761
	Rarely	21 (6)	13 (6)	8 (6)	
	Sometimes	77 (21)	49 (21)	28 (21)	
	Usually	122 (33)	77 (34)	45 (33)	
	Always	127 (35)	76 (33)	51 (37)	
How often do you plan meals before shopping for groceries?	Never	13 (4)	8 (4)	5 (4)	0.312
	Rarely	30 (8)	18 (8)	12 (9)	
	Sometimes	112 (31)	71 (31)	41 (30)	
	Usually	131 (36)	78 (34)	53 (39)	
	Always	75 (21)	51 (23)	24 (18)	
How often do you use a shopping list when grocery shopping?	Never	14 (4)	7 (3)	7 (5)	0.016
	Rarely	25 (7)	15 (6)	10 (7)	
	Sometimes	70 (19)	45 (20)	25 (19)	
	Usually	99 (27)	50 (22)	49 (36)	
	Always	156 (43)	111 (49)	45 (33)	
How often do you check food on hand before making a shopping list? *	Never	7 (2)	3 (1)	4 (3)	0.249
	Rarely	15 (4)	12 (5)	3 (2)	
	Sometimes	55 (15)	33 (15)	22 (16)	
	Usually	117 (32)	69 (30)	48 (35)	
	Always	170 (47)	111 (49)	59 (44)	
How often do you use grocery store flyers to plan meals?	Never	67 (19)	42 (18)	25 (18)	0.922
	Rarely	63 (17)	38 (17)	25 (18)	
	Sometimes	121 (33)	74 (32)	47 (35)	
	Usually	56 (15)	38 (17)	18 (13)	
	Always	57 (16)	36 (16)	21 (16)	
How often do you identify foods on sale or use coupons to save money? *	Never	26 (7)	14 (6)	12 (9)	0.453
	Rarely	21 (6)	16 (7)	5 (4)	
	Sometimes	108 (30)	64 (28)	44 (32)	
	Usually	105 (29)	65 (29)	40 (29)	
	Always	104 (28)	69 (30)	35 (26)	

[1] Chi-square test was conducted to determine differences between categorical variables and binary food security status. * For expected cell counts less than 5, p-value from Fisher's exact test was reported.

Significant differences were observed between food secure and food insecure households for all FRM self-confidence items (p-value < 0.05). More specifically, caregivers in food secure households were more likely to report being very confident in their abilities to "choose best priced fruits and vegetables" (42% vs. 27%), "buy healthy foods for their families" (41% vs. 21%), "cook healthy foods on a budget" (45% vs. 25%), "make a shopping list and stick to it" (43% vs. 26%), and "compare prices of similar foods when shopping to get the best value" (47% vs. 32%) when compared to their food insecure counterparts. On the other hand, only one item from the FRM behaviors was found to be significantly different between food secure and food insecure households in our study sample. A greater proportion of caregivers in food secure households reported that they always "use a shopping list when grocery shopping" as compared to their food insecure counterparts (49% vs. 33%, Table 2).

3.3. Financial Situation, Practices, and Difficulties and Household Food Insecurity

When caregivers were asked to describe the household's financial situation, 37% of the total sample reported being "very comfortable and secure" or "able to make ends meet without much difficulty", 34% "occasionally have some difficulty making ends meet", and the remaining 29% reported it is "tough to make ends meet but keeping your head above water" or they are "in over their heads". In terms of financial practices, the majority of caregivers in the study sample responded they usually or always "review bills for accuracy" (75%) and "pay bills on time" (79%), yet less than one-third of participants responded they "pay more than the "minimum payment due" on credit card bills" as frequently. With respect to financial difficulties, 39% of caregivers in our study reported going through a time "when they could not pay mortgage or rent, electricity or gas utilities, or important medical expenses", and 44% reported going through periods when they "could not pay the full amount of gas, oil, or electricity bills" (Table 3).

Table 3. Financial situation, practices and difficulties of Head Start caregivers in the study sample and by household food insecurity ($n = 365$) [1].

	Responses	Total Sample ($n = 365$)	Food Secure ($n = 229$)	Food Insecure ($n = 136$)	*p*-Value
Which of the following best describes your family's financial situation? * n (%)	Very comfortable & secure	31 (9)	27 (12)	4 (3)	<0.001
	Able to make ends meet without much difficulty	98 (28)	88 (40)	10 (7)	
	Occasionally have some difficulty making ends meet	121 (34)	69 (31)	52 (40)	
	Tough to make ends meet but keeping head above water	91 (26)	32 (14)	59 (45)	
	In over your head	13 (3)	7 (3)	6 (5)	
Financial practices n (%)					
How often do you review your bills for accuracy? *	Never	14 (4)	13 (6)	1 (1)	0.112
	Rarely	31 (8)	16 (7)	15 (11)	
	Sometimes	47 (13)	29 (13)	18 (13)	
	Usually	132 (36)	85 (37)	47 (35)	
	Always	140 (39)	85 (37)	55 (40)	
How often do you pay your bills on time? *	Never	5 (1)	3 (1)	2 (1)	<0.001
	Rarely	13 (4)	4 (2)	9 (7)	
	Sometimes	59 (16)	30 (13)	29 (21)	
	Usually	140 (38)	78 (34)	62 (46)	
	Always	148 (41)	114 (50)	34 (25)	
How often do you pay more than the "minimum payment due" on your credit card bills?	Never	109 (33)	66 (32)	43 (37)	0.001
	Rarely	46 (14)	19 (9)	27 (23)	
	Sometimes	70 (22)	47 (22)	23 (20)	
	Usually	46 (14)	35 (17)	11 (9)	
	Always	55 (17)	42 (20)	13 (11)	
Financial difficulties n (%)					
Has there been a time when you could not pay your mortgage or rent, electricity or gas utilities, or important medical expenses?	Yes	141 (39)	55 (24)	86 (63)	**<0.001**
Were you evicted from a home or apartment for not paying the rent or mortgage? *	Yes	6 (2)	2 (1)	4 (3)	0.201
Has there been a time when you could not pay the full amount of gas, oil, or electricity bills?	Yes	159 (44)	72 (32)	87 (64)	**<0.001**
Have you used a cash advance service on any of your credit cards? *	Yes	15 (4)	5 (2)	40 (7)	**0.013**
Have you used a payday loan or other high interest loan?	Yes	11 (3)	4 (2)	7 (5)	0.107

* For cells with counts less than 5 in the chi-square analysis, *p*-value from Fisher's exact test was reported.

In addition, Table 3 presents the financial situation, difficulties, and financial practices of caregivers in the study sample by HFI. Overall, food insecure households were more likely to report their financial situation as "occasionally have some difficulty making ends meet" (40% vs. 31%) or "tough to make ends meet but keeping head above water" compared to their food secure counterparts (45% vs. 14%). In terms of financial practices, a higher proportion of caregivers in food secure households reported they *always* "pay bills on time" (50% vs. 25%) and "pay more than the minimum payment due on credit card bills" (20% vs. 11%) compared to their food insecure counterparts. On the other hand, food insecure households were significantly more likely to report facing financial difficulties compared to food secure ones: "has there been a time when you could not pay your mortgage or rent, electricity or gas utilities, or important medical expenses?" (63% vs. 24%) and "has there been a time when you could not pay the full amount of gas, oil, or electricity bills" (64% vs. 32%), p-value < 0.001.

3.4. Food Resource Management, Financial Practices, and Household Food Insecurity

The associations between FRM self-confidence, FRM behaviors, and financial practices with HFI were also explored in the present study (Table 4). Results from the logistic regression analyses showed that caregivers with high FRM self-confidence had lower odds of HFI (OR = 0.54, 95% CI: 0.33, 0.87, p = 0.012), even after adjusting for financial practices and participation in food assistance programs (SNAP and WIC). Although the association between financial practices and HFI was significant in the simple regression analysis, this association lost its statistical significance in the adjusted model (OR = 0.77, 95%CI: 0.46, 1.3, p = 0.338). Results from the models remained robust after conducting sensitivity analyses and adjusting for significant and non-significant sociodemographic variables, including parent's age, employment, household income (imputed and not imputed values), and participation in food assistance programs in the past 12 months (Supplemental tables—Tables S1 and S2).

Table 4. Simple and multiple logistic regression analyses of food resource management (FRM) self-confidence, FRM behaviors, and financial practices of Head Start caregivers with household food insecurity (n = 365).

	Simple Logistic Regression	Multiple Logistic Regression [1]
FRM self-confidence		
Low	1.0	1.0
High	0.50 (0.32, 0.77)	0.54 (0.33, 0.87)
p-value	p = 0.002	p = 0.012
FRM behaviors		
Low	1.0	-
High	0.98 (0.64, 1.5)	-
p-value	p = 0.913	
Financial practices		
Low	1.0	1.0
High	**0.52 (0.32, 0.85)**	0.77 (0.46, 1.3)
p-value	**p = 0.010**	p = 0.338

[1] The model was adjusted for socio-economic characteristics found to be significant correlates of household food insecurity, namely participation in any assistance program (in the past 12 months) including SNAP/Food Stamps or WIC.

4. Discussion

Food insecurity remains a social and public health problem for low-income families with young children in the US that has serious consequences on children's overall health and wellbeing. To our knowledge, the present study is the first to examine the associations between FRM self-confidence, FRM behaviors, and financial practices by HFI status in a sample of low-income households with young children. Using a sample of SNAP-Ed-eligible Head Start families, our study findings showed that caregiver's self-confidence in their FRM was associated with lower odds of HFI. Nevertheless, the associations between the FRM behaviors and financial practices of Head Start caregivers by HFI were not statistically significant in the adjusted models.

As hypothesized, caregivers with high FRM self-confidence had lower odds of HFI in the present study, even after adjusting for other correlates including FRM behaviors, financial practices and participation in other federal assistance programs. When individual FRM questions were explored, all FRM self-confidence questions were also found to significantly differ by HFI status. More specifically, caregivers in food secure households were more likely to report being *"very confident"* in their abilities to choose the best priced fruits and vegetables, compare prices of similar foods when shopping to get the best value, as well as buy and cook healthy foods for their families on a budget as compared to their food insecure counterparts. These results were in concordance with those reported earlier by Begley et al. (2019) showing that food secure participants, who were assessed at the enrollment stage of an adult food literacy program in Australia, reported being *"always confident"* about managing money for healthy food compared to food insecure participants (41.2% vs. 9%) and *"always confident"* in their ability to cook a variety of healthy meals (21.9% vs. 15.4%) [31]. Our findings were also consistent with a few studies conducted to date that highlight how greater self-efficacy in shopping and preparing healthy food, based on nutrition education programs targeting low income adults, has been associated with lower risk of food insecurity [16,29]. According to Martin et al. (2016), self-efficacy in managing food resources was found to be associated with a decrease in very low food security levels among food pantry clients participating in the *Freshplace* intervention. This was an 18-month innovative food pantry intervention that combined several strategies to boost the confidence of participants, such as motivational interviewing and serving food in client-choice format to increase their confidence in planning meals ahead of time, making a shopping list before going to the store, and making food money last all month [16]. Another study evaluating the impact of *Cooking Matters for Adults* nutrition education program showed significant improvements in the FRM skills and self-confidence in managing food resources of low-income households up to six months after the program completion. In addition, participants in the Cooking Matters intervention were worried less that food would run out before they could get money to buy more [29]. It is worth noting that these nutrition education programs were focused primarily on improving the self-efficacy of low-income adults as integral components for the uptake and maintenance of FRM skills to maximize the use of limited food dollars.

Although self-efficacy represents a key construct within theories of behavioral change and has been shown to be effective in promoting healthy behaviors for weight loss, exercise, and chronic disease management [32,33], only a few studies to date, as described earlier, have explored the association between self-confidence in FRM with food insecurity among low-income households [16,29]. To our knowledge, the present study is the first to examine these associations in low-income households, focusing primarily on those with young children. Our study findings suggest that increased confidence in resource management skills among caregivers may be associated with lower risk of HFI. These results may be promising for families with young children, who may have increased concerns about smart shopping, stretching their food dollars, as well as cooking tasty and low-cost food to feed their children [20,34]. Food insecure individuals may be also influenced by financial, social, and personal stressors that can further affect their confidence in their ability to shop, prepare, and plan a healthy meal on a limited budget [35,36]. Thus, federal assistance and nutrition education programs targeting families with young children, such as Head Start and SNAP-Ed, may need to give particular attention to strategies that can help improve the self-confidence and efficacy of caregivers in their resource management skills. These programs can also help participants in accessing community-level resources and in overcoming common misconceptions and barriers to enrolling in other federal assistance programs, including WIC [37].

Nevertheless, when exploring FRM behaviors, only one of the six behaviors of caregivers were shown to differ significantly by HFI in the present study. In addition, the association between FRM behaviors and HFI was not found to be statistically significant in the regression models. Contrary to our study findings, food secure families were previously observed to have overall better FRM skills, such as shopping for sales, researching for best prices on particular products, traveling to multiple stores, and planning meals around their limited budgets [35,38]. According to Begley et al. (2019), individuals who reported at the onset of a food literacy program a low frequency of adopting certain planning and food preparation behaviors, such as planning meals ahead of time and making a list before they shop, were significantly more likely to be food insecure than those who reported adopting more frequently these behaviors [31]. The limited differences in FRM behaviors by HFI, as observed in the present study, can be attributed in part to the overall low proportion of caregivers who reported planning their meals prior to grocery shopping, using grocery store flyers to plan their meals, or identifying foods on sale and using coupons to save money. Another reason could be differences in questions raised when assessing caregivers' FRM confidence and behaviors in the present study. For example, questions relevant to buying and cooking healthy foods were only present in the FRM self-confidence questionnaire, whereas questions related to using shopping lists and planning meals prior to shopping were common among both scales. Caregivers participating in the present study may have also received family-centered services that cover topics related to child nutrition, growth, and development as part of the Head Start programs [39–42], which could have influenced their perceived confidence in providing healthy foods for their children. Nevertheless, confidence alone might be insufficient to alleviate HFI, and households with higher confidence may not be able to adopt adequate FRM behaviors when other environmental, financial, and personal barriers exist, such as limited availability and/or access to food stores with healthy and nutritious food, lack of kitchen appliances, as well as time and money constraints [31,38,43]. Poor physical and mental health can also affect the FRM skills and capabilities of food insecure individuals [38,44] and are worth further exploration when examining the association between resource management skills and HFI.

A growing body of evidence suggests that households facing economic hardships and with limited knowledge of basic financial concepts (i.e., financial literacy) are also more likely to experience food insecurity compared to those with higher financial management skills [22,25]. In line with former research, results from the present study showed significant differences in the financial situation, difficulties, and financial practices of caregivers by HFI status. Compared to caregivers from food insecure households, those from food secure households were more likely to report better financial situation and lower financial difficulties reflected through their ability to pay their mortgages or other basic expenses (such as rent, electricity, gas, and medical expenses). In addition, caregivers from food secure households were also more likely to report frequently adopting certain financial practices, such as paying bills on time and paying more than the "minimum payment due" on credit card bills. Nevertheless, the association between higher financial practices and HFI lost its statistical significance in the adjusted models. These results may be explained by the lower income levels of households enrolled in federal assistance programs, such as SNAP and WIC, who represent approximately three-quarters of the study sample, and who may be facing heightened financial hardships that could have attenuated the association between caregivers' better financial management practices and their HFI status. Our study findings highlight the need to further explore the association between financial literacy (knowledge and capabilities) and HFI, particularly in low-income households with children. The latter group may be at increased risk of facing economic hardships, and thus may adopt risky coping strategies that can further increase their risk for HFI and its adverse health consequences [22,45].

Strengths and Limitations

To our knowledge, this study is the first to explore the associations between FRM self-confidence, FRM behaviors and financial practices by HFI among a sample of low-income Head Start households with young children. Nevertheless, the present study has a number of limitations worth considering. First, the study is cross-sectional in nature, thus causality cannot be determined when exploring the associations between FRM self-confidence, FRM behaviors, and financial practices by HFI. The association between FRM self-confidence and food insecurity, as reported in the present study, may have been bidirectional in nature. Caregivers in food insecure households may have poor conditions that affect their self-confidence in their resource management skills as compared to food secure households; on the other hand, having higher self-confidence may also improve one's capabilities to access and utilize food, which can influence their food security and feeling of self-sufficiency [31]. Another limitation of the present study is that data were self-reported, thus we cannot rule out response bias. Our study findings may also have limited representativeness with a moderate survey response rate (30%) and the study population limited to only four rural areas in central Pennsylvania. Thus, results cannot be generalizable and the external validity of our findings may be limited to certain low-income families. Albeit modest, the response rate in the present study was still similar to other surveys conducted with rural Head Start families in Colorado (28.5%) and Appalachian Ohio (42%) [46,47]. Future research considering more diverse and larger samples of Head Start families are still needed to further examine the associations explored in the present study.

5. Conclusions

Our study findings suggest that increased self-confidence in FRM among caregivers of young children is associated with lower odds of HFI among low-income Head Start families. Nutrition and health education programs, such as SNAP-Ed and WIC, that are designed to assist low-income households in alleviating their HFI status may need to give more emphasis to the self-efficacy and confidence of caregivers in stretching their food dollars and adopting adequate FRM skills. The strategies may help caregivers in offering healthy food and improve the food choices offered to their children. Caregivers can also play a pivotal role in structuring their children's early experiences with food through child feeding practices, social modeling of healthy eating behaviors, and regulating the quality and quantity of food provided to the child [48–50]. Thus, future research should examine the extent to which nutrition education programs that focus on improving FRM self-confidence and behaviors can contribute (directly or indirectly) to the feeding practices of caregivers and, subsequently, to the diet quality and nutrition outcomes of young children in low-income households. It is also important to further investigate the role that financial literacy and practices of caregivers can play in improving the food security of low-income households.

Supplementary Materials: The following are available online at http://www.mdpi.com/2072-6643/12/8/2304/s1. Table S1. Sensitivity analysis to evaluate the association between food resource management (FRM) self-confidence with household food insecurity adjusting for significant and non-significant sociodemographic variables as potential confounders in the logistic regression models, and using imputed and non-imputed income values. Table S2: Sensitivity analysis to evaluate the associations between food resource management (FRM) self-confidence, FRM behaviors, and financial practices of Head Start caregivers by household food insecurity using simple and multiple linear regression analyses.

Author Contributions: Conceptualization, L.J., M.N., S.G.E., J.S.S.; methodology, L.J., M.N., S.G.E., M.D.-E.-H., J.S.S.; software, S.G.E., M.D.-E.-H.; validation, L.J., S.G.E., M.D.-E.-H.; formal analysis, L.J. and M.D.-E.-H.; investigation, J.S.S.; resources, J.S.S.; data curation, S.G.E.; writing—original draft preparation, L.J.; writing—review and editing, L.J., M.N., S.G.E., M.D.-E.-H., J.S.S.; visualization, L.J. and M.D.-E.-H.; supervision, J.S.S.; project administration, J.S.S.; funding acquisition, J.S.S. All authors have read and agreed to the published version of the manuscript.

Funding: This project was funded by USDA's Supplemental Nutrition Assistance Program (SNAP) through the PA Department of Human Services (DHS).

Conflicts of Interest: The authors declare no conflicts of interest.

References

1. Coleman-Jensen, A.; Rabbitt, M.; Gregory, C.; Singh, A. Household Food Security in the United States in 2018. Available online: https://www.ers.usda.gov/webdocs/publications/94849/err-270.pdf?v=963.1 (accessed on 28 May 2020).
2. Bickel, G.; Nord, M.; Price, C.; Hamilton, W.; Cook, J. Guide to Measuring Household Food Security. Available online: https://fns-prod.azureedge.net/sites/default/files/FSGuide.pdf (accessed on 29 May 2020).

3. U.S. Department of Agriculture (USDA). Key Statistics & Graphics:Food Security Status of U.S. Households in 2018. Available online: https://www.ers.usda.gov/topics/food-nutrition-assistance/food-security-in-the-us/key-statistics-graphics.aspx (accessed on 13 February 2020).
4. Thomas, M.M.; Miller, D.P.; Morrissey, T.W. Food insecurity and child health. *Pediatrics* **2019**, *144*, e20190397. [CrossRef] [PubMed]
5. Gundersen, C.; Ziliak, J.P. Food insecurity and health outcomes. *Health Aff.* **2015**, *34*, 1830–1839. [CrossRef] [PubMed]
6. Na, M.; Eagleton, S.G. Jomaa, L.; Lawton, K.; Savage, J.S. Food insecurity is associated with suboptimal sleep quality, but not sleep duration, among low-income Head Start children of pre-school age. *Public Health Nutr.* **2020**, *23*, 701–710. [CrossRef] [PubMed]
7. Ke, J.; Ford-Jones, E.L. Food insecurity and hunger: A review of the effects on children's health and behaviour. *Paediatr. Child Health* **2015**, *20*, 89–91. [CrossRef] [PubMed]
8. Shankar, P.; Chung, R.; Frank, D.A. Association of food insecurity with children's behavioral, emotional, and academic outcomes: A systematic review. *J. Dev. Behav. Pediatr.* **2017**, *38*, 135–150. [CrossRef] [PubMed]
9. Kirkpatrick, S.I.; McIntyre, L.; Potestio, M.L. Child hunger and long-term adverse consequences for health. *Arch. Pediatr. Adolesc. Med.* **2010**, *164*, 754–762. [CrossRef]
10. Kaiser, L.; Chaidez, V.; Algert, S.; Horowitz, M.; Martin, A.; Mendoza, C.; Neelon, M.; Ginsburg, D.C. Food resource management education with SNAP participation improves food security. *J. Nutr. Educ. Behav.* **2015**, *47*, 374–378 e1. [CrossRef]
11. U.S. Department of Agriculture (USDA). The Supplemental Nutrition Assistance Program Education (SNAP-ED) Toolkit: Obesity Interventions and Evaluation Framework. Available online: https://snapedtoolkit.org/framework/components/mt2/ (accessed on 4 February 2020).
12. U.S. Department of Agriculture (USDA). SNAP-Ed Toolkit: Glossary Terms. Available online: https://snapedtoolkit.org/glossary/#food_resource_management_frm (accessed on 10 March 2020).
13. Dollahite, J.; Olson, C. Scott-Pierce, M. The impact of nutrition education on food insecurity among low-income participants in EFNEP. *Fam. Consum. Sci. Res. J.* **2003**, *32*, 127–139. [CrossRef]
14. Farrell, J.A. The Impact of Nutrition Education on Food Security Status and Food-Related Behaviors. Available online: https://scholarworks.umass.edu/cgi/viewcontent.cgi?article=2204&context=theses (accessed on 8 May 2020).
15. Rivera, R.L.; Maulding, M.K.; Abbott, A.R.; Craig, B.A.; Eicher-Miller, H.A. SNAP-Ed (Supplemental Nutrition Assistance Program–Education) increases long-term food security among Indiana households with children in a randomized controlled study. *J. Nutr.* **2016**, *146*, 2375–2382. [CrossRef]
16. Martin, K.S.; Colantonio, A.G.; Picho, K.; Boyle, K.E. Self-efficacy is associated with increased food security in novel food pantry program. *SSM Popul. Health* **2016**, *2*, 62–67. [CrossRef]
17. Bandura, A. Health promotion by social cognitive means. *Health Educ. Behav.* **2004**, *31*, 143–164. [CrossRef] [PubMed]
18. Nezami, B.T.; Lang, W.; Jakicic, J.M.; Davis, K.K.; Polzien, K.; Rickman, A.D.; Hatley, K.E.; Tate, D.F. The effect of self-efficacy on behavior and weight in a behavioral weight-loss intervention. *Health Psychol.* **2016**, *35*, 714. [CrossRef] [PubMed]
19. Breland, J.Y.; Wong, J.J.; McAndrew, L.M. Are Common Sense Model constructs and self-efficacy simultaneously correlated with self-management behaviors and health outcomes: A systematic review. *Health Psychol. Open* **2020**, *7*, 2055102919898846. [CrossRef] [PubMed]
20. Hoisington, A.; Shultz, J.A.; Butkus, S. Coping strategies and nutrition education needs among food pantry users. *J. Nutr. Educ. Behav.* **2002**, *34*, 326–333. [CrossRef]
21. Kempson, K.; Keenan, D.P.; Sadani, P.S.; Adler, A. Maintaining food sufficiency: Coping strategies identified by limited-resource individuals versus nutrition educators. *J. Nutr. Educ. Behav.* **2003**, *35*, 179–188. [CrossRef]
22. Gundersen, C.G.; Garasky, S.B. Financial management skills are associated with food insecurity in a sample of households with children in the United States. *J. Nutr.* **2012**, *142*, 1865–1870. [CrossRef]
23. Chang, Y.; Chatterjee, S.; Kim, J. Household finance and food insecurity. *J. Fam. Econ. Issues.* **2014**, *35*, 499–515. [CrossRef]
24. Brewer, M. Household Debt and Children's Risk of Food Insecurity. *Soc. Probl.* **2018**, *67*, 565–584. [CrossRef]
25. Carman, K.G; Zamarro, G. Does Financial Literacy Contribute to Food Security? *Int. J. Food Agric. Econ.* **2016**, *4*, 1–19.

26. Office of Head Start. Facts about the Child and Adult Care Food Program: Food and Nutrition Service. Available online: http://eclkc.ohs.acf.hhs.gov/hslc/tta-system/health/Health/Nutrition/Nutrition%20Program%20Staff/health_mul_00592_090605.html (accessed on 29 May 2020).
27. Benjamin-Neelon, S.E. Position of the Academy of Nutrition and Dietetics: Benchmarks for nutrition in child care. *J. Acad. Nutr. Diet.* **2018**, *118*, 1291–1300. [CrossRef]
28. Fleary, S.; Heffer, R.W.; McKyer, E.L.; Taylor, A. A parent-focused pilot intervention to increase parent health literacy and healthy lifestyle choices for young children and families. *ISRN Fam. Med.* **2013**, *2013*. [CrossRef] [PubMed]
29. Pooler, J.A.; Morgan, R.E.; Wong, K.; Wilkin, M.K.; Blitstein, J.L. Cooking matters for adults improves food resource management skills and self-confidence among low-income participants. *J. Nutr. Educ. Behav.* **2017**, *49*, 545–553.e1. [CrossRef] [PubMed]
30. U.S. Department of Agriculture (USDA). National Food Study: Final Interview. Available online: https://www.ers.usda.gov/media/8619/finalinterview.pdf (accessed on 4 February 2020).
31. Begley, A.; Paynter, E.; Butcher, L.M.; Dhaliwal, S.S. Examining the association between food literacy and food insecurity. *Nutrients* **2019**, *11*, 445. [CrossRef] [PubMed]
32. Walpole, B.; Dettmer, E.; Morrongiello, B.A.; McCrindle, B.W.; Hamilton, J. Motivational interviewing to enhance self-efficacy and promote weight loss in overweight and obese adolescents: A randomized controlled trial. *J. Pediatr. Psychol.* **2013**, *38*, 944–953. [CrossRef] [PubMed]
33. Lyles, C.R.; Wolf, M.S.; Schillinger, D.; Davis, T.C.; DeWalt, D.; Dahlke, A.R.; Curtis, L.; Seligman, H.K. Food insecurity in relation to changes in hemoglobin A1c, self-efficacy, and fruit/vegetable intake during a diabetes educational intervention. *Diabetes Care* **2013**, *36*, 1448–1453. [CrossRef]
34. Wiig, K.; Smith, C. The art of grocery shopping on a food stamp budget: Factors influencing the food choices of low-income women as they try to make ends meet. *Public Health Nutr.* **2009**, *12*, 1726–1734. [CrossRef]
35. Edin, K.; Boyd, M.; Mabli, J.; Ohls, J.; Worthington, J.; Greene, S.; Redel, N.; Sridharan, S. SNAP Food Security in-Depth Interview Study: Final Report. Available online: https://www.fns.usda.gov/snap-food-security-depth-interview-study (accessed on 29 May 2020).
36. Gorman, K.S.; McCurdy, K.; Kisler, T.; Metallinos-Katsaras, E. Maternal strategies to access food differ by food security status. *J. Acad. Nutr. Diet.* **2017**, *117*, 48–57. [CrossRef]
37. FRAC. Making WIC Work Better: Strategies to Reach More Women and Children and Strengthen Benefits Use. Available online: https://frac.org/wp-content/uploads/Making-WIC-Work-Better-Full-Report.pdf (accessed on 22 July 2020).
38. Grutzmacher, S.; Braun, B. Food security status and food resource management skills over time among rural, low-income mothers. *J. Hunger Environ. Nutr.* **2008**, *2*, 81–92. [CrossRef]
39. Early Childhood Learning & Knowledge Center. Family Engagement. Available online: https://eclkc.ohs.acf.hhs.gov/family-engagement (accessed on 17 June 2020).
40. Whiteside-Mansell, L.; Swindle, T.M. Evaluation of Together We Inspire Smart Eating: Pre-school fruit and vegetable consumption. *Health Educ. Res.* **2019**, *34*, 62–71. [CrossRef]
41. Gurajada, N.; Reed, D.B.; Taylor, A.L. Jump2Health Website™ for Head Start parents to promote a healthy home environment: Results from formative research. *J. Public Health Res.* **2017**, *6*, 1054. [CrossRef]
42. Hindin, T.J.; Contento, I.R.; Gussow, J.D. A media literacy nutrition education curriculum for head start parents about the effects of television advertising on their children's food requests. *J. Am. Diet. Assoc.* **2004**, *104*, 192–198. [CrossRef] [PubMed]
43. Alaimo, K. Food insecurity in the United States: An overview. *Top. Clin. Nutr.* **2005**, *20*, 281–298. [CrossRef]
44. Melchior, M.; Caspi, A.; Howard, L.M.; Ambler, A.P.; Bolton, H.; Mountain, N.; Moffitt, T.E. Mental health context of food insecurity: A representative cohort of families with young children. *Pediatrics* **2009**, *124*, e564–e572. [CrossRef] [PubMed]
45. Bartfeld, J.; Collins, J.M. Food insecurity, financial shocks, and financial coping strategies among households with elementary school children in Wisconsin. *J. Consum. Aff.* **2017**, *51*, 519–548. [CrossRef]
46. McCloskey, M.; Johnson, S.L.; Benz, C.; Thompson, D.A.; Chamberlin, B.; Clark, L.; Bellows, L.L. Parent perceptions of mobile device use among preschool-aged children in rural head start centers. *J. Nutr. Educ. Behav.* **2018**, *50*, 83–89.e1. [CrossRef]
47. Holben, D.H.; McClincy, M.C.; Holcomb, J.P., Jr.; Dean, K.L.; Walker, C.E. Food security status of households in Appalachian Ohio with children in Head Start. *J. Am. Diet. Assoc.* **2004**, *104*, 238–241. [CrossRef]

48. Savage, J.S.; Fisher, J.C.; Birch, L.L. Parental influence on eating behavior: Conception to adolescence. *J. Law Med. Ethics* **2007**, *35*, 22–34. [CrossRef]
49. Birch, L.L.; Ventura, A.K. Preventing childhood obesity: What works? *Int. J. Obes.* **2009**, *33*, S74–S81. [CrossRef]
50. Wood, A.C.; Blissett, J.M.; Brunstrom, J.M.; Carnell, S.; Faith, M.S.; Fisher, J.O.; Hayman, L.L.; Khalsa, A.S.; Hughes, S.O.; Miller, A.L. Caregiver influences on eating behaviors in young children: A scientific statement from the American Heart Association. *J. Am. Heart Assoc.* **2019**, *9*, e014520. [CrossRef]

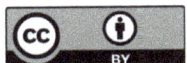

© 2020 by the authors. Licensee MDPI, Basel, Switzerland. This article is an open access article distributed under the terms and conditions of the Creative Commons Attribution (CC BY) license (http://creativecommons.org/licenses/by/4.0/).

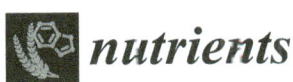 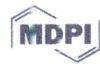

Article

Supplemental Nutrition Assistance Program-Education Improves Food Security Independent of Food Assistance and Program Characteristics

Heather A. Eicher-Miller [1,*], Rebecca L. Rivera [1,2], Hanxi Sun [3], Yumin Zhang [3], Melissa K. Maulding [4,5] and Angela R. Abbott [4]

1. Department of Nutrition Science, Purdue University, West Lafayette, IN 47907, USA; rerivera@iu.edu
2. Richard M. Fairbanks School of Public Health and the Regenstrief Institute, Inc., Indiana University, Indianapolis, IN 46202, USA
3. Department of Statistics, Purdue University, West Lafayette, IN 47907, USA; sun652@purdue.edu (H.S.); zhan2013@purdue.edu (Y.Z.)
4. Health and Human Sciences Cooperative Extension, Purdue University, West Lafayette, IN 47907, USA; Mkmaulding2@eiu.edu (M.K.M.); abbottar@purdue.edu (A.R.A.)
5. College of Health and Human Services, Eastern Illinois University, Charleston, IL 61920, USA
* Correspondence: heichrm@purdue.edu; Tel.: +1-765-494-6815; Fax: +1-765-494-0906

Received: 4 August 2020; Accepted: 27 August 2020; Published: 29 August 2020

Abstract: The purpose of this project was to determine whether consistent food assistance program participation or changes in participation over time mediated or moderated the effect of federal nutrition education through the Supplemental Nutrition Assistance Program-Education (SNAP-Ed) on food security and determine the associations of SNAP-Ed program delivery characteristics with change in food security. This secondary analysis used data from a randomized controlled trial from September 2013 through April 2015. SNAP-Ed-eligible participants (n = 328; ≥18 years) in households with children were recruited from 39 counties in Indiana, USA. The dependent variable was one year change in household food security score measured using the United States Household Food Security Survey Module. Assessment of mediation used Barron-Kenny analysis and moderation used interactions of food assistance program use and changes over time with treatment group in general linear regression modeling. Program delivery characteristics were investigated using mixed linear regression modeling. Results showed that neither consistent participation nor changes in food assistance program participation over time mediated nor moderated the effect of SNAP-Ed on food security and neither were SNAP-Ed program delivery characteristics associated with change in food security over the one year study period. SNAP-Ed directly improved food security among SNAP-Ed-eligible Indiana households with children regardless of food assistance program participation and changes over time or varying program delivery characteristics.

Keywords: supplemental nutrition assistance program-education; SNAP-Ed; nutrition education; food assistance; SNAP; food stamps; WIC; food security; food pantry; emergency food programs

1. Introduction

Members of low-income households face a high burden of food insecurity, poor nutrition, and undesirable health outcomes [1–5]. The Supplemental Nutrition Assistance Program-Education (SNAP-Ed) is a program of the United States Department of Agriculture (USDA) Food and Nutrition Service (FNS) that offers education on nutrition, budgeting, and resource management to low-income households to improve dietary intake and food security [6,7]. SNAP-Ed has been shown to improve household and adult food security in previous longitudinal randomized controlled trials [8,9]. Approximately 73% of households interested in receiving SNAP-Ed also report participating in at least one of three other food assistance programs [9] directed to alleviate food insecurity in qualifying low-income households [10], including the Supplemental Nutrition Assistance Program (SNAP), the Special Supplemental Nutrition Program for Women, Infants, and Children (WIC), and The Emergency Food Assistance Program (TEFAP). SNAP and WIC provide financial and food resources to help individuals and families obtain foods to supplement their nutritional needs [11,12] while TEFAP provides foods to state agencies who partner with private and local organizations to distribute emergency foods to food banks and food pantries where individuals in need may access foods at no cost [13]. Mutual participation in SNAP-Ed and SNAP is not required; some SNAP-Ed participants may not qualify for SNAP benefits or choose not to participate in SNAP. Further, sometimes SNAP-Ed lessons are used to fulfill WIC education requirements.

Previous evidence of improvement in food security because of SNAP [2], WIC [14], and associations with emergency program use [15], taken with knowledge of the common practice of simultaneous participation in food assistance programs and nutrition education programs, suggests that the changes observed in food security previously attributed to nutrition education [9] may actually be accounted for by participation or change in participation of food assistance (mediation). It may also be likely that the effect of nutrition education on food security may be differential by food assistance participation or changes in food assistance (moderation). SNAP-Ed educators commonly help participants with eligibility and encourage their application for local, state, and federal food assistance as part of the resource management education offered, making salient the reality that participation status in food assistance programs may frequently change during nutrition education participation [16]. Previous investigation of nutrition education program effectiveness on food insecurity has focused on singular program use and has not considered mediation or moderation by food assistance participation or changes in their use, specifically regarding the three most common food assistance programs, SNAP, WIC, and TEFAP [17]. Only one previous non-experimental short-term study evaluated joint use of two of these programs and showed that SNAP-Ed participants who were also receiving SNAP benefits and made more improvement in resource management skills, reported the greatest decrease in running out of food (measured by only one question) compared with participants who were not receiving SNAP benefits and who had less improvement in resource management skills [18]. Additional factors of relevance in SNAP-Ed effect on participant food security improvement are SNAP-Ed program delivery characteristics, such as the number of lessons, group or individual lessons, or SNAP-Ed educator. In Indiana, over sixty educators deliver up to ten SNAP-Ed lessons using group and individual lesson delivery. Program variability presented by these characteristics are inherent to SNAP-Ed and may potentially be associated with an effect on food security. For example, food security improvement may be influenced by participants receiving 10 rather than 4 lessons, individualized compared with group lessons, or by interaction with a particular SNAP-Ed educator.

Therefore, determining the potential mediating or moderating role of food assistance participation and changes in participation over time on nutrition education program participation would clarify knowledge of impacts to food security. Examination of the role of SNAP-Ed program characteristics number of lessons, delivery format, and variability of educator to food security improvement would inform program and policy of important programmatic aspects of success. The objectives of this paper were investigated among adults ≥18 years from Indiana in a dataset where a decrease of 1.2 ± 0.4 (mean $\pm$ SE) units in household food security score over the one year study period, indicating a meaningful longitudinal improvement in food security among the intervention compared to the control group, was previously discovered [9], and included:

1. Determine whether participation and changes in participation status in food assistance programs SNAP, WIC, and food pantries over one year mediated the effect of a SNAP-Ed intervention on one year change in household food security.

2. Determine whether participation and changes in participation status in food assistance programs SNAP, WIC, and food pantries over one year moderated the effect of a SNAP-Ed intervention on one year change in household food security.
3. Determine whether the number of SNAP-Ed lessons received as an intervention, SNAP-Ed lesson delivery format, or variability of SNAP-Ed educator was associated with one year change in household food security (independent of food assistance program participation).

2. Materials and Methods

2.1. Study Population

For this secondary data analysis, all data were obtained from The Indiana SNAP-Ed Long-term Study, a longitudinal (one year) parallel-arm randomized controlled nutrition education intervention trial conducted between August 2013 and April 2015 [9]. Thirty-five county-level Indiana SNAP-Ed nutrition education paraprofessionals (SNAP-Ed educators) recruited adult participants ($n = 575$) aged ≥18 years from August 2013 to March 2014 and administered baseline assessments. Participants were recruited from locations such as WIC clinics, food pantries, or Indiana Cooperative Extension county offices. The one year follow-up assessments were completed from September 2014 through April 2015. Data to address the hypotheses of this study are expected to maintain relevance to current program and participants as food insecurity in Indiana from 2013–2015 was not statistically significantly different from 2016–2018 estimates [5], and the data represent a unique opportunity to comprehensively address hypotheses using a singular sample. Only participants who completed the study (i.e., baseline and one year follow-up assessments) were included in the analysis presented here (total $n = 328$, control $n = 163$, intervention $n = 165$). SNAP-Ed educators were trained to determine participant study eligibility and randomly assigned participants to either the non-active control group or intervention group using an allocation ratio of ~1:1. A random number allocated the first participant or group recruited simultaneously (to prevent knowledge of different treatment) to the intervention or control group and then an alternating assignment was followed. After treatment group assignment, SNAP-Ed educators delivered lessons to the intervention group participants as per program protocol over the following four to ten weeks, at approximately 1 lesson per week, and facilitated all survey assessments to both treatment groups. Eligible study participants included Indiana adult residents who had one or more children living in the household, had not received a SNAP-Ed lesson in the past one year, were able to speak, read, and write in English, and were willing to wait one year to receive nutrition education lessons.

2.2. Intervention

The intervention consisted of the first four (out of ten) lessons in the Indiana SNAP-Ed curriculum [19] as these lessons comprise SNAP-Ed guidance and cover the USDA key behavioral outcomes of maintaining caloric balance over time for a healthy weight and consumption of nutrient-dense foods and beverages. Additionally, lessons included instruction on budgeting food resources through the following lesson topics: applying USDA MyPlate to build healthy meals, using food labels to make healthy choices, identifying the importance of whole grains, and adding more fruits and vegetables to meals [19,20]. The Purdue Institutional Review Board approved the trial protocol and all participants provided written informed consent. The trial was registered at www.clinicaltrials.gov as NCT03436589.

2.3. Food Security Measures

Household food security score was measured using the 18-item USDA U.S. Household Food Security Survey Module (US HFSSM) with scores ranging from 0 (food secure) to 18 (very low food secure) and a 12-month reference period [21,22]. Categorical classification of food security at baseline was also constructed as food secure, marginally food secure, and food insecure according to prior guidance [22]. Change in food security score was the response variable in this secondary data analysis to determine a more specific change compared with using food security categories, and was quantified by subtracting the baseline score from the one year follow-up score for each participant.

2.4. Food Assistance Program Measures Used in Objectives 1 and 2

Study participants self-reported participation status in SNAP, WIC, and food pantries over the 30 days prior to both baseline and one year follow-up assessments because the food assistance provided through these programs are generally distributed on a monthly basis. One month or 30 days was considered the minimal amount of time that these programs may exert influence on a participant household and on SNAP-Ed effectiveness. Missing values were 8% ($n = 27$) at baseline and 15% ($n = 50$) at follow-up. A sensitivity analysis was conducted where missing values were coded as participation and compared to coding values as non-participation. The results did not change so coding as non-participation was applied. Participation in local, state, or national food assistance programs other than SNAP, WIC, or food pantries was not recorded.

Three individual four-level categorical variables referred to as "change in one year participation status" were created for SNAP, WIC, and food pantries, respectively, to represent any changes or no changes in food assistance participation status between the 30 days prior to baseline and the 30 days prior to one year follow-up assessments. "Change in one year participation status" variables were created by concatenating the baseline and one year follow-up binary variables to simultaneously represent the participation status for each of the food assistance programs at baseline and at one year follow-up in addition to change in participation status if it occurred (00 = no participation; 10 = participation at baseline only; 01 = participation at one year follow-up only; 11 = participation at both baseline and one year follow-up). These variables were used as a categorical independent variable to address the first and second research objectives, whether change in food assistance program participation status or consistency mediated or moderated the impact of SNAP-Ed on one year change in food security score.

2.5. SNAP-Ed Program Characteristics Measures Used in Objective 3

The number of SNAP-Ed lessons a participant received, the lesson delivery format, and which SNAP-Ed educator delivered the lessons were investigated as the SNAP-Ed program characteristics among intervention group participants who completed the required four lessons to address the third research objective. Participants assigned to the intervention group that did not complete the four required intervention lessons, lost contact with SNAP-Ed educators, or did not follow the study protocol were considered withdrawn from the study ($n = 87$). The number of lessons (4–10 lessons) a participant received was recorded by the SNAP-Ed educator at each lesson and summed at the one year follow-up assessment. Lesson delivery format was a categorical variable with three levels representing how the participant received lessons (one-to-one lessons, group lessons, combination of one-to-one and group lessons) and was based on the preference of the participant to attend group lessons, educator facilitation, and the schedule of group or individual lessons. Assignment of SNAP-Ed educator ($n = 37$) was determined by the participant's county of residence at recruitment.

2.6. Other Covariates

A binary variable for treatment group (control, intervention) was used to address the first and second research objectives. Time was included as a binary variable in mixed regression modeling (baseline, follow-up) to address the third research objective. Self-reported baseline participant characteristics identified as potential confounders through Chi-square comparisons between the intervention and control groups were investigated: sex (female, male); age in years (18–30, 31–50, ≥51); race/ethnicity (non-Hispanic white, other); highest level of education among the household (no high school diploma, high school diploma, or General Educational Development certification indicating high school level skills; some college/associate's degree; ≥bachelor's degree); marital status (living with partner/married, never married, divorced/separated/widowed); household employment (household member employed, no household member employed); household poverty status (<federal poverty guideline, ≥federal poverty guideline); household size (two, three, four, or ≥five household members); SNAP, WIC, or food pantry participation status 30 days prior to baseline (not participating, participating); and food security category at baseline (food secure, marginally food secure, food insecure). Two categories for race/ethnicity were used in this study because reports other than non-Hispanic white were very few: 3 participants reported American Indian, 1 reported Asian, and 7 reported non-Hispanic black. Maintaining separate categories would threaten the robustness of the analysis and model fit so categories were combined to a single category.

2.7. Statistical Methods

To address the first research objective, the Baron-Kenny causal mediation approach was used to investigate whether the suspected mediator "change in one year participation status" in SNAP, WIC, or food pantries mediated the effect of the exposure, SNAP-Ed intervention, on the outcome, change in household food security score over the one year study period [23]. Additional covariates are not included in the Baron-Kenny three variable system regression approach (Figure 1, below); investigation of the role of other covariates are outside of the scope of the hypotheses of this paper.

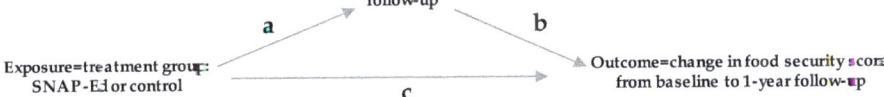

Step 1. Determine c. Results described in text in Section 3.1, Step 1.
Step 2. Determine a. Results described in text in Section 3.1, Step 2 and in Tables 1 and 2.
Step 3. Determine b: Results described in text in Section 3.1, Step 3.
Step 4. Determine c and b if there are significant relationships from Steps 1-3: Mediation is supported when the effect of the suspected mediator is significant after controlling for the exposure. Results described in text in Section 3.1, Step 4.

Figure 1. Hypothesized Baron-Kenny causal mediation model of the Supplemental Nutrition Assistance Program-Education (SNAP-Ed) intervention effect by the "change in one year participation status" in Supplemental Nutrition Assistance Program (SNAP), Women, Infants, and Children (WIC), or food pantries on the change in one year food security score among Indiana SNAP-Ed Study participants. a = the relationship of the exposure on the suspected mediator using regression, b = the relationship of the suspected mediator on the outcome using regression, c = the relationship of the exposure on the outcome using regression.

To address the second research objective, interactions between "change in one year participation status" (SNAP, WIC, and food pantries) and treatment group variables were used in general linear regression modeling to determine whether the change in food assistance program participation, consistent participation, or non-participation moderated the effect of SNAP-Ed on the change in food security score over the one year study period. SNAP, WIC, and food pantry interactions with treatment group were investigated in separate models; the reference group was consistent non-participation during the 30 days prior to baseline and one year follow-up. Other participant characteristics (sex, age, race/ethnicity, education, poverty status, employment status, marital status, household size) were initially included in the models as potential confounders but removed because they were not influential ($p < 0.2$). Statistical power to detect a difference at a significance level of $\alpha = 0.05$ with power at 0.90, for a one unit improvement in food security based on previous study data [9,18,24] was confirmed using a power analysis procedure for general linear regression models. A treatment effect of one unit on the food security scale was chosen for the power analysis because of the practical relevance and potential of a one unit decrease to transition a participant between two food security statuses and the associated positive benefit. In addition, an approximate one unit change was discovered in the study from which this data was derived and considered reasonable. Tukey adjustment for multiple comparisons was applied.

To address the third research objective, a mixed linear regression model was used to determine the association of the number of lessons, lesson delivery format, and variability between SNAP-Ed educators with change in food security score over one year among the intervention group ($n = 165$). Time, number of lessons, and lesson delivery format were included as fixed effects in the model. Participants and SNAP-Ed educator were considered random effects. The covariance structure was specified as compound symmetry after using the Sawa Bayesian information criterion (BIC) to compare various covariance structures. None of the potential participant characteristic confounders were found influential ($p > 0.2$), except for age ($p = 0.02$) which was included as a covariate in the model. Statistical power to detect a difference at a significance level of $\alpha = 0.05$ with power at 0.90 and one unit improvement in food security was confirmed using a power analysis procedure for mixed linear regression models.

Model assumptions were checked by plotting residuals against predicted means, Q-Q plots, and histograms of residuals for general and mixed linear regression modeling and applied to each study objective. All analyses were completed using SAS® software version 9.4 (SAS Institute Inc., Cary, NC, USA).

3. Results

The characteristics and food security of participants in the intervention and control groups are shown in Table 1.

Table 1. Comparison of baseline sociodemographic characteristics by treatment group of Indiana SNAP-Ed participants among households with children using Chi-Square analysis.

		Control		Intervention		χ^2 p-Value
		N	%	N	%	
Total		163	50	165	50	
Sex						0.7
	Female	148	93	148	92	
	Male	11	7	13	8	
Age Group						0.3
	18–30 Years	77	47	93	56	
	31–50 Years	73	45	60	36	
	51 Years or Older	13	8	12	7	
Race/Ethnicity						0.7
	Non-Hispanic White	145	96	149	97	
	Other	6	4	5	3	
Household Education						0.1
	No High School Diploma	7	4	13	8	
	High School Diploma	29	18	45	27	
	General Educational Development	31	19	27	16	
	Some College	53	33	46	28	
	Associate's Degree	23	14	25	15	
	Bachelor's Degree or Higher	17	11	8	5	
Marital Status						0.2

Table 1. Cont.

		Control		Intervention		χ^2 p-value
		N	%	N	%	
	Never Married	28	17	40	24	
	Married/with partner	94	58	94	57	
	Separated/Divorced	41	25	31	19	
Household Employment						0.01 *
	Not Employed	82	50	60	36	
	Employed	81	50	105	64	
Household Poverty Status (Income to Poverty Ratio)						0.3
	≥Federal Guideline	44	27	37	22	
	<Federal Guideline	119	73	128	78	
Household Size						0.5
	2	12	7	6	4	
	3	38	23	38	23	
	4	42	26	47	28	
	5 or more	70	43	74	45	
SNAP Participation (past 30 days)						0.1
	No	76	47	62	38	
	Yes	87	53	103	62	
WIC Participation (past 30 days)						<0.01 *
	No	81	50	58	35	
	Yes	82	50	107	65	
Food Pantry Participation (past 30 days)						<0.01 *
	No	138	85	156	95	
	Yes	25	15	9	5	
Baseline Household Food Security						0.9
	Food Secure	44	27	41	25	
	Marginal	64	39	65	39	
	Food Insecure	55	34	59	36	

Values are counts, percentages, and p-values from Chi-square comparisons of the distributions among sociodemographic characteristics between control and intervention group participants. Total numbers do not always add to sample size due to missing values and percentages do not always add to 100 due to rounding. * $p \leq 0.05$ Abbreviations: SNAP-Ed, Supplemental Nutrition Assistance Program-Education; SNAP, Supplemental Nutrition Assistance Program; WIC, Special Supplemental Nutrition Program for Women, Infants, and Children.

Participation in WIC, food pantries, and employment were the only characteristics with significantly different distributions among intervention and control groups at baseline.

3.1. Research Objective 1: Test for Food Assistance Program Mediation of SNAP-Ed Effect on Food Security

Step 1: Food security score did not differ between treatment groups at baseline using regression ($\beta = -0.4$, SE = 0.3, $p = 0.4$). The SNAP-Ed treatment group exposure had a significantly improved food security change from baseline to 12 months later ($\beta = 1.2$, SE = 0.4, $p = 0.001$).

Step 2: Participation status in WIC and food pantry use, but not for SNAP, 30 days prior to baseline differed ($p < 0.01$) between the intervention and control groups in Chi-square analyses (Table 1). Additionally, "change in one year participation status" (30 days prior to baseline and one year follow-up) in WIC and food pantry use differed ($p = 0.03$) between the intervention and control groups using Chi-square analysis (Table 2), but again, not for SNAP ($p = 0.3$). Logistic regression showed similar results of an association with treatment group and the potential for mediation for WIC ($p = 0.04$) and food pantry use ($p = 0.05$) but not SNAP ($p = 0.3$) (Table 2).

Step 3: Using general linear regression modeling, "change in one year participation status" in SNAP ($p = 0.3$), WIC ($p = 0.4$), or food pantry use ($p = 0.5$) were not associated with the long-term change in food security score.

Step 4: Since significant relationships were present in steps 1 and 2, multiple linear regression modeling of the relationship of treatment group and "change in one year participation status" in SNAP, WIC, and food pantries on the outcome was completed. Results showed that neither SNAP ($p = 0.2$), WIC ($p = 0.2$), nor food pantries ($p = 0.3$) were significant after treatment group was included in the model, yet treatment group remained significant ($p \leq 0.001$).

In conclusion of research objective 1, no mediation was found between the SNAP-Ed intervention and "change in one year participation status" in SNAP, WIC, or food pantries on the change in food security score over the one year study period in the intervention compared to the control group using the Baron-Kenny causal mediation approach.

Table 2. Change in one year participation status comparison of SNAP, WIC, and food pantries by treatment group among Indiana SNAP-Ed participants using Chi-Square and logistic regression.

		Total		Control		Intervention		χ2 p-Value	Logistic Regression p-Value
		n	%	N	%	n	%		
Total		328	100	163	50	165	50		
	Change in One Year Participation Status								
SNAP								0.3	0.3
	No Participation	105	32	58	36	47	28		
	Baseline Participation Only	39	12	21	13	18	11		
	Follow-up Participation Only	33	10	18	11	15	9		
	Baseline and Follow-up Participation	151	46	66	40	85	52		
WIC								0.03 *	0.04 *
	No Participation	122	37	73	45	49	30		
	Baseline Participation Only	61	19	24	15	37	22		
	Follow-up Participation Only	17	5	8	5	9	6		
	Baseline and Follow-up Participation	128	39	58	35	70	42		
Food Pantry								0.03 *	0.05 *
	No Participation	278	85	130	80	148	90		
	Baseline Participation Only	18	5	13	8	5	3		
	Follow-up Participation Only	16	5	8	5	8	5		
	Baseline and Follow-up Participation	16	5	12	7	4	2		

Values are counts, percentages, and p-values from Chi-square and logistic regression comparisons of the distributions among "change in one year food assistance participation status" between control and intervention group participants. Total numbers do not always add to sample size due to missing values and percentages do not always add to 100 due to rounding. Reference period for one year participation status covered the 30 days prior to baseline and 30 days prior to one year follow-up. * $p \leq 0.05$. Abbreviations: SNAP-Ed, Supplemental Nutrition Assistance Program-Education; SNAP, Supplemental Nutrition Assistance Program; WIC, Special Supplemental Nutrition Program for Women, Infants, and Children.

3.2. Research Objective 2: Test for Food Assistance Program Moderation of SNAP-Ed Effect on Food Security

The interactions of "change in one year participation status" in SNAP, WIC, or food pantries with the treatment group did not moderate the mean difference (mean ± SEM) in food security scores in the intervention compared to the control over the one year study period using general linear regression modeling (SNAP −0.8 ± 0.4, $p = 0.2$; WIC −1.1 ± 0.5, $p = 0.1$; food pantries −1.2 ± 0.8, $p = 0.7$) (Table 3).

Table 3. Change in food security score over one year study period for the interaction of "change in one year participation status" and treatment group among Indiana SNAP-Ed participants using general linear regression modeling.

		Mean Change in Household Food Security Score						
		Control $n = 165$		Intervention $n = 165$		Intervention-Control		
		Mean	SE	Mean	SE	Mean Difference ‡	SE	p-Value §
SNAP	SNAP × Treatment Group	−0.9	0.3	−1.7	0.3	−0.8	0.4	0.2
	No Participation	−0.8	0.4	−1.3	0.5	−0.5	0.6	1.0
	Baseline Participation Only	−2.1	0.7	−2.4	0.8	−0.3	1.0	1.0
	Follow-up Participation Only	−0.8	0.8	−1.3	0.8	−0.5	1.1	1.0
	Baseline and Follow-up Participation	0	0.4	−2.0	0.3	−2.0	0.5	<0.01
WIC	WIC × Treatment Group	−0.9	0.4	−1.9	0.3	−1.1	0.5	0.1
	No Participation	−0.6	0.4	−2.7	0.5	−2.1	0.6	<0.01
	Baseline Participation Only	−1.0	0.7	−0.8	0.5	0.2	0.8	1.0
	Follow-up Participation Only	−1.5	1.1	−2.7	1.1	−1.2	1.6	1.0
	Baseline and Follow-up Participation	−0.4	0.4	−1.5	0.4	−1.1	0.6	0.5
Food Pantry	Food Pantry × Treatment Group	−0.9	0.4	−2.1	0.6	−1.2	0.8	0.7
	No Participation	−0.5	0.3	−1.8	0.3	−1.3	0.4	0.03
	Baseline Participation Only	−0.4	0.9	−3.2	1.5	−2.8	1.7	0.7
	Follow-up Participation Only	−0.6	1.1	−0.9	1.1	−0.3	1.6	1.0
	Baseline and Follow-up Participation	−2.3	0.9	−2.8	1.6	−0.5	1.9	1.0

Least squares means were calculated using general linear regression models with change in food security as the response variable. SNAP, WIC, and food pantries were investigated in separate models including interactions with treatment group. ‡ A decrease in food security score from baseline to 1 year follow-up indicates improved food security. § Tukey adjustment for multiple comparisons in stratified analyses in each model. Interactions of each food assistance program with treatment were significant when interaction term $p \leq 0.05$. Abbreviations: SE, Standard Error of the Least Squares Mean; SNAP-Ed, Supplemental Nutrition Assistance Program-Education; SNAP, Supplemental Nutrition Assistance Program; WIC Special Supplemental Nutrition Program for Women, Infants, and Children.

3.3. Research Objective 3: Test for SNAP-Ed Program Characteristics Relationship with SNAP-Ed on Food Security

The majority of intervention group participants ($n = 165$, 78%) received more than the minimum of four lessons with a mean of 6.8 lessons (Table 4). Approximately half of participants ($n = 85$, 57%) received lessons in a one-to-one or individualized format, followed by group ($n = 38$, 26%), and combination the two types ($n = 25$, 17%). There was no statistical evidence of an association between lesson delivery format ($p = 0.3$), the number of lessons received ($p = 0.6$), or variation between SNAP-Ed educators ($p = 0.4$) and the mean increase in food security score over time using a mixed multiple linear regression model.

Table 4. Evaluation of lesson delivery format, SNAP-Ed educator, and number of lessons received by Indiana SNAP-Ed Study participants on change in food security score over one year study period using mixed multiple linear regression modeling.

Program Characteristic	Control Group N	Control Group %	Intervention Group n	Intervention Group %	p-Value [§]
Total	163	50	165	50	
Lesson Delivery Format					0.3
Individual	-	-	85	57	
Group	-	-	38	26	
Combination	-	-	25	17	
Number of Lessons					0.6
0	163	100	-	-	
4	-	-	37	22	
5	-	-	25	15	
6	-	-	25	15	
7	-	-	9	6	
8	-	-	12	7	
9	-	-	23	14	
10	-	-	34	21	
SNAP-Ed Educator					0.4

Lesson delivery format was reported at baseline assessment. Number of lessons was reported at the one year follow-up assessment. The control group did not receive lessons. A minimum of 4 lessons was required to have completed the intervention. Only treatment group participants were included in the mixed multiple linear regression modeling. Cells do not always add to total sample size due to missing data. [§] p-values reported for lesson delivery format and number of lessons are from the type 3 test of fixed effects. The p-value reported for SNAP-Ed educator is from the random effect covariance parameter estimate. Abbreviations: SNAP-Ed, Supplemental Nutrition Assistance Program-Education.

4. Discussion

The major finding from this secondary data analysis indicated an improvement in household food security among the SNAP-Ed intervention group compared to the control group regardless of participation and changes in participation in food assistance programs SNAP, WIC, or food pantries 30 days prior to baseline and one year after the intervention. The mediation and moderation analyses addressing research objectives one and two revealed that SNAP-Ed directly improved food security rather than exerting or magnifying improvement through food assistance participation or changes in participation over one year.

One previous study found greater improvements in food security among SNAP-Ed participants who also received SNAP [18] indicating that for certain populations and shorter time periods, SNAP may assist SNAP-Ed to further improve food security. However, the present results using experimental data, determined no significant difference between the treatment groups for change in food security across the four types of one year SNAP participation status. Together, previous and current study results build evidence that SNAP-Ed is effective in directly improving food security over a one year period [9].

In addition to improving food security, SNAP-Ed may have caused changes in participation status in food assistance programs throughout the study period for the following reasons. As part of the normal program delivery, SNAP-Ed educators may have encouraged and assisted intervention group participants who were not receiving food assistance at baseline to apply for financial benefits through SNAP or WIC or to maximize nutrition resources available through food pantries or other resources. On the other hand, improvements in food security directly from SNAP-Ed may have led intervention group participants who reported receiving food assistance at baseline to attain and maintain sufficient nutrition resources and withdraw participation in SNAP, WIC, or use of food pantries by the one year follow-up. Alternatively, participation in other local, state, or federal food assistance programs or resources that were not recorded in this study may have impacted food security.

For example, policy, systems, environment, and other nutrition and lifestyle related resources may be influential in the success of SNAP-Ed and should continue to be investigated in the future [25]. Investigation to the reasons for changes in food assistance participation were outside of the scope of this research but present an opportunity for the future. Due to the observational nature of food assistance designation in this study, the results do not provide causal evidence of SNAP-Ed influence on changes in food assistance participation status. This limitation provides an important research opportunity, yet ethical constraints may hinder randomization of food assistance resources and require pragmatic study designs in future research [18].

In addition to finding no mediation or moderation of changes or consistency in food assistance program participation on SNAP-Ed effectiveness on food security, nutrition education program characteristics such as the number of lessons, delivery format (group or individual lessons), and SNAP-Ed educator were not associated with the magnitude of SNAP-Ed effectiveness on food security. A study describing the effect of online compared to in-person SNAP-Ed lesson delivery [26], on nutrition knowledge, intentions to change behavior, and self-efficacy, is the only previously published SNAP-Ed study to evaluate similar SNAP-Ed program characteristics. No previously published studies have addressed the question of a dose-response effect of the number of SNAP-Ed lessons on food security. In the study described herein, more than four lessons did not result in a significantly larger improvement in food security. The minimum lessons comprising SNAP-Ed guidance, four in this case, were a sufficient intervention to improve food security, reinforcing the notion that these limited lessons cover the most important behavioral recommendations for SNAP-Ed set by the USDA FNS at least in regard to food security [21]. The results suggest that participation in the minimally adherent intervention lessons is more critical to food security gains than the frequency and amount of additional time spent in lessons. Other beneficial outcomes that were not quantified here, such as sustainability of food security gains over a period longer than one year, increased nutrition knowledge, or dietary changes, may potentially be influenced by additional lessons; however, those outcomes have yet to be investigated.

The format of lesson delivery was also not significantly associated with change in food security over the one year study period among the intervention group. A current Indiana SNAP-Ed priority set forth by the USDA FNS encourages a transition to mostly group lesson delivery format rather than one-to-one format. This policy decision is supported by these study results in regard to food security improvements. Group lessons reach a greater number of participants at less cost and time, and, in this study, were as effective as individual lessons. Yet, reach to participants with special needs was not evaluated here and the provision of individual lessons may remain relevant for this group.

The third program characteristic assessed in this study, variability in one year food security score due to different educators, was not statistically significant. Variable characteristics inherent to the educator that may potentially influence outcomes include age, race, ethnicity, language, gender, education level, years of experience, depth of nutrition education knowledge, personality, knowledge and connection with community resources, among many others. These characteristics may affect the delivery and acceptance of the program to participants by potentially influencing SNAP-Ed educators' and participants' abilities to connect and relate to each other. Investigating the educator as a random effect in the model did not allow for comparisons specifically based on the educator characteristics mentioned or between specific educators yet, did allow insight to educator significance with regard to SNAP-Ed effectiveness. The study results suggest that the SNAP-Ed educators delivered a program effective at improving participants' household food security irrespective of educator.

A few studies have evaluated the impact of SNAP-Ed on food security; however, there is a paucity of SNAP-Ed literature specifically evaluating the impact of program delivery characteristics on food security outcomes [8,9,18]. A small body of literature has evaluated a second federally-supported nutrition education program, the Expanded Food and Nutrition Education Program (EFNEP) [27–30]. Since the two programs are similar in terms of aligning program goals with the Dietary Guidelines for Americans and target population, research results from EFNEP provide relevant background. Studies evaluating EFNEP reported an increase in food security using a variety of food security measures including one survey question [27] and the 6-item [28] and 18-item [30] US HFSSM. The number of lessons needed to increase food security greatly varied across the studies. In one study, program completers (mean number of lessons 8.5 ± 0.02) compared to drop-outs (mean number of lessons 6.8 ± 0.11) showed a positive dose-response in food security with increasing number of lessons [27]. Additionally, food security was higher in participants who received lessons in a one-to-one format compared to those who received lessons in a group format or a combination of group and individual lessons [27]. In other studies, participants improved food security after receiving seven EFNEP lessons [28] or with just two or more lessons compared to a comparison group receiving one or no lessons [30]. Lesson delivery format was not always defined in these studies. The results of the present study strengthen the evidence that effectiveness of nutrition education to improve food security does not depend on the number of lessons exceeding the program completion criteria, nor format of lessons (group or one-to-one), despite the mixed results from the small body of EFNEP and SNAP-Ed literature.

Results from the present study provide a foundation for further research that improves upon some limitations, but others are presented. Treatment groups were not originally designed to test participation in singular or concurrent food assistance programs or program characteristics as main effects in the analysis. The implication of the simple randomization technique in conjunction with the large number of potential confounding characteristics presents a possibility for uneven distribution of characteristics across treatment groups, which could result in overestimation their effects. Although no significant effect was detected in this study, designing future studies to further stratify the control and intervention groups by food assistance participation status may enhance evaluation of simultaneous food assistance program participation and changes in participation and nutrition education on target outcomes. Potential for misclassification was present; however, non-response was low (baseline 8% ($n = 27$), follow-up 15% ($n = 50$)) and did not influence the results based on the sensitivity analysis, but the hesitation for some participants to answer these types of sensitive survey questions is important to consider when calculating future study sample sizes and mitigation of bias. Specifically, responses on the HFSSM were made for the entire household by one adult in the household (as per guidance [22]) and entail the reporting adult's perceptions on the other household member's food security. The 30-day reference periods before baseline and one year follow-up may not have captured all changes in food assistance. Collecting additional information on the consistency and timing of food assistance use in future studies could elucidate the temporality of the relationship between food assistance program participation, SNAP-Ed, and food security improvement. Interpretation of the results should be carefully limited to the hypothesis focused on SNAP-Ed as the main independent variable and do not inform the role of SNAP as the main independent variable on food security status.

A major strength of this study was the use of longitudinal data derived from a randomized controlled impact evaluation showing an improvement in one year food security due to SNAP-Ed [9]. Participants included in these analyses represented the greater Indiana SNAP-Ed population except for less racial diversity (89% of Indiana SNAP-Ed participants compared to 95% of study participants were non-Hispanic White; Chi-square $p < 0.01$). This difference in racial diversity is likely due to not having SNAP-Ed educators from more racially diverse geographic areas volunteer to assist with the study. Participants who withdrew from the trial were less likely to be married or living with a partner, resided in smaller households, and reported lower incomes compared to study completers [9]. The results of this study may not be generalizable to SNAP-Ed participants who have similar characteristics as the participants who withdrew from the trial and do not classify themselves as non-Hispanic white. Quantification of the change in food security score using the US HFSSM contributed a second major strength to the study. This tool is considered to be the gold standard that is used in national surveys and other research studies, permitting comparisons of results across other populations and enhancing external validity. Use of the score allows a more specific understanding of the change in food security and relationships evaluated.

5. Conclusions

This study highlights nutrition education as a critical, independent component to improving food security in the US low-income population by showing SNAP-Ed directly and sustainably improves food security with or without the presence of food assistance. Neither group, individual or mixed type lessons nor SNAP-Ed educator were related to the effectiveness of SNAP-Ed on food security. Neither were provision of lessons additional to those fulfilling SNAP-Ed guidance related to the magnitude of SNAP-Ed effectiveness. The current study results, along with previous documentation of food assistance effectiveness on food security, support a need for future investigation into the longitudinal effect of participation in multiple food assistance programs, including SNAP-Ed, to maximize improvements in food security and other USDA FNS targeted health outcomes.

Author Contributions: Conceptualization, R.L.R. and H.A.E.-M.; methodology, R.L.R., H.A.E.-M., H.S., Y.Z.; formal analysis, R.L.R. and H.A.E.-M.; data curation, R.L.R., H.A.E.-M., M.K.M., A.R.A.; writing—original draft preparation, R.L.R.; writing—review and editing, H.E.-M., R.L.R., H.S., Y.Z., M.K.M., A.R.A. All authors have read and agreed to the published version of the manuscript.

Funding: This research was funded by the Purdue University Frederick N. Andrews Fellowship, Purdue University Nutrition Education Program, the USDA National Institute of Food and Agriculture Hatch Project grant (IND030489), a North Central Nutrition Education Center of Excellence grant (IND030473G), a U.S. National Library of Medicine training grant (T15LM012502), and the University of Kentucky Center for Poverty Research (UKCPR) through funding by the U.S. Department of Agriculture, Food and Nutrition Service (AG-3198-S-12-0044). The opinions and conclusions expressed herein are solely those of the author(s) and should not be construed as representing the opinions or policies of the UKCPR or any agency of the Federal Government.

Acknowledgments: The authors would like to thank Bruce Craig from the Purdue Department of Statistics for providing oversight for the analyses.

Conflicts of Interest: The authors declare no conflict of interest. The funders had no role in the design of the study; in the collection, analyses, or interpretation of data; in the writing of the manuscript, or in the decision to publish the results.

References

1. Hanson, K.L.; Connor, L.M. Food insecurity and dietary quality in US adults and children: A systematic review. *Am. J. Clin. Nutr.* **2014**, *100*, 684–692. [CrossRef] [PubMed]
2. Gundersen, C.; Ziliak, J.P. Food insecurity and health outcomes. *Health Aff.* **2015**, *34*, 1830–1839. [CrossRef]
3. Lee, J.S.; Gundersen, C.; Cook, J.; Laraia, B.; Johnson, M.A. Food insecurity and health across the lifespan. *Adv. Nutr.* **2012**, *3*, 744–745. [CrossRef]
4. Gundersen, C.; Kreider, B.; Pepper, J. The economics of food insecurity in the United States. *Appl. Econ. Perspect. Policy* **2011**, *33*, 281–303. [CrossRef]
5. Coleman-Jensen, A.; Rabbitt, M.P.; Gregory, C.A.; Singh, A. *Household Food Security in the United States in 2018*; ERR-237; U.S. Department of Agriculture, Economic Research Service: Washington, DC, USA, 2019.
6. United States Department of Agriculture, National Institute of Food and Agriculture. Supplemental Nutrition Education Program-Education (SNAP-Ed). Available online: https://nifa.usda.gov/program/supplemental-nutrition-education-program-education-snap-ed (accessed on 29 April 2020).
7. United States Department of Agriculture, Food and Nutrition Service. Supplemental Nutrition Assistance Program-Education (SNAP-Ed). Available online: https://www.fns.usda.gov/snap/SNAP-Ed (accessed on 29 April 2020).
8. Eicher-Miller, H.A.; Mason, A.C.; Abbott, A.R.; McCabe, G.P.; Boushey, C.J. The effect of Food Stamp Nutrition Education on the food insecurity of low-income women participants. *J. Nutr. Educ. Behav.* **2009**, *41*, 161–168. [CrossRef]
9. Rivera, R.L.; Maulding, M.K.; Abbott, A.R.; Craig, B.A.; Eicher-Miller, H.A. SNAP-Ed (Supplemental Nutrition Assistance Program-Education) increases long-term food security among Indiana households with children in a randomized controlled study. *J. Nutr.* **2016**, *146*, 2375–2382. [CrossRef]
10. United States Department of Agriculture, Food and Nutrition Service. Available online: https://www.fns.usda.gov/ (accessed on 29 April 2020).

11. United States Department of Agriculture, Food and Nutrition Service. Supplemental Nutrition Assistance Program (SNAP). Available online: https://www.fns.usda.gov/snap/supplemental-nutrition-assistance-program (accessed on 29 April 2020).
12. United States Department of Agriculture, Food and Nutrition Service. Special Supplemental Nutrition Program for Women, Infants, and Children (WIC). Available online: https://www.fns.usda.gov/wic (accessed on 29 April 2020).
13. United States Department of Agriculture, Food and Nutrition Service. The Emergency Food Assistance Program (TEFAP). Available online: https://www.fns.usda.gov/tefap/emergency-food-assistance-program-tefap. (accessed on 29 April 2020).
14. Kreider, B.; Pepper, J.V.; Roy, M. Identifying the effects of WIC on food insecurity among infants and children. *South. Econ. J.* **2016**, *82*, 1106–1122. [CrossRef]
15. Wright, B.N.; Bailey, R.L.; Craig, B.A.; Mattes, R.D.; McCormack, L.; Stluka, S.; Franzen-Castle, L.; Henne, B.; Mehrle, D.; Remley, D.; et al. Daily dietary intake patterns improve after visiting a food pantry among food-insecure rural Midwestern adults. *Nutrients* **2018**, *10*, 583. [CrossRef]
16. United States Department of Agriculture, Food and Nutrition Service, Office of Research and Analysis. Building a healthy America: A Profile of the Supplemental Nutrition Assistance Program. Washington, DC. 2012. Available online: http://www.fns.usda.gov/sites/default/files/BuildingHealthyAmerica.pdf (accessed on 29 April 2020).
17. United States Department of Agriculture, Food and Nutrition Service. *Assessing the Food Security and Diet Quality Impacts of FNS Program Participation: Final Report*; Report No. 53-3198-2-0262007; United States Department of Agriculture, Food and Nutrition Service: Washington, DC, USA, 2007. Available online: https://www.fns.usda.gov/assessing-food-security-and-diet-quality-impacts-fns-program-participation (accessed on 29 April 2020).
18. Kaiser, L.; Chaidez, V.; Algert, S.; Horowitz, H.; Martin, A.; Mendoza, C.; Neelon, M.; Ginsburg, D.C. Food resource management education with SNAP participation improves food security. *J. Nutr. Educ. Behav.* **2015**, *47*, 374–378. [CrossRef]
19. Maulding, M.K. Family Nutrition Program. In *Small Steps to Health Curriculum*; Purdue University Health and Human Sciences Cooperative Extension. Purdue Agricultural Communication Media Distribution Center: West Lafayette, IN, USA, 2013.
20. United States Department of Agriculture, Food and Nutrition Service. Supplemental Nutrition Assistance Program Education Plan Guidance FY 2018: Nutrition Education and Obesity Prevention Program. Published March 2018. Available online: https://snaped.fns.usda.gov/snap/Guidance/FY2018SNAP-EdPlanGuidance.pdf (accessed on 29 April 2020).
21. United States Department of Agriculture, Economic Research Service. Measurement. Published 2017. Available online: https://www.ers.usda.gov/topics/food-nutrition-assistance/food-security-in-the-us/measurement/ (accessed on 29 April 2020).
22. Bickel, G.; Nord, M.; Price, C.; Hamilton, W.; Cook, J. *Guide to Measuring Household Food Security*; United States Department of Agriculture, Food and Nutrition Service: Alexandria, VA, USA, 2000. Available online: https://fns-prod.azureedge.net/sites/default/files/FSGuide.pdf (accessed on 29 April 2020).
23. Baron, R.M.; Kenny, D.A. The moderator–mediator variable distinction in social psychological research: Conceptual, strategic, and statistical considerations. *J. Personal. Soc. Psychol.* **1986**, *51*, 1173–1182. [CrossRef]
24. Leung, C.W.; Cluggish, S.; Villamor, E.; Catalano, P.J.; Willett, W.C.; Rimm, E.B. Few changes in food security and dietary intake from short-term participation in the Supplemental Nutrition Assistance Program among low-income Massachusetts adults. *J. Nutr. Educ. Behav.* **2014**, *46*, 68–74. [CrossRef]
25. Rivera, R.; Dune, J.; Maulding, M.K.; Wang, Q.; Savaiano, D.A.; Nickols-Richardson, S.M.; Eicher-Miller, H.A. Exploring the association of urban or rural county status and environmental, nutrition and lifestyle-related resources with the efficacy of SNAP-Ed (Supplemental Nutrition Assistance Program-Education) to improve food security. *Public Health Nutr.* **2018**, *21*, 957–966. [CrossRef] [PubMed]
26. Neuenschwander, L.M.; Abbott, A.; Mobley, A.R. Comparison of a web-based vs in-person nutrition education program for low-income adults. *J. Acad. Nutr. Diet.* **2013**, *113*, 120–126. [CrossRef] [PubMed]
27. Dollahite, J.; Olson, C.; Scott-Pierce, M. The impact of nutrition education on food insecurity among low-income participants in EFNEP. *Fam. Consum. Sci.* **2003**, *32*, 127–139. [CrossRef]

28. Farrell, J.A.; Cordeiro, L.S.; Qian, J.; Sullivan-Werner, L.; Nelson-Peterman, J.L. Food affordability, food security, and the Expanded Food and Nutrition Education Program. *J. Hunger Environ. Nutr.* **2017**, *13*, 1–12. [CrossRef]
29. Crouch, E.L.; Dickes, L.A. Evaluating a nutrition education program in an era of food insecurity. *J. Hunger Environ. Nutr.* **2017**, *12*, 101–111. [CrossRef]
30. Greer, B.; Poling, R. *Impact of Participating in the Expanded Food and Nutrition Education Program on Food Insecurity*; Mississippi State University: Starkville, MS, USA, 2001; Available online: http://srdc.msstate.edu/ridge/projects/recipients/00_greer_final.pdf (accessed on 29 April 2020).

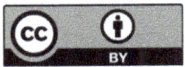

© 2020 by the authors. Licensee MDPI, Basel, Switzerland. This article is an open access article distributed under the terms and conditions of the Creative Commons Attribution (CC BY) license (http://creativecommons.org/licenses/by/4.0/).

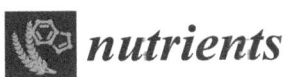

Review

Fruit and Vegetable Incentive Programs for Supplemental Nutrition Assistance Program (SNAP) Participants: A Scoping Review of Program Structure

Katherine Engel and Elizabeth H. Ruder *

Rochester Institute of Technology; Rochester, NY 14620, USA; katherine.engel4@gmail.com
* Correspondence: ehrihst@rit.edu; Tel.: +1-585-475-2402

Received: 29 April 2020; Accepted: 1 June 2020; Published: 4 June 2020

Abstract: The low intake of fruits/vegetables (FV) by Supplemental Nutrition Assistance Program (SNAP) participants is a persistent public health challenge. Fruit and vegetable incentive programs use inducements to encourage FV purchases. The purpose of this scoping review is to identify structural factors in FV incentive programs that may impact program effectiveness, including (i.) differences in recruitment/eligibility, (ii.) incentive delivery and timing, (iii.) incentive value, (iv.) eligible foods, and (v.) retail venue. Additionally, the FV incentive program impact on FV purchase and/or consumption is summarized. Using the Preferred Reporting Items for Systematic Reviews and Meta-Analyses (PRISMA) guidelines for scoping reviews, a search of four bibliographic databases resulted in the identification of 45 publications for consideration; 19 of which met the pre-determined inclusion criteria for full-length publications employing a quasi-experimental design and focused on verified, current SNAP participants. The data capturing study objective, study design, sample size, incentive program structure characteristics (participant eligibility and recruitment, delivery and timing of incentive, foods eligible for incentive redemption, type of retail venue), and study outcomes related to FV purchases/consumption were entered in a standardized chart. Eleven of the 19 studies had enrollment processes to receive the incentive, and most studies (17/19) provided the incentive in the form of a token, coupon, or voucher. The value of the incentives varied, but was usually offered as a match. Incentives were typically redeemable only for FV, although three studies required an FV purchase to trigger the delivery of an incentive for any SNAP-eligible food. Finally, most studies (16/19) were conducted at farmers' markets. Eighteen of the 19 studies reported a positive impact on participant purchase and/or consumption of FV. Overall, this scoping review provides insights intended to inform the design, implementation, and evaluation of future FV incentive programs targeting SNAP participants and demonstrates the potential effectiveness of FV incentive programs for increasing FV purchase and consumption among vulnerable populations.

Keywords: incentive programs; Supplemental Nutrition Assistance Program (SNAP); fruits and vegetables; low-income; farmers' markets; dietary quality; produce intake; produce purchasing

1. Introduction

Eating sufficient amounts of fruits/vegetables (FV) is vital for a healthy dietary pattern associated with a lower risk of cardiovascular disease and certain cancers [1]. However, Americans do not consume enough FV; only 12.2% and 9.3% of US adults meet the *2015–2020 Dietary Guidelines for Americans*' recommendations for daily fruit and vegetable consumption, respectively [2]. Among Americans, lower income groups consume less FV than higher income groups, and this is a key socioeconomic disparity in overall dietary quality [2–4]. Thus, it is important that low-income participants in federal food assistance programs in the United States, such as the Supplemental Nutrition Assistance Program (SNAP), have access to these foods.

SNAP is the largest federal food assistance program in the United States. It functions by providing participants with food purchasing resources in the form of an electronic benefit transfer (EBT, an electronic system that allows a recipient to authorize transfer of their government benefits from a federal account to a retailer) on a monthly cycle. Although SNAP eligibility requirements vary from state to state, households that are SNAP eligible have gross incomes of less than 130% of the federal poverty line [5]. Unlike other U.S. food assistance programs, like the Supplemental Nutrition Assistance Program for Women, Infants, and Children (WIC), SNAP benefits can be used for most food products with few exceptions (such as hot foods and foods that are intended to be eaten in stores) [6,7]. In contrast to SNAP, WIC benefits are limited to foods such as milk, cheese, yogurt, FV, canned fish, tofu, breakfast and infant cereal, whole wheat breads and grains, eggs, peanut butter, infant formula, and jarred baby foods [8]. Thus, although SNAP plays an integral role in ensuring that millions of people have the resources they need to access sufficient amounts of food, it lacks specific restrictions that dictate the nutritional quality of foods that participants can purchase. Importantly, it has been shown that individuals who receive SNAP benefits have poor diets relative to the overall population and other income-eligible non-participants [3]. In some cases, SNAP participation has been associated with negative health outcomes and inversely correlated to self-assessed health status [9]. Given the evidence that WIC participation is associated with health benefits [10], one proposed alteration to the SNAP program is creating restrictions around which foods can be purchased with benefits. However, key constituencies, ranging from members of U.S. Congress to hunger relief organizations, have rejected these proposals for reasons including concerns about limiting participants' ability to exercise autonomy in food choice and administrative burdens [11]. Moreover, restrictions on the types of food eligible for SNAP could contribute to worsening food security in areas where a variety of healthful foods is not sold by food retailers. Another alteration to the SNAP program that has been suggested is FV incentives, which provide participants with considerable autonomy in deciding what foods to purchase [12].

FV incentives include a variety of inducements to offer low-income participants funds to purchase these foods. They are potentially appropriate for improving dietary quality, because they are a tool for facilitating behavior change. The theory that incentives serve as a strategy for inducing changes in behavior centers on the standard direct price effect [13]. The standard direct price effect makes the incetivzed behavior more attractive by providing a financial reward. As a result, incentives have the capacity to instill new, positive habits, as well as end pre-existing, negative habits. Thus, when applied on a large enough scale, incentives may have the ability to shift cultural norms [13]. Incentives may be particularly useful for promoting healthy behaviors, such as consuming more FV, because the benefits of healthy behaviors are often uncertain and delayed, while the cost of these behaviors is immediate. Consumers tend to value current costs and benefits more than future costs and benefits, which in turn can lead to choosing not to engage in healthy behaviors, since the present value of these behaviors is low. Incentives create an immediate benefit because they lower the cost of healthy foods for consumers. By creating short-term rewards for healthy behaviors, incentives serve to make these behaviors more appealing by increasing their present value [14]. In general, the cost of food plays a critical role in how people make food choices [15,16]. Glanz and colleagues [17] found that behind taste, price is the second most important influence on food choice. For SNAP participants specifically, it has been demonstrated that the cost of healthy foods is a barrier for improving dietary quality [18,19]. Incentives expand the financial resources participants have available to purchase healthy foods, and thus address the barrier that the cost of these food poses to dietary quality [18–20].

FV incentive programs have been designed and implemented for a number of different populations, including WIC and SNAP participants, and venues, such as farmers' markets and grocery stores. In addition, the types and value of incentives that have been developed vary widely from point-of-sale (POS) discounts to coupons, vouchers, and tokens. A preliminary search for existing scoping reviews on this topic was conducted by searching the Cochrane Database of Systematic Reviews, Google Scholar, ProQuest, PubMed, and Sage Journals Online. No scoping reviews on this topic were identified. Given the emerging evidence related to FV incentive programs among SNAP participants and the diversity of structural factors within these programs, a scoping review was selected as the appropriate method. The objective of this scoping review is to characterize the factors in program structure which may impact the effectiveness of incentive programs. The scoping review research question is, "What are the differences in structural factors, including recruitment and eligibility criteria, delivery and timing of incentives, financial value of incentives, foods eligible for incentive redemption, and type of retail venue reported among FV incentive programs?" Finally, this review summarizes the outcomes of existing FV incentive programs with respect to the purchase and/or consumption of FV among SNAP participants, with specific attention to the quality of the assessment methods for FV purchase and/or consumption. This work provides insight intended to inform the design, implementation, and evaluation of future FV incentive programs targeting SNAP participants.

2. Materials and Methods

A scoping review was undertaken to systematically synthesize factors in program structure which may impact the effectiveness of FV incentive programs. This review was conducted as per the Arksey and O'Malley framework for scoping reviews [21] and integrated with the guidance from the Joanna Briggs Institute (JBI) [22] and the Preferred Reporting Items for Systematic Reviews and Meta-Analyses (PRISMA) guidelines for scoping reviews [23]. A protocol document is publically available online at: https://figshare.com/articles/Protocol_Document_pdf/12380669, and a completed PRISMA ScR checklist is included as Supplementary Table S1.

2.1. Search Strategy

Focused searches were conducted by one author (K.E.) using Google Scholar, ProQuest, PubMed, and Sage Journals Online. The search terms that were used include "SNAP incentives," "WIC incentive," "food benefits incentive," and "food assistance incentive." Results were limited to English language publications and indexed up to 7 November 2019. In addition to the use of these search terms, papers were identified by examining the articles cited by the papers found in the preliminary search.

2.2. Study Selection

Full-text articles identified in the search were imported into Mendeley reference management software and duplicates were manually removed. In total, 45 unique publications were identified and both authors independently reviewed the full-text documents for pre-determined inclusion/exclusion criteria. The inclusion criteria included: full-length publication in a peer-reviewed journal or government report, quasi-experimental design, and targeted focus on verified, current SNAP participants studies that solely examined the use of FV vouchers as part of the WIC foods package were excluded for the following reasons: (1.) FV vouchers became a standard part of the WIC Food Package following a final rule published in May 2014 [24] and (2.) WIC FV vouchers can only be used for FV and therefore are not used to incentivize the purchase of FV over other foods within the WIC Food Package. The authors conferenced regularly to ensure agreement and talked through any inconsistencies. Due to the relative lack of research on this topic, papers were not excluded based on their publication date.

2.3. Data Charting

Data were extracted from eligible papers into a standardized Google Doc chart developed by both authors. The two authors independently charted the data, discussed the results and continuously updated the data collection chart. The data ultimately collected included: study authors, year of publication, study objective, population and sample size, methodology, incentive program structure characteristics (participant eligibility and recruitment, delivery and timing of incentive, foods eligible for incentive redemption, type of retail venue), and study outcomes related to FV purchases and FV consumption. In addition, study methods for the assessment of FV purchase and/or consumption were charted. The charted data were summarized as counts where applicable.

3. Results and Discussion

Of the 45 publications initially reviewed, $n = 6$ were excluded for not falling within the scope of the review, $n = 8$ were excluded for not employing a quasi-experimental design, $n = 6$ were excluded because participation was not focused on current, verified SNAP participants, and $n = 2$ were excluded for being solely related to WIC FV vouchers prior to the implementation of the 2014 WIC Food Package. In addition, two poster presentations were excluded and two publications were excluded because they presented preliminary data that was included in a subsequent publication. In total, 19 publications were included in the final review (Table 1).

3.1. Incentive Program Structure

A variety of types of incentive programs have explored approaches for increasing the purchase and consumption of FV by SNAP participants. The following section details ways in which eligible individuals become participants in incentive programs, the delivery and timing of incentives, and differences in the financial value of incentives to participants.

Table 1. Summary of studies on fruit and vegetable incentives as an approach for encouraging and enabling Supplemental Nutrition Assistance Program (SNAP) participants in the United States to increase the purchase and/or consumption of healthy foods.

Author	Study Objective	Incentive Benefit	Food Eligible for Incentive Redemption	Venue Type	Program Scale	Sample Size	Relevant Findings
Alaofè et al. 2017 [25]	Examine the impact of the Double Up SNAP (DUSP) farmers' market incentive program on awareness and access to farmer's markets, and FV purchase and consumption in Pima County, AZ.	Token/Voucher/Coupon	Unspecified FV	Farmers' Market	One farmers' market	353 participants	DUSP customers reported greater consumption of FV compared to non-DUSP shoppers.
Amaro and Roberts 2017 [26]	Examine characteristics (e.g., demographics, household food security) and needs of families using SNAP incentive program and evaluate incentive program usage in terms of shopping habits, food consumption patterns, and household food security.	Token/Coupon/Voucher	Unspecified FV	Farmers' Market	One farmers' market	143 parents	Participants reported a positive impact of incentive program use and appeared to value fresh fruits and vegetables. The majority of participants reported that the incentive enabled them to afford to shop at the farmers' markets using their SNAP funds. Participants reported higher consumption of dark green vegetables, red/orange vegetables, and other vegetables, as well as fruits other than citrus, melons, and berries.
Bartlett et al. 2014 [7]	Assess the causal impact of incentive on FV consumption, and other key measures of dietary intake, by SNAP participants.	POS	Any SNAP eligible item	Farmers' Market and Grocery Stores	130 retailers in a single metropolitan area	7500 households	Participants reported their consumption of vegetables more than their consumption of fruit. Increased fruit and vegetable consumption drove an increased score on the 2010 Healthy Eating Index.
Bowling et al. 2016 [27]	Examine effects of program participation on participants' FV and soda consumption; investigate the program's effect on WIC/SNAP budget FV expenditure patterns and use of food assistance at participating farmers' markets, and explore the relative importance of financial (access) incentives and exposure interventions as drivers of participant enrollment and retention, as well as participants' perceptions of barriers, support, and benefits from participation.	POS and Token/Coupon/Voucher	Fresh FV	Farmers' Market	Six farmers' markets in a single metropolitan area	146 households	Participants reported significantly higher vegetable consumption and lower soda consumption post implementation of the incentive program.

Table 1. Cont.

Author	Study Objective	Incentive Benefit	Food Eligible for Incentive Redemption	Venue Type	Program Scale	Sample Size	Relevant Findings
Dimitri et al. 2013 [28]	Examine the association between monetary incentives given for the purchase of fresh FV and fresh produce consumption among federal food assistance participants, including SNAP.	Token/Voucher/Coupon	Fresh FV	Farmers' Market	73 farmers' markets	1227 participants	Participants perceived increased consumption of fresh FV because they shopped at the market when offered financial incentives. Participants living in areas with low FV access, and who were also income constrained, were the most likely to perceive higher FV consumption.
Dimitri et al. 2015 [29]	Assess the effectiveness of incentives on the intake of fresh vegetables among federal food assistance program participants.	Token/Voucher/Coupon	Fresh FV	Farmers' Market	Five farmers' markets in three metropolitan areas	138 households	Incentives increased FV consumption overall. Groups responded to incentives differently based on level of food insecurity and education.
Durward et al. 2019 [30]	Evaluate the effect of Utah Double Up Food Bucks (DUFB) program on FV intake and food security status among SNAP participants.	Token/Voucher/Coupon	Fresh FV	Farmers' Market	17 farmers' markets in Utah; evaluation data collected from a sample of eight markets	138 participants	Increase in median FV consumption and percentage of participants in the incentive program who were food secure increased.
Freedman et al. 2014 [31]	Examine the influence of FV incentive on intervention program on farmers' market revenue. The intervention included a federal monetary incentive to increase fruit and vegetable purchases at farmers' markets for food assistance recipients.	POS	Unspecified FV	Farmers' Market	One farmers' market	336 participants	Incentives increased farmers' market revenue and improved access to FV.
Lindsay et al. 2013 [32]	Examine patterns of enrollment and market visits, participants' self-reported dietary changes while participating in the program, and the economic benefits of the program.	Token/Voucher/Coupon	Fresh FV, eggs, bread, and meat	Farmers' Market	Five farmers' markets in a single metropolitan area	252 participants	Incentives increased daily FV consumption and weekly FV spending.
Marcinkevage et al. 2019 [33]	Examine strengths and weaknesses of the FV prescription program implementation; gain insight into successful programming activities for FV prescriptions; assess overall effectiveness of the program in improving affordability of healthy foods among low-income patients; and assess patient satisfaction with the program.	Token/Voucher/Coupon	Fresh, Frozen, Canned, and/or Dried FV	Grocery Store	169 grocery stores in a single state	144 participants	Incentives increased FV purchase and consumption, participants reported managing their health conditions better, and an improvement in meeting nutrition, diet-related, or meal plan goals.

Table 1. Cont.

Author	Study Objective	Incentive Benefit	Food Eligible for Incentive Redemption	Venue Type	Program Scale	Sample Size	Relevant Findings
Olsho et al. 2015 [34]	Assess the effectiveness of incentive program in increasing access to and awareness of farmers' markets, and increasing purchase and consumption of fruits and vegetables.	Token/Voucher/Coupon	Fresh FV	Farmers' Market	86 farmers' markets in a single metropolitan area	2287 participants	Health Bucks increased awareness of farmers' markets and FV purchases. No significant change in FV consumption was detected.
Pellegrino et al. 2018 [35]	Determine FV consumption among incentive program participants and identify demographic and behavioral factors associated with higher consumption.	Token/Voucher/Coupon	Fresh FV	Farmers' Market	Six farmers' markets in a single metropolitan area	228 participants	Participants reported higher median FV consumption than people with similar income levels, but still below recommended levels.
Ratigan et al. 2017 [36]	Examine the factors associated with the ongoing utilization of a farmers' market incentive program among federal food assistance participants.	Token/Voucher/Coupon	SNAP participants could use the incentive for any SNAP-eligible food, WIC participants could use the incentive for fresh produce only.	Farmers' Market	Five farmers' markets in a single metropolitan area	7298 participants	Increases in FV consumption and spending and improvement in perception of overall diet quality. Factors, including ethnicity, type of government assistance, age, disability status, enrolment market, season of enrolment, baseline FV serving, and perceived diet quality, affected program utilization and retention.
Rummo et al. 2019 [37]	Evaluate the effectiveness and feasibility of incentive program in grocery stores.	Token/Voucher/Coupon	Fresh FV	Grocery Store	16 grocery stores in a single metropolitan area	Unspecified number of participants	Incentives had a positive effect on FV sales but did not affect spending on sugar-sweetened beverages.
Savoie-Rosko et al. 2016 [38]	Determine whether participation in a farmers' market incentive pilot program had an impact on food security and FV intake of participants.	Token/Voucher/Coupon	Unspecified FV	Farmers' Market	One farmers' market	54 participants	Incentives decreased food insecurity-related behaviors and increased intake of select FV.
Savoie Roskos et al. 2017 [39]	Identify benefits and barriers to using a farmers' market incentive program.	Token/Voucher/Coupon	Any SNAP eligible item	Farmers' Market	One farmers' market	28 participants	Incentives reduced barriers associated with farmers' market use, including cost and accessibility, and provided more spending flexibility, as well as enabled the purchase of FV that previously did not fit into budget.
Steele-Adjognon et al. 2017 [40]	Analyze how FV expenditures, expenditure shares, variety, and purchase decisions were affected by the initiation and conclusion of an FV incentive program, as well as analyze any persistent effects of the program.	Token/Voucher/Coupon	Fresh FV	Grocery Store	One grocery store	156 participants	Incentives were associated with increased vegetable spending, FV expenditure shares, and variety of FV purchased, but the effects were minimal and unsustainable without the continuation of the program. Fruit spending and FV purchase decisions were not impacted by the program.

149

Table 1. Cont.

Author	Study Objective	Incentive Benefit	Food Eligible for Incentive Redemption	Venue Type	Program Scale	Sample Size	Relevant Findings
Wetherill et al. 2017 [41]	Describe the design, implementation, and consumer response to a coupon-style intervention aimed to increase SNAP use at a farmers' market among Temporary Assistance for Needy Families (TANF) participants.	Token/Voucher/Coupon	Unspecified FV	Farmers' Market	One farmers' market	254 participants	Very few participants (6.3%) redeemed the incentive coupons. Stand-alone coupon incentive programs may not be sufficient for encouraging farmers' market use among the population using TANF. Complementary strategies, such as education, to build vegetable preparation knowledge and skills are needed.
Young et al. 2013 [42]	Determine if FV incentive program was associated with increased FV consumption and SNAP sales at farmers' markets in low-income areas.	Token/Voucher/Coupon	Fresh FV	Farmers' Market	22 farmers' markets in a single metropolitan area	662 participants	Incentives were tied to increases in FV consumption and sales.

FV: fruits and vegetables, WIC: Special Supplemental Nutrition Program for Women, Infants, and Children, POS: point of sale.

3.1.1. Recruitment and Eligibility of Incentive Program Participants

In the studies under review, individuals became incentive program participants in a multitude of ways. Eleven programs had an enrollment process through which individuals had to complete some type of informal or formal sign-up process for the program to receive the incentive [7,26–28,31–33,36,38,40,41], while eight studies had no enrollment process and provided the incentive when participants visited and/or made a purchase at a retailer and provided evidence of their SNAP participation [25,28,30,34,35,37,39,42]. Bowling et al. provided all SNAP participants shopping at participating markets with an incentive and provided an additional incentive to a subset of this population that had specifically enrolled in the program [27]. It is important to note that the inclusion of an enrollment process may create additional administrative challenges, as well as barriers for participation. However, as enrollment processes often included a pre-test survey and/or a method of tracking participants' transactions throughout the implementation period, these programs may provide opportunities for more rigorous evaluation and therefore greater insight regarding the impact of incentive programs of FV purchases and consumption. One study assessed programs in which participants were given the incentive after visiting a health clinic [33]. Similar to the challenges with enrollment processes, this requirement may create a participation barrier, but may have a greater impact on dietary quality and health, as it is part of a broader focus on the health status of federal food assistance program participants.

3.1.2. Delivery and Timing of Incentive Benefits

Table 1 summarizes the types of incentive benefits that have been granted to participants. Two programs were structured such that the incentive was provided at the point-of-sale (POS) [7,31]. For the purposes of this review, POS incentives are defined as those that immediately discount participants' FV purchases at checkout. In contrast to this model, 17 programs provided participants with coupons, vouchers, or tokens [25–30,32–42]. The delivery of coupons, vouchers, or tokens (hereafter referred to as incentives) varied by program. Some programs provided the incentives when the participant enrolled in the program or following their enrollment, such as when they visited a farmers' market [28,32,35,41]. Other programs provided the incentives following or in conjunction with the purchase of FV [7,25,26,28,30,31,33,35–38,40]. Moreover, some programs required incentives to be redeemed immediately upon receipt [7,31], but others allowed the incentive to be used for a future transaction. Importantly, allowing participants to save the incentive and choose when they use it may be beneficial, due to the monthly "SNAP-cycle" spending pattern, where the majority of recipients spend most of their monthly benefits within two weeks after receiving them [43,44]. In all cases, the intent of these benefits is to induce participants to increase their FV purchases by providing them with financial rewards for these purchases and/or resources that enable them to purchase these foods at a lower price.

Most incentive programs included in this review required participants to make an FV purchase in order to "trigger" the delivery of the incentive benefit [7,25,26,28,30,31,33,36–38,40]. However, the types of FV that qualify as trigger foods differ. For example, the Healthy Incentives Pilot, a federally funded FV incentive program administered in Hampden County, MA, distributed incentive benefits after participants purchased targeted FV, which were defined as any fresh, canned, frozen, and dried fruit or vegetable FV without any added sugars, fats, oils, or sodium. In addition, the pilot excluded fruit juice, mature legumes, and white potatoes. These specifications were selected to mirror the restrictions of WIC-eligible produce items [7]. In contrast, for programs held at farmers' markets, participants often had to purchase fresh FV in order to receive the incentive.

A few programs had multiple points and locations at which incentive benefits were distributed to participants. In the program evaluated by Young et al. [42], a $2 bonus incentive coupon was provided for every $5 in SNAP benefits used at a farmers' market. Additionally, coupons were distributed at community organizations that serve SNAP-eligible populations, absent of any initial purchase by the participant. The program examined by Olsho et al. [34], was structured similarly, in that some participants received the incentive through a match after they made a purchase, while others received the incentive from community-based organizations absent of any purchase, usually after they attended a nutrition workshop or other health and fitness program. Similarly, two incentive distribution methods were employed in the program examined by Savoie-Roskos et al. [39]; participants received either "regular incentives", which were distributed at regular intervals without any purchase requirement, or matched incentives. Bowling et al. [27] employed both POS incentives and tokens; all SNAP recipients shopping at participating markets received a matched incentive when they used their EBT card at these markets, which could not be saved for future use, but at every third market, participants also received $20 in "Bonus Buck" tokens.

3.1.3. Financial Value of Incentive to Participants

The value of incentive benefits to participants differed widely. As stated previously, most programs required a purchase to receive the incentive [7,25–27,30–32,34,36–38,40,42]. In these programs, the value of the benefit was either pre-determined or determined by the value of the participants' purchases. For example, in the incentive program studied by Freedman et al. [31], participants received benefits valued at $5 regardless of the cost of their initial purchases. However, many incentive programs functioned such that the value of the benefit was determined by the magnitude of the participants' spending [7,25–27,29,30,32,34,36–40,42]. In these cases, the value of the benefit was either equal to the participants' spending or a percentage of their spending. In many instances, 100% of the participants' spending was matched, meaning that the value of the benefits was equal to the amount of money spent by participants [25,26,30,32,36–40]. In some cases, the value of the benefit was adjusted based on the size of participating families, as families with children were given additional value [38].

Among incentive programs that provided a match to participant spending, there was frequently a ceiling on the value of the match. In all, 11 of the studies [7,25–28,30,32,36–38,41] reviewed had some type of ceiling. For instance, in a Utah-based farmers' market incentive program, participants received $1 in incentives for every $1 they spent in SNAP benefits, with individuals and couples receiving $10 worth of incentives each week and families receiving an additional $5 per child, up to $30 each week [39]. Another type of ceiling was demonstrated, where participants could receive an extra $20 in bonus tokens every third farmers' market visit but were limited to receiving $120 of these bonus tokens during the program's implementation [27]. Other programs provided benefits that were valued as a percentage of the participants' spending. For instance, the Health Bucks and Philly Food Bucks programs provided $2 vouchers for every $5 participants spent, and thus acted as a 40% match of the participants' spending [32,42,45]. Notably, incentives that are granted in proportion to the participants' spending are designed to encourage participants to purchase more fruits and vegetables, because with these programs, the more participants spend on these foods, the more they are rewarded.

Some programs implemented multiple forms of incentives. For example, Savoie-Roskos et al. [39] provided one group of participants with incentive benefits that did not require them to make a purchase and another group with benefits, in the form of spending matches, that augmented the incentive. A comparison of the outcomes between the groups was not reported.

Overall, programs that match participants' spending may provide incentive benefits that have greater financial value than those that provide a benefit of a fixed value. In addition, programs with ceilings may create less value for participants than those without ceilings. Thus, certain programs may be more effective in inducing participants to purchase and consume more FV, because they expand participants' purchasing power to a greater degree. Differences in value may also be important, given that program retention is a challenge across the literature, and programs that provide less value may be less effective in encouraging ongoing participation. Notably, Wetherill et al. [41] posited that low incentive redemption rates may be tied to perceived differences in the value of different kinds of incentives, as incentives that function as discounts and expand buying power may be less valuable to participants than incentives that provide free products.

3.1.4. Eligible Foods

The foods that were eligible for purchase using incentive benefits also differed. While some of the programs provided benefits that could be utilized to purchase only FV, others were triggered by an FV purchase, but provided benefits redeemable for a diverse range of foods, such as any SNAP-eligible food [7,36,39]. A drawback of awarding incentives that can be used for any SNAP-eligible food is the possibility that incentive benefits are used to purchase foods with low nutrient density. For example, in the Healthy Incentives Pilot, an additional $0.30 was added to participants' EBT cards for every $1 of SNAP benefits spent on FV. There are few limitations on the types of foods and beverages that can be purchased with EBT, and some evidence suggests that reducing the price of healthful foods may result in the increased purchase of energy, which could contribute to obesity [46].

In contrast, other FV incentive benefits could be used only to purchase locally grown FV [27,29,31, 32,34,37,40,47]. In some cases, the foods included in the incentive program varied based on participant eligibility. For example, in the Fresh Funds program [36], participants could use the tokens they purchased with their SNAP benefits, and the tokens that they received as a match, to purchase fresh produce or packaged foods, such as jams/spreads, breads, eggs, pasta, cheese, and fish; however, the tokens they purchased using WIC benefits could only be spent at vendors selling fresh produce.

The characteristics and needs of the recipients must be considered when designing incentive programs and the types of FV eligible for incentive redemption. For example, FV may not be an appealing incentive to people with limited facilities and equipment for food preparation. However, for participants with access to food preparation facilities, frozen, canned, and dried FV have a longer shelf-life than fresh FV and may be useful for prolonging food security throughout the month and between monthly SNAP benefit distributions. Likewise, the capacity of the retail environment must also be considered. SNAP vendor eligibility implemented in January 2018 requires vendors to stock FV, but does not require those FV to be fresh if other perishable foods are stocked (i.e., meat or dairy), and only one type of perishable food needs to be offered (i.e., selling just one type of fruit would fulfill the fresh FV requirement) [48]. Low income communities tend to have more convenience stores and small markets [49,50] where the availability of FV tends to be lower [51–53]. Therefore, the retail capacity, including the availability of freezers/refrigeration, must be considered when designing fresh FV incentive programs.

3.1.5. Retail Venue

Table 1 illustrates that the majority (16/19) of the reviewed studies were implemented in part or in entirety at farmers' markets. Farmers' market incentive programs have the advantage of supporting local farmers and food vendors. Additionally, the literature indicates that shopping at farmers' markets positively impacts FV purchases and that by drawing participants to shop at these venues, incentive programs implemented at farmers' markets may positively impact FV purchase and consumption behaviors and attitudes beyond the time period in which the program is implemented [31,32,54].

Several studies indicate that farmers' market incentive programs attract SNAP participants who otherwise might not shop at these venues [30–32,35]. One incentive program study found that 57% of participants in a farmers' market incentive program had never been to a farmers' market [31]. Similarly, another study noted that SNAP participants' awareness of farmers' markets rose in relation to their exposure to the Health Bucks incentive program [35]. In addition, these researchers found that 54% of Health

Bucks participants who used their benefits at farmers' markets strongly agreed that "I shop at farmers' markets more often because of Health Bucks", and a Utah-based incentive program reported that 98% of baseline participants reported that the incentive made it more likely that they would shop at the farmers' market [30]. In the Farmers' Market Fresh Fund Incentive Program, 82% of participants had never attended a farmer's market prior to participating in the program, and 93% of participants reported that incentives were "important" or "very important" in their decision to shop at farmers' markets [32]. In addition to drawing more SNAP participants to farmers' markets, the Farmers' Market Fresh Fund Incentive Program demonstrated the potential to impact participants' long-term shopping behavior. In particular, the majority of participants reported that they would be "somewhat likely" or "completely likely" to shop at farmers' markets even without the continuation of the incentive program [32]. Increased awareness that EBT is accepted at many farmers' markets has also been noted among incentive program participants [39]. Accordingly, there is evidence that farmers' market incentive programs increase participants' exposure to markets as venues offering affordable, healthy food, and in turn have the potential to positively influence their long-term food purchasing behavior.

Another potential benefit of implementing incentive programs at farmers' markets is the potential for the increased consumption of FV. Shopping at farmers' markets is linked to increased FV consumption, and thus offering incentives at farmers' markets has the capacity to improve dietary quality beyond merely increasing the financial resources participants have to purchase FV [55]. Specifically, Olsho et al. [34] found that both incentive program participants and farmers' market shoppers who were not enrolled in the program reported higher FV consumption than other residents in their neighborhoods. However, incentive program participation per se was not related to an increase in daily FV servings.

Despite the potential benefits of implementing incentive programs at farmers' markets, it is important to consider access issues in this context. Specifically, farmers' markets are not as abundant as other types of food retailers, such as grocery stores, and may not exist in certain communities. Driving distance from residence to market has been inversely correlated with repeat use of farmer's market incentives [56]. However, other research suggests that the distance from food retailers does not significantly affect the extent to which incentives impact SNAP participants' FV spending [7,32]. Moreover, many markets are not open year-round and have limited hours of operation.

3.2. Outcome Assessment

All of the studies included in this review considered the impact of incentives on FV purchases and/or consumption. Four of the studies reviewed focused exclusively on FV purchases [25,30,36,39,41], five focused exclusively on FV consumption [28,29,34,37,40], and nine examined both FV purchase and consumption [7,24,26,27,31–33,35,38]. As explored later in this section, only one of the reviewed studies [41] did not report some positive impact on FV purchases and/or consumption in conjunction with incentive programs.

Studies employed a variety of approaches for measuring these outcomes, as shown in Tables 2 and 3. The majority of studies assessed FV purchase and/or consumption using a pre-/post-test design, where participants' FV purchase and consumption behaviors and attitudes were assessed prior to the implementation of the incentive program and then again at the program's conclusion [25–28,30–36,38,39,42]. In addition, the Healthy Incentives Program also assessed the program impact at various points throughout the implementation phase [7]. A few studies also used control or quasi-control groups to assess program impact [7,34,37,41,47]. The merits of quasi-control groups are somewhat limited if the comparison groups do not share important characteristics with the incentive program participants. For example, Olsho et al. [34], compared the FV purchase and consumption of incentive program participants with that of other non-participant neighborhood residents, but these residents were not necessarily federal food assistance program participants. Although the groups may have shared relevant demographic characteristics, the comparison is problematic because federal food assistance program participants have unique circumstances that may make incentive programs particularly salient, such as the challenge of managing food-purchasing resources in conjunction with the monthly SNAP distribution cycle. Another study compared SNAP transaction data from participating grocery stores to that of nonparticipating stores to determine whether the percentage of dollars spent on fresh produce in total SNAP transactions is higher in stores that implement incentives than in stores that do not [37]. Control stores were selected using a coarsened exact matching and linear probability match to match on store characteristics and sociodemographics. While this approach is not as rigorous as randomizing stores to the incentive or control condition, the use of matched controls is preferred to non-matched controls. Wetherill et al. [41] employed a quasi-experimental design to compare two coupon interventions: basic information and plain coupon distribution compared to tailored, targeted marketing coupon intervention. However, low coupon redemption by either group made comparisons difficult.

Table 2. Assessment of fruit and vegetable purchases in nutrition incentive programs.

Author	Assessment Method
Survey Assessment of FV Purchases	
Alaofè et al. (2017) [25]	Frequency of farmer's market shopping, purchasing amount, and types of purchases were assessed by the questions: 1. "Because of Double-Up SNAP Pilot (DUSP) program rebates, is your family buying a larger amount of … ?" 2. "Because of DUSP program rebates, is your family eating a greater amount of … ?", and 3. "Because of DUSP program rebates, have you or your family tried any new or unfamiliar fruits or vegetables?"
Amaro and Roberts (2017) [26]	Open-ended survey responses demonstrated that participants purchased FV at the farmers' market because the incentive program made it affordable for them to do so. Additionally, they were asked to indicate the degree to which they agreed or disagreed with "I can afford to buy fresh fruits and vegetables".
Bartlett et al. (2014) [7]	Specific survey items not provided but questions sought to discern general food shopping patterns and food expenditures.
Bowling et al. (2016) [27]	"How much of your family's weekly WIC/SNAP budget is spent on FVs?"
Dimitri et al. (2013) [28]	Survey assessed questions covering five aspects: (1) frequency of shopping at farmers' markets and the number of years receiving incentives, (2) perception of how much incentives influenced the decision to shop at the farmers' market, (3) perception of the impact that shopping at the market with incentives had on fresh FV consumption, (4) importance of farmers' market characteristics on the decision to shop at that market, and (5) access to the market and use of the market for fresh FV.
Lindsay et al. (2013) [32]	"How much on average do you spend on fresh fruits and vegetables per week?"
Marcinkevage et al. (2019) [33]	Perceptions of affordability, purchase of FV not previously tried.
Olsho et al. (2015) [34]	Specific survey items not provided but questions sought to discern changes in farmers' market spending, including whether FV were purchased each visit.
Ratigan et al. (2017) [36]	Perceptions of food purchasing behavior and affordability of FV, weekly spending on FV (<$10, $10–19, $20–29, $30–39, ≥$40.)
Interviews or Focus Groups to Assess FV purchases	
Bartlett et al. (2014) [7]	Experiences with the program, including financial impact on the household and changes in willingness to purchase FV.
Savoie-Roskos et al. (2017) [39]	Cost and budgeting as barriers to FV purchases prior to the incentive program emerged as themes and participants noted that the program helped them overcome these barriers, citing greater spending flexibility and decreased anxiety over the cost of food.
Bartlett et al. 2014) [7]	EBT transaction data to determine Healthy Incentive Program (HIP) incentive earnings by pilot participants, focusing on HIP-eligible purchases, the amount of incentives earned, and the percent of SNAP benefits spent on HIP-eligible purchases. Analysis of spending in different types of store, focusing on spending on targeted FV in supermarkets and superstores.

Table 2. *Cont.*

Author	Assessment Method
Sales Tracking to Assess FV Purchases	
Freedman et al. (2014) [31]	Sales tracking using unique identifier for each participant; transaction data, including date of transaction, customer type (patient, staff, or community member), total cost, and payment type; comparing venue revenue trends from the previous year with those during the implementation period.
Lindsay et al. (2013) [32]	Data were collected from vendors regarding total sales each day from incentive tokens as a percentage of total sales.
Marcinkevage et al. (2019) [33]	Quarterly and yearly redemption rates, dollar amount spent on FV per incentive redeemed.
Olsho et al. (2015) [34]	Comparison of average daily SNAP sales from farmers' markets accepting incentives with those not accepting incentives.
Ratigan et al. (2017) [36]	Records of market attendance and frequency of visits to booths where participants received incentives.
Rummo et al. (2019) [37]	FV spending as a percentage of total spending from individual transactions at grocery stores that implemented programs and that did not implement programs.
Steele-Adjognon et al. (2017) [40]	Loyalty card scanner data was acquired to assess: "FV expenditure; fruit expenditure; vegetable expenditure; FV expenditure share; FV variety; and FV purchase decision. FV expenditure is the aggregate dollar amount spent during the month on all fresh FV."
Wetherill et al. (2017) [41]	Differences in baseline sociodemographic, predisposing, enabling, and reinforcing factors related to FV attitudes and behaviors by incentive redemption.
Young et al. (2013) [42]	Comparison of market SNAP sales from implementation period to those from previous years; incentive redemption rates.

Table 3. Assessment of fruit and vegetable consumption in nutrition incentive programs.

Author	Description of Assessment Method
Alaofè et al. (2017) [25]	FV consumption frequency measured using Behavioral Risk Factor Surveillance System FV module.
Bartlett et al. (2014) [7]	24-h dietary recall interviews at multiple points in implementation period and followed up by focus groups, which included discussion of impact on FV consumption. Surveys on FV consumption (frequency and quantity) using Eating at America's Table Study (EATS) Fruit and Vegetable Screener.
Bowling et al. (2016) [27]	Survey questions including "On an average day, how many times do you have a vegetable to eat?" and "On an average day, how many times do you have a fruit to eat?"
Dimitri et al. (2015) [29]	National Health and Nutrition Examination Survey food frequencyquestionnaire: Number of times vegetables were consumed in the last six months, daily and weekly serving of FV.
Dimitri et al. (2013) [28]	Specific survey items not provided, but assessed participant perception that fresh FV consumption increased or did not increase.
Durward et al. (2019) [30]	FV consumption frequency measured using Behavioral Risk Factor Surveillance System FV module.
Lindsay et al. (2013) [32]	"On average, how many servings of fruits and/or vegetables do you usually eat each day?" and "In general, how healthy would you say your overall diet is?"
Marcinkevage et al. (2019) [33]	Survey included questions related to participant perceived improvement in the consumption of healthy foods, including FV, and perceived health benefit prescriptions (trying new FV, eating more FV, increases in FV consumption by family members.)
Olsho et al. (2015) [34]	New York City Community Health Survey: "total servings of fruits and vegetables eaten on the previous day" and "consumption today vs. consumption one year ago"; interviews included questions about the consumption of FV from farmers' markets.
Pellegrino et al. (2018) [35]	FV consumption frequency measured using Behavioral Risk Factor Surveillance System FV module.
Ratigan et al. (2017) [36]	Survey regarding number of servings of FV consumed daily, rank overall dietary quality (very healthy, healthy, average, unhealthy, very unhealthy).
Savoie-Roskos et al. (2016) [38] Savoie-Roskos et al. (2017) [39]	FV consumption frequency measured using Behavioral Risk Factor Surveillance System FV module. Interview: "How does your diet now compare to your diet before the study?"
Young et al. (2013) [42]	"Since becoming a customer at this market, do you eat more, less, or the same amount of fruits and vegetables?"

Assessment of FV consumption varied in the quality of methods used for dietary assessment. Of the 15 studies which assessed the change in FV consumption (Table 3), five studies employed the validated Behavioral Risk Factor Surveillance System FV module [57], and two other studies used other validated assessment tools [7,29]. The validity of the dietary assessment methods for the remaining eight studies was not clear.

All studies under review noted some degree of positive impact, with the exception of Wetherill et al. [41]. In that study, participants were all recipients of Temporary Assistance for Needy Families (TANF), a cash-assistance program in the United States for very low-income families with children. Generally, TANF participation automatically qualifies a household for SNAP. Given the severe income restriction of TANF households, these participants may not be representative of the general SNAP population. Moreover, few participants in this study ($n = 16$, 6.3%) redeemed the incentive coupons; making outcome assessment difficult, although the authors did note that that education surrounding food preparation skills may be necessary, in conjunction with incentives to alter food purchasing behaviors at farmers' markets. Among the remaining studies that reported some positive impact, limitations in the impact of the incentive programs were identified. Conclusions from the Michigan farmers' market-based Double Up Food Bucks program included that the impact of incentive programs was unsustainable and minimal [40], and a Washington, DC-based farmers' market evaluation noted that although participants reported higher FV consumption, their intake still fell below recommended levels [35]. Olsho et al. [34], reported an increase in purchases but concluded that there was no observable difference in consumption between incentive program participants and non-participants, and similarly, Bowling et al. [27] observed that while participants reported increased fruit and vegetable consumption, they did not change the amount of their WIC/SNAP budget spent on these foods.

Several demographic factors have been linked to incentive program retention and use frequency and thus may be important when considering outcome assessment. Specifically, Dimitri et al. [29] noted that participants who were more reliant on food banks, very income restrained, and lived in areas where access to food was limited were more likely to drop out of the incentive program they studied [29]. These findings suggest that the presence of these factors may impact the effectiveness of incentive programs, as participant retention is essential for incentives to influence FV purchases and consumption. Ratigan et al. found that participants who had unhealthier diets at the beginning of the program were more likely to use incentives a greater number of times in the short term, but incentive use waned after six months [36]. In addition, Ratigan et al. noted that elderly and disabled individuals were more likely to use incentive programs in the long term than those who were younger and noted that ethnicity, type of government food assistance program participation, income, season of incentive program enrollment, and baseline FV consumption were related to the frequency of incentive utilization and total duration of their retention in the incentive programs [36]. They also noted that ethnicity, type of government food assistance program participation, income, season of incentive program enrollment, and baseline FV consumption correlate with both the number of times participants utilize incentives in a given period of time, as well as the total duration of their retention in incentive programs. Together, these results suggest that additional work is needed to identify the characteristics of subgroups who are most responsive to incentive programs in order to target incentive programs.

4. Conclusions and Recommendations

This scoping review highlights the wide range of FV incentive program structures and demonstrates that, in general, these programs may be an effective approach for increasing FV purchase and consumption by SNAP participants, while preserving autonomy in food choice. However, it is unclear whether the potential positive effects of these programs are substantial and sustainable. Moreover, the assessment methods employed to evaluate these programs have often relied on self-reports and lack sufficient rigor to assess program impact. Specifically, dietary assessment, when performed, frequently failed to utilize validated methods, such as the 24-h recall. Additionally, there are limitations to the scoping review process itself. Namely, a professional librarian was not consulted to assist with developing the search strategy and the protocol was not published early enough in the process to allow input from the greater scientific community. These factors, in conjunction with the significant variation in program structure, makes it difficult to elucidate which programmatic elements may be most critical for designing and implementing effective programs.

Although the literature indicates that incentive programs may positively impact FV purchases and consumption by SNAP participants, several areas that require additional research in order to understand how to create effective programs are revealed. For instance, other interventions, such as nutrition education, cooking demonstrations, and food tastings, are often deployed in conjunction with incentives. These interventions not only equip participants with the knowledge they need to make healthy eating decisions and integrate healthy foods into their diets but may also contribute to participant use and retention. Participant use of available incentives and retention is a key determinant of program effectiveness, and additional research is needed to understand how to maximize participation and retention. Additional work is needed to elucidate how participant characteristics, such as food security status and demographics, may be associated with the use of incentives. Another area for future research is the impact of incentive program participation on objective measures of health. The studies reviewed in this scoping review demonstrated an improvement in program participants' perceptions of their health [7,32,33,36] and one study demonstrated an improvement in food security status [30], but none of the studies under review measured BMI or other health measures. Consequently, the actual impact of incentives on health remains unclear, and identifying the point at which incentives create a tangible difference in health outcomes is key for creating programs that promote participants' well-being. Lastly, more research is needed to understand the long-term effects of incentives. Some evidence suggests that the increases in FV purchases resulting from incentive program participation are not sustained following program termination [40]. Additionally, few studies have investigated the capacity of incentive programs to influence long-term food consumption and purchasing behavior. Thus, the long-term efficacy of incentives is uncertain [38,58]. Moreover, the research that has considered the long-term impacts of incentive programs has relied on self-reported predictions of future food purchasing behavior [32]. As no longitudinal studies of the impact of incentive programs have been performed, additional research is required to determine the long-term impact of these programs.

Overall, studies of FV incentive programs reveal a positive impact on both FV purchases and consumption. This scoping review provides insights intended to inform the design, implementation, and evaluation of future FV incentive programs targeting SNAP participants. Exploring these factors is critical for understanding how to effectively design and implement effective, sustainable incentive programs.

Supplementary Materials: The following are available online at http://www.mdpi.com/2072-6643/12/6/1676/s1, Table S1: Preferred Reporting Items for Systematic reviews and Meta-Analyses extension for Scoping Reviews (PRSIMA-ScR) Checklist.

Author Contributions: Conceptualization, K.E. and E.H.R.; methodology, K.E. and E.H.R., formal analysis, K.E. and E.H.R.; writing—original draft preparation, K.E. and E.H.R.; writing—review and editing, K.E. and E.H.R. All authors have read and agreed to the published version of the manuscript.

Funding: This research received no external funding.

Acknowledgments: This manuscript grew from Katherine Engel's Thesis in Science, Technology and Public Policy at the Rochester Institute of Technology. The authors would like to thank Kathryn Faulring and Claire Cook for administrative support.

Conflicts of Interest: The authors declare no conflict of interest.

References

1. U.S. Department of Health and Human Services; U.S. Department of Agriculture. *2015–2020 Dietary Guidelines for Americans*, 8th ed.; U.S. Department of Health and Human Services: Washington, DC, USA; U.S. Department of Agriculture: Washington, DC, USA, 2015. Available online: https://health.gov/our-work/food-nutrition/2015-2020-dietary-guidelines/guidelines/ (accessed on 3 June 2020).
2. Lee-Kwan, S.H.; Moore, L.V.; Blanck, H.M.; Harris, D.M.; Galuska, D. Disparities in State-Specific Adult Fruit and Vegetable Consumption—United States, 2015. *Morb. Mortal. Wkly. Rep.* **2017**, *66*, 1241–1247. [CrossRef] [PubMed]
3. Zhang, F.; Liu, J.; Rehm, C.D.; Wilde, P.; Mande, J.R.; Mozaffarian, D. Trends and Disparities in Diet Quality Among US Adults by Supplemental Nutrition Assistance Program Participation Status. *JAMA Netw. Open* **2018**, *1*, e180237. [CrossRef] [PubMed]
4. Rehm, C.D.; Peñalvo, J.L.; Afshin, A.; Mozaffarian, D. Dietary intake among US Adults, 1999–2012. *J. Am. Med. Assoc.* **2016**, *315*, 2542–2553. [CrossRef] [PubMed]
5. USDA Food and Nutrition Services Cost of Living Adjustment (COLA). Available online: https://www.fns.usda.gov/snap/allotment/COLA (accessed on 19 May 2020).
6. What Can SNAP Buy? USDA-FNS. Available online: https://www.fns.usda.gov/snap/eligible-food%20items (accessed on 5 March 2020).
7. Bartlett, S.; Klerman, J.; Olsho, L.; Logan, C.; Blocklin, M.; Beauregard, M.; Enver, A. *Evaluation of the Healthy Incentives Pilot (HIP) Final Report*; Food and Nutrition Service: Alexandria, VA, USA, 2014.
8. USDA. WIC Food Packages-Regulatory Requirements for WIC-Eligible Foods. Available online: https://www.fns.usda.gov/wic/wic-food-packages-regulatory-requirements-wic-eligible-foods (accessed on 21 May 2020).
9. Yen, S.T.; Bruce, D.J.; Jahns, L. Supplemental Nutrition Assistance Program participation and health: Evidence from low-income individuals in Tennessee. *Contemp. Econ. Policy* **2012**, *30*, 1–12. [CrossRef]
10. About WIC-How WIC Helps. USDA-FNS. Available online: https://www.fns.usda.gov/wic/about-wic-how-wic-helps (accessed on 5 March 2020).
11. Pros and Cons of restricting SNAP Purchases. Available online: https://www.govinfo.gov/content/pkg/CHRG-115hhrg24325/html/CHRG-115hhrg24325.htm (accessed on 3 June 2020).
12. United States Government Accountability Office. FOOD STAMP PROGRAM Options for Delivering Financial Incentives to Participants for Purchasing Targeted Foods 2008. Available online: https://www.gao.gov/new.items/d08415.pdf (accessed on 3 June 2020).
13. Gneezy, U.; Meier, S.; Rey-biel, P. When and Why Incentives (Don't) Work to Modify Behavior. *J. Econ. Perspect.* **2011**, *25*, 191–209. [CrossRef]
14. Loewenstein, G.; Brennan, T.; Volpp, K.G. Asymmetric paternalism to improve health behaviors. *J. Am. Med. Assoc.* **2007**, *298*, 2415–2417. [CrossRef] [PubMed]
15. Steenhuis, I.H.M.; Waterlander, W.E.; de Mul, A. Consumer food choices: The role of price and pricing strategies. *Public Health Nutr.* **2011**, *14*, 2220–2226. [CrossRef]
16. Andreyeva, T.; Long, M.W.; Brownell, K.D. The Impact of Food Prices on Consumption: A Systematic Review of Research on the Price Elasticity of Demand for Food. *Am. J. Public Health* **2010**, *100*, 216–222. [CrossRef]
17. Glanz, K.; Basil, M.; Maibach, E.; Goldberg, J.; Snyder, D. Taste Nutrition Cost Convenience and Weight Control Influence Food Consumption. *J. Am. Diet. Assoc.* **1998**, *98*, 1118–1126. [CrossRef]
18. Leung, C.W.; Hoffnagle, E.E.; Lindsay, A.C.; Lofink, H.E.; Hoffman, V.A.; Turrell, S.; Willett, W.C.; Blumenthal, S.J. A qualitative study of diverse experts' views about barriers and strategies to improve the diets and health of Supplemental Nutrition Assistance Program (SNAP) beneficiaries. *J. Acad. Nutr. Diet.* **2013**, *113*, 70–76. [CrossRef]
19. Blumenthal, S.J.; Hoffnagle, E.E.; Leung, C.W.; Lofink, H.; Jensen, H.H.; Foerster, S.B.; Cheung, L.W.Y.; Nestle, M.; Willett, W.C. Strategies to improve the dietary quality of Supplemental Nutrition Assistance Program (SNAP) beneficiaries: An assessment of stakeholder opinions. *Public Health Nutr.* **2013**, *17*, 2824–2833. [CrossRef] [PubMed]

20. Richards, M.R.; Sindelar, J.L. Rewarding healthy food choices in SNAP: Behavioral economic applications. *Milbank Q.* **2013**, *91*, 395–412. [CrossRef] [PubMed]
21. Arksey, H.; O'Malley, L. Scoping studies: Towards a methodological framework. *Int. J. Soc. Res. Methodol. Theory Pract.* **2005**, *8*, 19–32. [CrossRef]
22. Peters, M.D.J.; Godfrey, C.; McInerney, P.; Munn, Z.; Tricco, A.C.; Khalil, H. Chapter 11: Scoping Reviews. (2020 Version); In *Joanna Briggs Institute Reviewer's Manual*; Aromataris, E., Munn, Z., Eds.; The Joanna Briggs Institute: Adelaide, Australia, 2020; Available online: https://reviewersmanual.joannabriggs.org/ (accessed on 3 June 2020).
23. Tricco, A.C.; Lillie, E.; Zarin, W.; O'Brien, K.K.; Colquhoun, H.; Levac, D.; Moher, D.; Peters, M.D.J.; Horsley, T.; Weeks, L.; et al. PRISMA extension for scoping reviews (PRISMA-ScR): Checklist and explanation. *Ann. Intern. Med.* **2018**, *169*, 467–473. [CrossRef] [PubMed]
24. Federal Register: Special Supplemental Nutrition Program for Women, Infants and Children (WIC): Revisions in the WIC Food Packages. Available online: https://www.federalregister.gov/documents/2014/03/04/2014-04105/special-supplemental-nutrition-program-for-women-infants-and-children-wic-revisions-in-the-wic-food (accessed on 4 March 2020).
25. Alaofè, H.; Freed, N.; Jones, K.; Plano, A.; Taren, D. Impacts of Double Up SNAP Farmers' Market Incentive Program on Fruit and Vegetable Access, Purchase and Consumption. *J. Nutr. Health Sci.* **2017**, *4*, 304. [CrossRef]
26. Amaro, C.M.; Roberts, M.C. An Evaluation of a Dollar-for-Dollar Match Program at Farmers' Markets for Families Using Supplemental Nutrition Assistance Program Benefits. *J. Child Fam. Stud.* **2017**, *26*, 2790–2796. [CrossRef]
27. Bowling, A.B.; Moretti, M.; Ringelheim, K.; Tran, A.; Davison, K. Healthy Foods, Healthy Families: Combining incentives and exposure interventions at urban farmers' markets to improve nutrition among recipients of US federal food assistance. *Health Promot. Perspect.* **2016**, *6*, 10–16. [CrossRef]
28. Dimitri, C.; Oberholtzer, L.; Nischan, M. Reducing the Geographic and Financial Barriers to Food Access: Perceived Benefits of Farmers' Markets and Monetary Incentives. *J. Hunger Environ. Nutr.* **2013**, *8*, 429–444. [CrossRef]
29. Dimitri, C.; Oberholtzer, L.; Zive, M.; Sandolo, C. Enhancing food security of low-income consumers: An investigation of financial incentives for use at farmers markets. *Food Policy* **2015**, *52*, 64–70. [CrossRef]
30. Durward, C.M.; Savoie-Roskos, M.; Atoloye, A.; Isabella, P.; Jewkes, M.D.; Ralls, B.; Riggs, K.; LeBlanc, H. Double Up Food Bucks Participation is Associated with Increased Fruit and Vegetable Consumption and Food Security Among Low-Income Adults. *J. Nutr. Educ Behav.* **2019**, *51*, 342–347. [CrossRef]
31. Freedman, D.A.; Mattison-Faye, A.; Alia, K.; Guest, M.A.; Hébert, J.R. Comparing farmers' market revenue trends before and after the implementation of a monetary incentive for recipients of food assistance. *Prev. Chronic Dis.* **2014**, *11*, E87. [CrossRef] [PubMed]
32. Lindsay, S.; Lambert, J.; Penn, T.; Hedges, S.; Ortwine, K.; Mei, A.; Delaney, T.; Wooten, W.J. Monetary matched incentives to encourage the purchase of fresh fruits and vegetables at farmers markets in underserved communities. *Prev. Chronic Dis.* **2013**, *10*, E188. [CrossRef] [PubMed]
33. Marcinkevage, J.; Auvinen, A.; Nambuthiri, S. Washington State's Fruit and Vegetable Prescription Program: Improving Affordability of Healthy Foods for Low-Income Patients. *Prev. Chronic Dis.* **2019**, *16*. [CrossRef] [PubMed]
34. Olsho, L.E.; Holmes Payne, G.; Klein Walker, D.; Baronberg, S.; Jernigan, J.; Abrami, A. Impacts of a farmers' market incentive programme on fruit and vegetable access, purchase and consumption. *Public Health Nutr.* **2015**, *18*, 2712–2721. [CrossRef] [PubMed]
35. Pellegrino, S.; Bost, A.; McGonigle, M.; Rosen, L.; Peterson-Kosecki, A.; Colon-Ramos, U.; Robien, K. Fruit and vegetable intake among participants in a District of Columbia farmers' market incentive programme. *Public Health Nutr.* **2018**, *21*, 601–606. [CrossRef]
36. Ratigan, A.R.; Lindsay, S.; Lemus, H.; Chambers, C.D.; Anderson, C.A.M.; Cronan, T.A.; Browner, D.K.; Wooten, W.J. Factors associated with continued participation in a matched monetary incentive programme at local farmers' markets in low-income neighbourhoods in San Diego, California. *Public Health Nutr.* **2017**, *20*, 2786–2795. [CrossRef]

37. Rummo, P.E.; Noriega, D.; Parret, A.; Harding, M.; Hesterman, O.; Elbel, B.E. Evaluating A USDA Program That Gives SNAP Participants Financial Incentives To Buy Fresh Produce In Supermarkets. *Health Aff.* **2019**, *38*, 1816–1823. [CrossRef]
38. Savoie-Roskos, M.; Durward, C.; Jeweks, M.; LeBlanc, H. Reducing Food Insecurity and Improving Fruit and Vegetable Intake Among Farmers' Market Incentive Program Participants. *J. Nutr. Educ. Behav.* **2016**, *43*, 70–76. [CrossRef]
39. Savoie Roskos, M.R.; Wengreen, H.; Gast, J.; LeBlanc, H.; Durward, C. Understanding the Experiences of Low-Income Individuals Receiving Farmers' Market Incentives in the United States: A Qualitative Study. *Health Promot. Pract.* **2017**, *18*, 869–878. [CrossRef]
40. Steele-Adjognon, M.; Weatherspoon, D. Double Up Food Bucks program effects on SNAP recipients' fruit and vegetable purchases. *BMC Public Health* **2017**, *17*, 946. [CrossRef]
41. Wetherill, M.S.; Williams, M.B.; Gray, K.A. SNAP-Based Incentive Programs at Farmers' Markets: Adaptation Considerations for Temporary Assistance for Needy Families (TANF) Recipients. *J. Nutr. Educ. Behav.* **2017**, *49*, 743–751. [CrossRef] [PubMed]
42. Young, C.R.; Aquilante, J.L.; Solomon, S.; Colby, L.; Kawinzi, M.A.; Uy, N.; Mallya, G. Improving fruit and vegetable consumption among low-income customers at farmers markets: Philly food bucks, Philadelphia, Pennsylvania, 2011. *Prev Chronic Dis.* **2013**, *10*, E166. [CrossRef] [PubMed]
43. Wilde, P.E.; Ranney, C.K. The Monthly Food Stamp Cycle: Shopping Frequency and Food Intake Decisions in an Endogenous Switching Regression Framework. *Am. J. Agric. Econ.* **2000**, *82*, 200–213. [CrossRef]
44. Whiteman, E.D.; Chrisinger, B.W.; Hillier, A. Diet Quality Over the Monthly Supplemental Nutrition Assistance Program Cycle. *Am. J. Prev. Med.* **2018**, *55*, 205–212. [CrossRef] [PubMed]
45. Payne, G.H.; Wethington, H.; Olsho, L.; Jernigan, J.; Farris, R.; Walker, D.K. Implementing a farmers' market incentive program: Perspectives on the New York City Health Bucks Program. *Prev. Chronic Dis.* **2013**, *10*, E145. [CrossRef] [PubMed]
46. Epstein, L.H.; Dearing, K.K.; Roba, L.G.; Finkelstein, E. The influence of taxes and subsidies on energy purchased in an experimental purchasing study. *Psychol. Sci.* **2010**, *21*, 406–414. [CrossRef]
47. Herman, D.R.; Harrison, G.G.; Afifi, A.A.; Jenks, E. Effect of a targeted subsidy on intake of fruits and vegetables among low-income women in the Special Supplemental Nutrition Program for Women, Infants, and Children. *Am. J. Public Health* **2008**, *98*, 98–105. [CrossRef]
48. Retailer Eligibility-Clarification of Criterion A and Criterion B Requirements. USDA-FNS. Available online: https://www.fns.usda.gov/snap/retailer-eligibility-clarification-of-criterion (accessed on 2 February 2020).
49. Laska, M.N.; Caspi, C.E.; Pelletier, J.E.; Friebur, R.; Harnack, L.J. Lack of healthy food in small-size mid-size retailers participating in the Supplemental Nutrition Assistance Program, Minneapolis-St. Paul, Minnesota, 2014. *Prev. Chronic Dis.* **2015**, *12*, E135. [CrossRef]
50. Rigby, S.; Leone, A.F.; Kim, H.; Betterley, C.; Johnson, M.A.; Kurtz, H.; Lee, J.S. Food Deserts in Leon County, FL: Disparate Distribution of Supplemental Nutrition Assistance Program-Accepting Stores by Neighborhood Characteristics. *J. Nutr. Educ. Behav.* **2012**, *44*, 539–547. [CrossRef]
51. Racine, E.F.; Kennedy, A.; Batada, A.; Story, M. Foods and Beverages Available at SNAP-Authorized Drugstores in Sections of North Carolina. *J. Nutr. Educ. Behav.* **2017**, *49*, 674–683. [CrossRef]
52. Racine, E.F.; Batada, A.; Solomon, C.A.; Story, M. Availability of Foods and Beverages in Supplemental Nutrition Assistance Program–Authorized Dollar Stores in a Region of North Carolina. *J. Acad. Nutr. Diet.* **2016**, *116*, 1613–1620. [CrossRef] [PubMed]
53. Hosler, A.S.; Cong, X. Effect of change in the supplemental nutrition assistance program guidelines on vendor participation and availability of fresh produce. *Prev. Chronic Dis.* **2019**, *16*, E115. [CrossRef] [PubMed]
54. Oberholtzer, L.; Dimitri, C.; Schumacher, G. Linking Farmers, Healthy Foods, and Underserved Consumers: Exploring the Impact of Nutrition Incentive Programs on Farmers and Farmers' Markets. *J Agric. Food Syst. Community Dev.* **2012**, *2*, 63–77. [CrossRef]

55. Jilcott Pitts, S.B.; Gustafson, A.; Wu, Q.; Mayo, M.L.; Ward, R.K.; McGuirt, J.T.; Rafferty, A.P.; Lancaster, M.F.; Evenson, K.R.; Keyserling, T.C.; et al. Farmers' market use is associated with fruit and vegetable consumption in diverse southern rural communities. *Nutr. J.* **2014**, *13*, 1. [CrossRef]
56. Cohen, A.J.; Lachance, L.L.; Richardson, C.R.; Mahmoudi, E.; Buxbaum, J.D.; Noonan, G.K.; Murphy, E.C.; Roberson, D.N.; Hesterman, O.B.; Heisler, M.; et al. "Doubling Up" on Produce at Detroit Farmers Markets: Patterns and Correlates of Use of a Healthy Food Incentive. *Am. J. Prev. Med.* **2018**, *54*, 181–189. [CrossRef]
57. Surveillance of Fruit and Vegetable Intake Using the Behavioral Risk Factor Surveillance System. Available online: https://www.cdc.gov/brfss/pdf/fruits_vegetables.pdf (accessed on 23 April 2020).
58. Olsho, L.E.W.; Klerman, J.A.; Wilde, P.E.; Bartlett, S. Financial incentives increase fruit and vegetable intake among Supplemental Nutrition Assistance Program participants: A randomized controlled trial of the USDA Healthy Incentives Pilot. *Am. J. Clin. Nutr.* **2016**, *104*, 423–435. [CrossRef]

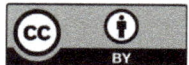

© 2020 by the authors. Licensee MDPI, Basel, Switzerland. This article is an open access article distributed under the terms and conditions of the Creative Commons Attribution (CC BY) license (http://creativecommons.org/licenses/by/4.0/).

MDPI
St. Alban-Anlage 66
4052 Basel
Switzerland
Tel. +41 61 683 77 34
Fax +41 61 302 89 18
www.mdpi.com

Nutrients Editorial Office
E-mail: nutrients@mdpi.com
www.mdpi.com/journal/nutrients

www.ingramcontent.com/pod-product-compliance
Lightning Source LLC
LaVergne TN
LVHW070639100526
838202LV00013B/835